Evidence-Based Neonatal Pharmacotherapy

Guest Editors

ALAN R. SPITZER, MD
DAN L. ELLSBURY, MD

CLINICS IN PERINATOLOGY

www.perinatology.theclinics.com

Consulting Editor

LUCKY JAIN, MD, MBA

March 2012 • Volume 39 • Number 1

SAUNDERS an imprint of ELSEVIER, Inc.

W.B. SAUNDERS COMPANY
A Division of Elsevier Inc.

Elsevier, Inc. • 1600 John F. Kennedy Blvd. • Suite 1800 • Philadelphia, PA 19103-2899

http://www.theclinics.com

CLINICS IN PERINATOLOGY Volume 39, Number 1
March 2012 ISSN 0095-5108, ISBN-13: 978-1-4557-3911-0

Editor: Kerry Holland
Developmental Editor: Donald Mumford

Clinics in Perinatology (ISSN 0095-5108) is published quarterly by Elsevier Inc., 360 Park Avenue South, New York, NY 10010-1710. Months of issue are March, June, September, and December. Business and Editorial Offices: 1600 John F. Kennedy Blvd., Ste. 1800, Philadelphia, PA 19103-2899. Customer Service Office: 3251 Riverport Lane, Maryland Heights, MO 63043. Periodicals postage paid at New York, NY and additional mailing offices. Subscription prices are $273.00 per year (US individuals), $401.00 per year (US institutions), $326.00 per year (Canadian individuals), $509.00 per year (Canadian institutions), $400.00 per year (foreign individuals), $509.00 per year (foreign institutions), $130.00 per year (US students), and $187.00 per year (Canadian and foreign students). Foreign air speed delivery is included in all Clinics subscription prices. All prices are subject to change without notice. **POSTMASTER:** Send address changes to *Clinics in Perinatology*, Elsevier Health Sciences Division, Subscription Customer Service, 3251 Riverport Lane, Maryland Heights, MO 63043. **Customer Service: Telephone: 1-800-654-2452** (U.S. and Canada); **1-314-447-8871** (outside U.S. and Canada). **Fax: 1-314-447-8029.** E-mail: **journalscustomerservice-usa@elsevier.com** (for print support); **journalsonlinesupport-usa@elsevier.com** (for online support).

Reprints. For copies of 100 or more, of articles in this publication, please contact the Commercial Reprints Department, Elsevier Inc., 360 Park Avenue South, New York, NY 10010-1710. Tel. (212) 633-3812; Fax: (212) 482-1935; E-mail: reprints@elsevier.com.

Clinics in Perinatology is also pubilshed in Spanish by McGraw-Hill Interamericana Editores S.A., P.O. Box 5-237, 06500 Mexico D.F., Mexico.

Clinics in Perinatology is covered in *MEDLINE/PubMed (Index Medicus) Current Contents, Excepta Medica, BIOSIS* and *ISI/BIOMED.*

Printed in the United States of America.

Contributors

CONSULTING EDITOR

LUCKY JAIN, MD, MBA
Richard Blumberg Professor and Executive Vice Chairman, Department of Pediatrics, Emory University School of Medicine, Atlanta, Georgia

GUEST EDITORS

ALAN R. SPITZER, MD
Senior Vice President, The Center for Research, Education, and Quality MEDNAX, Inc./Pediatrix Medical Group/American Anesthesiology, Sunrise, Florida

DAN L. ELLSBURY, MD
Director of Continuous Quality Improvement, The Center for Research, Education, and Quality MEDNAX, Inc./Pediatrix Medical Group/American Anesthesiology, Sunrise, Florida

AUTHORS

MARTA AGUAR, MD
Division of Neonatology, University & Polytechnic Hospital La Fe, Valencia, Spain

DANIEL K. BENJAMIN Jr, MD, PhD, MPH
Faculty Associate Director, Duke Clinical Research Institute; Professor, Department of Pediatrics, Duke University, Duke University Medical Center, Durham, North Carolina

MARÍA CERNADA, MD
Neonatal Research Unit, Health Research Institute Hospital La Fe, Valencia, Spain

ROBERT D. CHRISTENSEN, MD
The Women and Newborns Program, Intermountain Healthcare, Salt Lake City; McKay-Dee Hospital Center, Ogden, Utah

C. ANDREW COMBS, MD, PhD
Associated Director of Research for Obstetrix, Pediatrix Medical Group, Sunrise, Florida; Obstetrix Medical Group, San Jose, California

C. MICHAEL COTTEN, MD, MHS
Assistant Professor, Division of Neonatal-Perinatal Medicine, Department of Pediatrics, Duke University, Durham, North California

DAN L. ELLSBURY, MD
Director of Continuous Quality Improvement, The Center for Research, Education, and Quality MEDNAX, Inc./Pediatrix Medical Group/American Anesthesiology, Sunrise, Florida

JAVIER ESCOBAR, PhD
Neonatal Research Unit, Health Research Institute Hospital La Fe, Valencia, Spain

RAQUEL ESCRIG, MD
Division of Neonatology, University & Polytechnic Hospital La Fe, Valencia, Spain

M. PAIGE FULLER, PharmD, BCPS
Neonatal ICU Clinical Pharmacist, Department of Pharmacy, Monroe Carell Jr. Children's Hospital at Vanderbilt, Nashville, Tennessee

THOMAS J. GARITE, MD
Professor Emeritus, Retired E.J. Quilligan Chair of Obstetrics and Gynecology, University of California Irvine, College of Medicine, Irvine, California; Director of Research and Education for Obstetrics, Pediatrix Medical Group, Sunrise, Florida

GEORGE P. GIACOIA, MD
Program Scientist, Obstetric and Pediatric Pharmacology Branch; Eunice Kennedy Shriver National Institute of Child Health and Human Development (NICHD), Rockville, Maryland

MARIA GILLAM-KRAKAUER, MD
Assistant Professor, Division of Neonatology, Department of Pediatrics, Vanderbilt University Medical Center, Nashville, Tennessee

R. WHIT HALL, MD
Professor, Division of Neonatology, University of Arkansas for Medical Sciences, Arkansas Children's Hospital and Center for Translational Neuroscience, Little Rock, Arkansas

PALMER G. JOHNSTON, MD
Fellow, Neonatal-Perinatal Medicine, Division of Neonatology, Department of Pediatrics, Vanderbilt University Medical Center, Nashville, Tennessee

WILLIAM F. MALCOLM, MD
Assistant Professor, Division of Neonatal-Perinatal Medicine, Department of Pediatrics, Duke University, Durham, North California

SHAHAB NOORI, MD
Associate Professor of Pediatrics, Center for Fetal and Neonatal Medicine and the USC Division of Neonatal Medicine, Children's Hospital Los Angeles and the LAC+USC Medical Center, Keck School of Medicine, University of Southern California, Los Angeles, California

NICOLAS F.M. PORTA, MD
Assistant Professor, Department of Pediatrics, Children's Memorial Hospital, Northwestern University, Chicago, Illinois

JEFF REESE, MD
Associate Professor, Division of Neonatology, Department of Pediatrics; Department of Cell and Developmental Biology, Vanderbilt University Medical Center, Nashville, Tennessee

MATTHEW A. SAXONHOUSE, MD
Attending Neonatologist, Pediatrix Medical Group, Jeff Gordon Children's Hospital, Carolinas Medical Center, Concord, North Carolina

JEFFREY L. SEGAR, MD
Professor, Director, Division of Neonatology, Department of Pediatrics, University of Iowa Children's Hospital, Iowa City, Iowa

ISTVAN SERI, MD, PhD
Professor of Pediatrics, Center for Fetal and Neonatal Medicine and the USC Division of Neonatal Medicine, Children's Hospital Los Angeles and the LAC+USC Medical Center, Keck School of Medicine, University of Southern California, Los Angeles, California

P. BRIAN SMITH, MD, MHS, MPH
Duke Clinical Research Institute; Department of Pediatrics, Duke University Medical Center, Duke University, Durham, North Carolina

ALAN R. SPITZER, MD
Senior Vice President, The Center for Research, Education, and Quality MEDNAX, Inc./Pediatrix Medical Group/American Anesthesiology, Sunrise, Florida

ROBIN H. STEINHORN, MD
Professor and Vice-Chair, Department of Pediatrics, Children's Memorial Hospital, Northwestern University, Chicago, Illinois

PERDITA TAYLOR-ZAPATA, MD
Medical Officer, Obstetric and Pediatric Pharmacology Branch; Eunice Kennedy Shriver National Institute of Child Health and Human Development (NICHD), Rockville, Maryland

DANIELA TESTONI, MD
Duke Clinical Research Institute, Duke University Medical Center, Durham, North Carolina

NIDHI TRIPATHI, BS
Duke University School of Medicine; Duke Clinical Research Institute, Durham, North Carolina

ROBERT URSPRUNG, MD
Associate Director, Clinical Quality Improvement MEDNAX Services/Pediatrix Medical Group/American Anesthesiology, Sunrise, Florida

MÁXIMO VENTO, MD, PhD
Professor of Pediatrics, Director of the Neonatal Research Unit, Division of Neonatology, University & Polytechnic Hospital La Fe; Health Research Institute Hospital La Fe, Valencia, Spain

KRISTI WATTERBERG, MD
Professor of Pediatrics/Neonatology, Department of Pediatrics, University of New Mexico School of Medicine, Albuquerque, New Mexico

RICHARD J. WHITLEY, MD
Distinguished Professor, Loeb Scholar in Pediatrics, Professor of Pediatrics, Microbiology, Medicine and Neurosurgery, The University of Alabama at Birmingham, Birmingham, Alabama

THOMAS E. YOUNG, MD
WakeMed Faculty Physicians - Neonatology, Raleigh, North Carolina; Professor of Pediatrics, University of North Carolina, Chapel Hill, North Carolina

ANNE ZAJICEK, MD
Branch Chief, Obstetric and Pediatric Pharmacology Branch; Eunice Kennedy Shriver National Institute of Child Health and Human Development (NICHD), Rockville, Maryland

Contents

Despite many years of heavy use in premature and critically ill newborns, surprisingly few medications have been rigorously tested in neonatal multicenter randomized clinical trials. Little is known about the pharmacology of these drugs at various birth weights, gestational ages, and chronologic ages. This article describes a quality improvement approach to evaluating and improving neonatal intensive care unit (NICU) medication use, with an emphasis on adaptation of drug use to the specific clinical NICU context and use of system-based changes to minimize harm and maximize clinical benefit.

Although some drugs have been developed for the neonate, drug development for the least mature and most vulnerable pediatric patients is lacking. Most of the drugs are off-label or off-patent and are empirically administered to newborns once efficacy has been demonstrated in adults and usefulness is suspected or demonstrated in the older pediatric population. Few drugs are approved by the Food and Drug Administration for use in this population. The factors that prevent the demonstration of efficacy and safety in the newborn are discussed and a change in the current approach for neonatal drug studies is suggested.

Neonates and young infants are in a unique and dynamic pharmacokinetic state, in which they undergo relatively rapid maturational changes in drug absorption, distribution, metabolism, and excretion. In addition to these maturational changes, most drug pharmacokinetic studies in neonates show wide interindividual variability despite similar gestational and postnatal ages. Therapeutic drug monitoring is a necessary tool in the neonatal intensive care unit, despite the relative lack of outcome data. This article discusses therapeutic drug monitoring for several frequently used drugs in neonates.

Thomas J. Garite and C. Andrew Combs

Although improvements in neonatal care have continued to result in reduced mortality and morbidity of prematurely delivering newborns for decades, the results of a myriad of obstetric efforts and interventions have failed to reduce the overall rate of prematurity or prolong pregnancy at any gestational age. A few new developments or refinements of established interventions give increased hope for an improved obstetric contribution to the problem of prematurity. These include a better understanding of how best to use antenatal corticosteroids, and the newer options of magnesium sulfate to ameliorate or avoid cerebral palsy associated with prematurity and maternal progesterone administration to selected at-risk populations to decrease the likelihood of premature delivery.

Kristi Watterberg

Corticosteroids are used in the neonatal intensive care unit primarily to treat two conditions: bronchopulmonary dysplasia (BPD) and hypotension (cardiovascular insufficiency). Historically, high-dose dexamethasone was used for BPD, but its use was later associated with adverse neurodevelopmental outcomes and decreased substantially. Data from randomized controlled trials regarding efficacy and safety of lower-dose dexamethasone therapy are insufficient to recommend its use. Hydrocortisone may be an alternative to dexamethasone, but again data are insufficient to support use. Hydrocortisone therapy is increasingly used to treat hypotension in critically ill newborns; however, the outcomes of this therapy must be evaluated in randomized trials.

Nidhi Tripathi, C. Michael Cotten, and P. Brian Smith

Neonatal sepsis causes significant morbidity and mortality, especially in preterm infants. Clinicians are compelled to treat with empiric antibiotics at the first signs of suspected sepsis. Broad-spectrum antibiotics and prolonged treatment with empiric antibiotics are associated with adverse outcomes. Most common neonatal pathogens are susceptible to narrow-spectrum antibiotics. The choice of antibiotic and duration of empiric treatment are strongly associated with center-based risk factors. Clinicians should treat with short courses of narrow-spectrum antibiotics whenever possible, choosing the antibiotics and treatment duration to balance the risks of potentially untreated sepsis against the adverse effects of treatment in infants with sterile cultures.

Richard J. Whitley

Parenteral therapy of viral infections of the newborn and infant began with vidarabine (adenine arabinoside) for the treatment of neonatal herpes simplex virus (HSV) infections in the early 1980s. Acyclovir has become the treatment of choice for neonatal HSV infections and a variety of other herpesvirus infections. Ganciclovir is beneficial for the treatment of congenital cytomegalovirus (CMV) infections involving the central nervous system (CNS). This article reviews the use of acyclovir and ganciclovir in the treatment of neonatal HSV and congenital CMV infections. A brief summary precedes a detailed discussion of available established and alternative therapeutics.

Invasive fungal infections remain a significant cause of infection-related mortality and morbidity in preterm infants. Central nervous system involvement is the hallmark of neonatal candidiasis, differentiating the disease's impact on young infants from that among all other patient populations. Over the past decade, the number of antifungal agents in development has grown, but most are not labeled for use in newborns. We summarize the findings of several antifungal studies that have been completed to date, emphasizing those including infant populations. We conclude that more studies are required for antifungals to be used safely and effectively in infants.

Pharmacotherapy for gastroesophageal reflux (GER) in neonates, aimed at interfering with this physiologic process and potentially reducing the negative sequelae that providers often attribute to GER, consists primarily of drugs that increase the viscosity of feeds, reduce stomach acidity, or improve gut motility. Medications used to treat clinical signs thought to be from GER, such as apnea, bradycardia, or feeding intolerance, are among the most commonly prescribed medications in neonatal intensive care units in the United States, despite the lack of evidence of safety and efficacy in this population.

Indomethacin and ibuprofen are potent inhibitors of prostaglandin synthesis. Neonates have been exposed to these compounds for more than 3 decades. Indomethacin is commonly used to prevent intraventricular hemorrhage (IVH), and both drugs are prescribed for the treatment or prevention of patent ductus arteriosus (PDA). This review examines the basis for indomethacin and ibuprofen use in the neonatal intensive care population. Despite the call for restrained use of each drug, the most immature infants are likely to need pharmacologic approaches to reduce high-grade IVH, avoid the need for PDA ligation, and preserve the opportunity for an optimal outcome.

The introduction of methylxanthines, especially caffeine, for the treatment of apnea of prematurity has been one of the most important and effective therapies in the neonatal intensive care unit (NICU) to date. Several trials have demonstrated its effectiveness in most NICU infants. It remains a cost-effective intervention with minimal short- and long-term risks when used appropriately. Caffeine also seems to be effective for reducing the risk of bronchopulmonary dysplasia and patent ductus arteriosus, and for decreasing the need for reintubation. For the infant with apnea, currently there does not seem to be any more effective treatment, and caffeine is also more effective and safer than any other methylxanthine.

The perinatal transition from fetal to extrauterine life requires a dramatic change in the circulatory pattern as the organ of gas exchange switches from the placenta to the lungs. Pulmonary hypertension can occur during early newborn life, and present as early respiratory failure or as a complication of more chronic diseases, such as bronchopulmonary dysplasia. The most effective pharmacotherapeutic strategies for infants with persistent pulmonary hypertension of the newborn are directed at selective reduction of pulmonary vascular resistance. This article discusses currently available therapies for pulmonary hypertension, their biologic rationales, and evidence for their clinical effectiveness.

This article describes aerobic metabolism, oxygen free radicals, antioxidant defenses, oxidative stress, inflammatory response and redox signaling, the fetal to neonatal transition, arterial oxygen saturation, oxygen administration in the delivery room, oxygen during neonatal care in the NICU, evolving oxygen needs in the first few weeks of life, and complications that can occur when infants go home from the hospital on oxygen.

This article focuses on the use of rEpo, IVIG, and rG-CSF in the NICU. It discusses the most recent studies and the most definitive and clinically relevant evidence, rather than summarizing all published studies. The last section was written for NICU practice groups that choose to use any of these medications and are seeking a consistent approach for doing so. The section provides the author's approach to the use of rEpo, IVIG, and rG-CSF, revealing personal preferences, interpretations, and experiences, and is based on the dictum, "if you are going to use it, use it the same way each time."

Neonates have one of the highest risks for thromboembolism among pediatric patients. This risk is attributable to a combination of multiple genetic and acquired risk factors. Despite a significant number of these events being either life threatening or limb threatening, there is limited evidence on appropriate management strategy. Most of what is recommended is based on uncontrolled studies, case series, or expert opinion. This review begins with a discussion of the neonatal hemostatic system, focusing on the common sites and imaging modalities for the detection of neonatal thrombosis. Perinatal and postnatal risk factors are presented and management options discussed.

Jeffrey L. Segar

Diuretics are commonly used to treat infants with oxygen-dependent chronic lung disease. However, there are limited data suggesting a beneficial effect of long-term diuretic therapy on pulmonary function or clinical outcome in this population. Furthermore, data available for review were primarily obtained before the widespread use of antenatal steroids or surfactant replacement therapy, before recognition of the new bronchopulmonary dysplasia. If used in this population, limitations of diuretic therapy as well as significant side effects need to be understood and a rationale approach to clinical use developed on a patient-centered basis.

Shahab Noori and Istvan Seri

A solid understanding of the mechanisms of action of cardiovascular medications used in clinical practice along with efforts to develop comprehensive hemodynamic monitoring systems to improve the ability to accurately identify the underlying pathophysiology of cardiovascular compromise are essential in the management of neonates with shock. This article reviews the mechanisms of action of the most frequently used cardiovascular medications in neonates. Because of paucity of data from controlled clinical trials, evidence-based recommendations for the clinical use of these medications could not be made. Careful titration of the given medication with close monitoring of the cardiovascular response might improve the effectiveness and decrease the risks associated with administration of these medications.

R. Whit Hall

Painful procedures in the neonatal intensive care unit are common, undertreated, and lead to adverse consequences. A stepwise approach to treatment should include pain recognition, assessment, and treatment, starting with nonpharmacologic and progressing to pharmacologic methods for increasing pain. The most common nonpharmacologic techniques include nonnutritive sucking with and without sucrose, kangaroo care, swaddling, and massage therapy. Drugs used to treat neonatal pain include the opiates, benzodiazepines, barbiturates, ketamine, propofol, acetaminophen, and local and topical anesthetics. The indications, advantages, and disadvantages of the commonly used analgesic drugs are discussed. Guidance and references for drugs and dosing for specific neonatal procedures are provided.

GOAL STATEMENT

The goal of *Clinics in Perinatology* is to keep practicing neonatologists and maternal-fetal medicine specialists up to date with current clinical practice in perinatology by providing timely articles reviewing the state of the art in patient care.

ACCREDITATION

The *Clinics in Perinatology* is planned and implemented in accordance with the Essential Areas and Policies of the Accreditation Council for Continuing Medical Education (ACCME) through the joint sponsorship of the University of Virginia School of Medicine and Elsevier. The University of Virginia School of Medicine is accredited by the ACCME to provide continuing medical education for physicians.

The University of Virginia School of Medicine designates this enduring material activity for a maximum of 15 *AMA PRA Category 1 Credit*(s)™ for each issue, 60 credits per year. Physicians should only claim credit commensurate with the extent of their participation in the activity.

The American Medical Association has determined that physicians not licensed in the US who participate in this CME enduring material activity are eligible for a maximum of 15 *AMA PRA Category 1 Credit*(s)™ for each issue, 60 credits per year.

Credit can be earned by reading the text material, taking the CME examination online at http://www.theclinics.com/home/cme, and completing the evaluation. After taking the test, you will be required to review any and all incorrect answers. Following completion of the test and evaluation, your credit will be awarded and you may print your certificate.

FACULTY DISCLOSURE/CONFLICT OF INTEREST

The University of Virginia School of Medicine, as an ACCME accredited provider, endorses and strives to comply with the Accreditation Council for Continuing Medical Education (ACCME) Standards of Commercial Support, Commonwealth of Virginia statutes, University of Virginia policies and procedures, and associated federal and private regulations and guidelines on the need for disclosure and monitoring of proprietary and financial interests that may affect the scientific integrity and balance of content delivered in continuing medical education activities under our auspices.

The University of Virginia School of Medicine requires that all CME activities accredited through this institution be developed independently and be scientifically rigorous, balanced and objective in the presentation/discussion of its content, theories and practices.

All authors/editors participating in an accredited CME activity are expected to disclose to the readers relevant financial relationships with commercial entities occurring within the past 12 months (such as grants or research support, employee, consultant, stock holder, member of speakers bureau, etc.). The University of Virginia School of Medicine will employ appropriate mechanisms to resolve potential conflicts of interest to maintain the standards of fair and balanced education to the reader. Questions about specific strategies can be directed to the Office of Continuing Medical Education, University of Virginia School of Medicine, Charlottesville, Virginia.

The faculty and staff of the University of Virginia Office of Continuing Medical Education have no financial affiliations to disclose.

The authors/editors listed below have identified no professional or financial affiliations for themselves or their spouse/partner:
Marta Aguar, MD; Robert Boyle, MD (Test Author); Maria Cernada, MD; Robert D. Christensen, MD; C. Michael Cotten, MD, MHS; Javier Escobar, PhD; Raquel Escrig, MD; M. Paige Fuller, PharmD, BCPS; George P. Giacoia, MD; Maria Gillam-Krakauer, MD; R. Whit Hall, MD; Kerry Holland, (Acquisitions Editor); Lucky Jain, MD, MBA (Consulting Editor); Palmer G. Johnston, MD; Nicolas F.M. Porta, MD; Jeff Reese, MD; Matthew A. Saxonhouse, MD; Jeffrey L. Segar, MD; Shahab Noori, MD; Robin H. Steinhorn, MD; Perdita Taylor-Zapata, MD; Daniela Testoni, MD; Nidhi Tripathi, BS; Máximo Vento, MD, PhD; Kristi Watterberg, MD; and Anne Zajicek, MD.

The authors/editors listed below identified the following professional or financial affiliations for themselves or their spouse/partner:
Daniel K. Benjamin, Jr, MD, PhD, MPH is a consultant for Astellas Pharma US, Johnson & Johnson, Pfizer, Inc., Biosynexus, and Cerexa, Inc.; and is an industry funded research/investigator for Astellas Pharma US, Astra Zeneca, and UCB Pharma, Inc.
C. Andrew Combs, MD, PhD is an industry funded research/investigator for KV Pharmaceuticals.
Dan L. Ellsbury, MD (Guest Editor) is employed and owns stock with Pediatrix Medical Group.
Thomas J. Garite, MD is employed by the Pediatrix Medical Group.
William F. Malcolm, MD is on the Speakers' Bureau for Abbott Nutrition.
Istvan Seri, MD, PhD receives grant support from Somanetics, Inc.
P. Brian Smith, MD, MPH, MHS is a consultant for Astellas Pharma, Johnson and Johnson, and Cubist Pharmaceuticals; and is on the Advisory Committee/Board for Pfizer, Inc.
Alan R. Spitzer, MD (Guest Editor) is employed by and owns stock in MEDNAX, Inc.

Robert Ursprung, MD is employed by Pediatrix Medical Group, and is on the Speakers' Bureau and Advisory Board for Vermont Oxford Network.

Richard J. Whitley, MD is on the Advisory Committee/Board for Gilead Sciences, Inc., and is a consultant for Chimerix, Inc.

Thomas E. Young, MD is a consultant for Cornerstone Therapeutics.

Disclosure of Discussion of Non-FDA Approved Uses for Pharmaceutical Products and/or Medical Devices

The University of Virginia School of Medicine, as an ACCME provider, requires that all faculty presenters identify and disclose any off-label uses for pharmaceutical and medical device products. The University of Virginia School of Medicine recommends that each physician fully review all the available data on new products or procedures prior to clinical use.

TO ENROLL

To enroll in the Clinics in Perinatology Continuing Medical Education program, call customer service at 1-800-654-2452 or visit us online at www.theclinics.com/home/cme. The CME program is available to subscribers for an additional fee of $196.00

THE CLINICS ARE NOW AVAILABLE ONLINE!

Access your subscription at:
www.theclinics.com

Foreword

The Challenge of Managing Drugs Safely in the Newborn

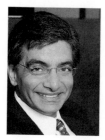

Lucky Jain, MD, MBA
Consulting Editor

The challenge of safe and appropriate use of drugs in the neonatal period is a daunting one and is complicated by the glaring lack of evidence-based data that should guide decision-making. Clinicians struggle with a meager choice of drugs that have not been rigorously tested in the tiniest newborns; they often complicate this issue with their own unacceptably high variation in drug usage, which precludes collection of meaningful outcomes data. The result is an unsatisfactory state of either too much or too little use of drugs, and an industry that has yet to embrace pediatric drug development as an essential part of their overall strategy.[1] Newborns worldwide continue to suffer with plenty of blame to be passed around and few ready to shoulder the responsibility.

These significant issues notwithstanding, clinicians have an obligation to optimize drug therapy in neonates and track outcomes. Many institutions have begun this process using advanced quality improvement methodology tools, but the vast majority of practitioners are far removed from any such exercise. This multistep process begins with a thorough review of available literature pertaining to a particular drug use and generation of practice guidelines. These guidelines are then followed by all practitioners participating in the quality improvement (QI) project for a specified period of time with rigorous collection of data pertaining to safety and efficacy of the medication. The information gathered is then used to modify the original protocol as necessary, and the cycle of plan-do-check-act (**Fig. 1**) continues.[2] Such a process has yielded enormous benefits for pediatric oncology groups worldwide.[3]

As mentioned above, an essential first step in this QI approach requires a thorough review of the literature by experts who can then recommend practice guidelines. This issue of the *Clinics in Perinatology* represents an impressive body of work by experts in the field of neonatal pharmacotherapy. Drs Spitzer and Ellsbury are to be congratulated for assembling an impressive array of articles pertaining to neonatal drug therapy. The reader is now challenged to take these recommendations and

Clin Perinatol 39 (2012) xv–xvi
doi:10.1016/j.clp.2011.12.020
0095-5108/12/$ – see front matter © 2012 Elsevier Inc. All rights reserved.

perinatology.theclinics.com

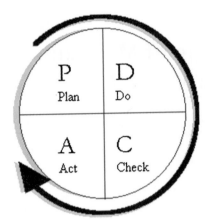

Fig. 1. The Demming Wheel of Quality Improvement.

engage in the plan-do-check-act cycle locally using consensus-driven practice guide-lines and data monitoring.

I want to thank the editors and authors for a superb collection of articles and Kerry Holland at Elsevier for supporting their publication. With nanomedicine and genetically engineered drugs knocking on our doors, and with computerized ordering/electronic medical records readily available to minimize errors and track outcomes, the driver's seat in this journey convincingly belongs to the prescribing clinician!

Lucky Jain, MD, MBA
Department of Pediatrics
Emory University School of Medicine
2015 Uppergate Drive
Atlanta, GA 30322, USA

E-mail address:
ljain@emory.edu

REFERENCES

1. Van den Anker JN. Managing drugs safely. Semin Fetal Neonatal Med 2005;10: 73–81.
2. Demming WE. Out of the crisis. Cambridge (MA): MIT Press; 1986.
3. Unguru Y. The successful integration of research and care: how pediatric oncology became the subspecialty in which research defines the standard of care. Pediatr Blood Cancer 2011;56:1019–25.

Preface

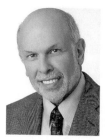 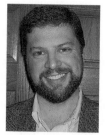

Alan R. Spitzer, MD   Dan L. Ellsbury, MD
Guest Editors

It has become increasingly apparent in the practice of modern medicine that evidence-based practices and quantitation of patient outcomes have become critical foundations of clinical care. While clinical judgment and experience will always be highly valued qualities of any practicing physician, even the most competent physician will now be asked for specific outcome results in discussing care with patients. As we noted in our March 2010 issue of *Clinics in Perinatology* devoted to Continuous Quality Improvement in Neonatal-Perinatal Medicine, "patients and families expect to be informed not only of the options in care, but the likely outcomes of those options so that they can become active participants in the decision-making process. In order to evaluate outcomes, therefore, the clinician now requires information that was previously often only anecdotally collected, namely accurate outcomes of specific conditions for large groups of patients and comparative results of different treatments of those conditions in significant patient populations." Perhaps nowhere are evidence-based approaches and clinical outcomes more important than in the use of medications in the neonatal intensive care unit (NICU).

One of the great problems in current neonatal practice is the fact that many of the drugs commonly used in the NICU have never been approved for neonatal care. The newborn infant has long been a true therapeutic orphan, exposed to therapies that have never been properly studied or evaluated by appropriate randomized trials. As a result, many pharmacological treatments have slipped into neonatal practice that have little merit to support their continued use. Nevertheless, many of these therapies continue to be employed, even when the evidence strongly suggests that the treatment has little or no value for the patient. It has long been our belief that the exposure of critically ill infants to medications that do little to enhance their outcome must be emphatically discontinued as quickly as possible. It is therefore our hope that this issue of *Clinics in Perinatology* leads the way in this respect and illuminates the appropriate use of many important neonatal medications.

Fortunately, the contributors to this issue of *Clinics in Perinatology* agree with this concept and have done a marvelous job in outlining some of the most controversial areas of medication therapy for the neonate. With a strong emphasis on the prospective randomized trial, the authors for this volume have critically evaluated the literature

Clin Perinatol 39 (2012) xvii–xviii
doi:10.1016/j.clp.2011.12.019
0095-5108/12/$ – see front matter © 2012 Elsevier Inc. All rights reserved.
perinatology.theclinics.com

and have presented their own research work as well, in order to provide the reader with the most current evidence that exists in many areas of modern drug use in the NICU. Their efforts in this respect have been exceptional and we believe that the reader should pay careful attention to the recommendations contained in this volume.

This is a very exciting time in the history of medicine, as we increasingly identify the molecular basis for disease and specifically tailor therapy to the individual needs of a patient. "Shotgun" therapy, where anything that can be tried will be tried, has now become part of the history of medicine. The continuing advances that we see daily in pharmacological therapy represent the future of medical care, and the contributors to this issue of *Clinics in Perinatology* are leading the way in our understanding of how drugs can best be used for the benefit of the patient. We are delighted to have the opportunity to bring their ideas to you, and it is our wish that these articles generate new ideas about medications that one day will make what is written here seem "old hat." Here's to the future of medical care!

Alan R. Spitzer, MD
The Center for Research, Education, and Quality
MEDNAX Services/Pediatrix Medical Group/American Anesthesiology
1301 Concord Terrace
Sunrise, FL 33323, USA

Dan L. Ellsbury, MD
Clinical Quality Improvement
MEDNAX Services/Pediatrix Medical Group/American Anesthesiology
1301 Concord Terrace
Sunrise, FL 33323, USA

E-mail addresses:
alan_spitzer@pediatrix.com (A.R. Spitzer)
Dan_Ellsbury@pediatrix.com (D.L. Ellsbury)

A Quality Improvement Approach to Optimizing Medication Use in the Neonatal Intensive Care Unit

Dan L. Ellsbury, MD*, Robert Ursprung, MD

KEYWORDS
• Neonatology • Iatrogenesis • Medication
• Quality improvement

THE KNOWLEDGE AND IMPLEMENTATION GAP IN NEONATAL INTENSIVE CARE UNIT MEDICATION USE

Despite many years of heavy use in premature and critically ill newborns, surprisingly few medications have been rigorously tested in neonatal multicenter randomized clinical trials. Little is known about the pharmacology of these drugs at various birth weights, gestational ages, and chronologic ages.[1,2] Data regarding potential short-term and long-term adverse effects are largely unknown, and benefits are often unproven. Even when medications have been rigorously studied and found to be of benefit, their widespread use is often slowly adopted or incomplete.[3,4]

The knowledge and implementation gap in use of these medications represents an ongoing source of neonatal iatrogenesis, the full impact of which will be felt by countless children and families in years to come. Given the magnitude of potential harm in the misuse of these drugs, all neonatologists are obligated to take a critical look at which medications they use and how they use them. This article describes a quality improvement approach to evaluating and improving neonatal intensive care unit (NICU) medication use, with an emphasis on adaptation of drug use to the specific clinical NICU context and use of system-based changes to minimize harm and maximize clinical benefit (**Fig. 1**).

FIRST, DO NO HARM

Extrapolation of benefits and safety from adult studies of NICU medications is common, as is a sense of perceived safety derived from a long history of a drug's

Clinical Quality Improvement MEDNAX Services/Pediatrix Medical Group/American Anesthesiology, 1301 Concord Terrace, Sunrise, FL 33323, USA
* Corresponding author.
E-mail address: Dan_Ellsbury@pediatrix.com

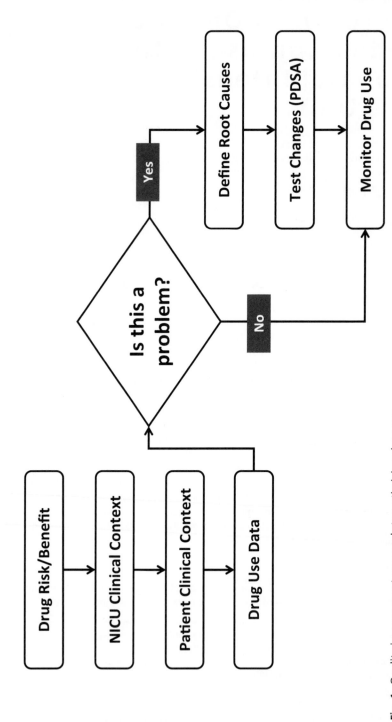

Fig. 1. Quality improvement approach to optimizing drug use.

use in neonatal care. This creeping comfort with medication use has generated an infamous track record of iatrogenic injury in neonatology (**Table 1**).[5–7]

WHAT ARE THE RISKS AND BENEFITS

The risks and benefits of any NICU medication should be continuously assessed. Has the medication been studied in randomized clinical trials? Were these trials done in premature infants? What were the short-term and long-term benefits; what were the short-term and long-term risks? Were there important drug interactions, cost issues, medication administration difficulties, and/or therapeutic drug monitoring concerns? Was the magnitude of benefit or harm clinically relevant? Was the treatment benefit or risk related to a specific gestational age or chronologic age? For what patient population and indication is the drug labeled? Is there a Food and Drug Administration black box warning regarding the drug? Is there an evidence-based clinical practice guideline available to direct the medication's use?

DOES THE NICU CLINICAL CONTEXT MODIFY THE RISKS AND BENEFITS

The risk/benefit profile of a medication should be modified to fit the specific clinical context of its use. The pattern of mortality and morbidities in an individual NICU may significantly alter the risk/benefit ratio of a given drug. The well-described center-to-center variations in clinical outcomes may result in a significantly altered risk/benefit ratio for the same medication when used in different NICUs.[8,9] Failure to appreciate this point may lead to needless adverse effects, suboptimal outcomes, and waste of valuable resources. Indeed, a mental filter of "if it's not broke, don't fix it" and "if it is broke, fix it" may be useful to consider when weighing the risks and benefits of a particular medication in a particular NICU.

Example: Antenatal Steroids and Surfactant

In an NICU with a low rate of antenatal steroid use, the benefit from use of prophylactic surfactant administration may be quite high. In an NICU with a high use of antenatal steroids, a rescue approach may be just as effective as prophylaxis and may reduce

Table 1
History of medication iatrogenesis in neonatology

Years	Drug	Adverse Effects
1941–present	Oxygen	ROP
1945–1961	Synthetic vitamin K	Kernicterus
1953–1956	Sulfisoxazole	Kernicterus
1956–1960	Chloramphenicol	Gray baby syndrome
1952–1971	Hexachlorophene	Brain lesions
1964–1965	Epsom salts enemas	Magnesium toxicity
1976–1999	Erythromycin	Pyloric stenosis
1981–1983	Propylene glycol	Seizures
Uncertain–1982	Benzyl alcohol	Gasping syndrome
1983–1984	Intravenous vitamin E	Multiorgan damage
1985–present	Postnatal corticosteroids	Cerebral palsy

Data from Refs.[5–7]

unnecessary intubation and surfactant administration in a substantial proportion of infants.[10–12]

Example: Prophylactic Indomethacin

In an NICU with a low rate of severe intraventricular hemorrhage (IVH), the risk of prophylactic indomethacin would seem to outweigh the benefit. However, in an NICU with a moderate to high rate of severe IVH, prophylactic indomethacin would be beneficial for reducing the short-term outcome of severe IVH. The decision to use indomethacin prophylaxis could also be favorably influenced by the NICU's baseline rate of pulmonary hemorrhage, symptomatic patent ductus arteriosus (PDA), and PDA ligation.[13–15]

Example: Erythropoietin

In an NICU seeking to reduce blood transfusions, use of erythropoietin (EPO) would seem like a logical drug to consider for routine use. However, although several meta-analyses concluded that EPO did reduce transfusions slightly, the small reduction was considered to be of minimal clinical importance. Of greater concern was an increase in severe retinopathy of prematurity (ROP) with EPO use.[16–19] In this context, use of EPO in an NICU with a low rate of severe ROP would seem of minimal benefit at best, and use in an NICU with a moderate or high rate of severe ROP would be counterproductive.

DOES THE INDIVIDUAL PATIENT'S CLINICAL CONTEXT MODIFY THE RISKS AND BENEFITS

After assessing the risk/benefit ratio of a medication in the NICU's clinical context of morbidity and mortality and after establishing a general approach to the drug's use, the individual baby's clinical status should be considered. The risk/benefit ratio of a drug may be further altered by the child's gestational age, chronologic age, presence of organ dysfunction, previous and current use of other medications, availability of vascular access, and a host of other clinical variables.[20–25] Blind use of a drug protocol without consideration of these important clinical variables may inadvertently result in ineffective or counterproductive results.

Example: Dexamethasone

Dexamethasone has been used in premature infants to reduce or prevent bronchopulmonary dysplasia (BPD). Great concern has been raised regarding the dose, duration of treatment, timing of treatment (early vs later in the hospitalization), and adverse effects such as bowel perforations and cerebral palsy. Routine use seems contraindicated, but some data suggest that infants at high risk of developing BPD have an improved neurologic outcome if treated with dexamethasone, compared with infants with a lower risk of BPD.[26–29] So although an NICU may not routinely use dexamethasone and may even enjoy a low rate of BPD, an occasional infant may be found that is at high risk for developing BPD and could warrant treatment.

PERCEPTION VERSUS THE REALITY OF NICU MEDICATION USE

A major cause of failure to use medications appropriately in the NICU is lack of awareness of actual drug use data. The data may not be routinely collected, reported, or reviewed by the NICU team. This lack of critical self-assessment may lead to years of drug misuse. Some NICU drug use data are available in certain NICU databases such as the Pediatrix Clinical Data Warehouse and the Vermont Oxford Network database.[30,31] Benchmarking the use of key drugs against a large network database can provide valuable insight into one's own drug use. Review of these data in the context of gestational age or birth weight or by use of risk adjustment models is important to avoid misinterpretation. Thorough review of the risks and benefits of a medication's use, including NICU and patient level modifiers, and comparison against NICU drug databases enables the NICU team to answer the question "do we have a problem?"

IDENTIFYING THE ROOT CAUSES OF MEDICATION MISUSE

When a clinical practice problem is identified in the NICU, the immediate response may be an ultimatum to the clinical staff (eg, we are not going to use dexamethasone). This approach may be transiently effective, but improvement is often not sustained. Evaluation of the root causes of the specific use of an NICU medication reveals the system factors that are driving the current pattern of medication use. Once these system factors are identified, system-based changes can be implemented that have a much greater chance of producing sustainable change.

Root cause analysis (RCA) can be done using complex formal methodology or by more simple methods. In its simplest form, RCA is done by assembling a multidisciplinary team (physicians, nurse practitioners, nurses, pharmacists) that is involved in the use of the drug.[32] This team analyzes the process of how and why the medication is used or not used. Initial proximate causes are identified. The team then drills down further by repeatedly asking "why" at each step. Root causes that are driving the drug use are identified, providing the team with specific targets for intervention (**Fig. 2**).

Example: Antireflux Medications

Antireflux medications, such as metoclopramide, histamine 2 blockers, and proton pump inhibitors are highly used in some NICUs and virtually never used in other NICUs.[33,34] A NICU clinical team reviews its use of antireflux medications and identifies itself as a heavy user. A RCA reveals that the physicians and nurses have viewed

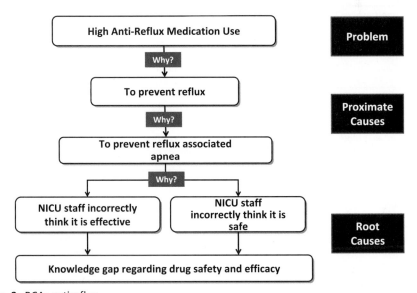

Fig. 2. RCA: antireflux.

these medicines as both safe and effective in reducing apnea related to gastroesophageal reflux. Review of the literature on the topic shows no definitive link between reflux and apnea and further shows little evidence of these drugs being safe or effective in premature infants. Indeed, adverse effects, including necrotizing enterocolitis, pneumonia, and central nervous system and endocrine abnormalities, have been associated with use of these drugs.[35–41] An educational intervention is devised to bridge this knowledge gap and create acceptance for stopping use of what was previously considered to be a safe and effective therapy.

MAKING AND TESTING CHANGES

Once the root causes of the medication's misuse have been identified, specific system changes can be devised and tested. Testing changes requires an iterative process of change, measurement, evaluation of impact, and redesign of change or full implementation of change depending on the results. This process is at the heart of quality improvement methodology and is commonly referred to as the plan-do-study-act (PDSA) cycle.[42,43] Once changes have successfully been made, it is imperative to track the medication's use on a continuous basis. System disruptions or modifications are frequent in the NICU setting and may affect medication use. Surveillance of drug use enables timely identification of aberrations in drug use, allowing for rapid correction and avoidance of adverse drug effects.

Example: Reversal of Improvement in Antireflux Medication Reduction

Continuing the earlier-mentioned example, the NICU team successfully implements the educational intervention and the use of antireflux drugs dramatically decreases. However, within 2 years antireflux drug use increases back to previous levels. A repeat

Table 2
NICU medications of concern

Drug	Potential Risks	Benefits
Dexamethasone[26,28,29,44]	Cerebral palsy, cardiomyopathy, hyperglycemia, hypertension	Improved lung function
Cefotaxime[45–48]	Mortality, fungal infection, development of drug resistance, extended-spectrum β-lactamase	Good penetration into cerebrospinal fluid
Prolonged antibiotic use[48–50]	Mortality, necrotizing enterocolitis, antibiotic resistance, fungal infection	Uncertain
Histamine 2 blockers[39–41]	Necrotizing enterocolitis, sepsis, alteration of gut microflora, fungal infection	Treatment of reflux esophagitis, gastritis
Metoclopramide[33,51–53]	Extrapyramidal effects, tardive dyskinesia	Uncertain
EPO[16–19]	ROP	Slight decrease in transfusions
Spironolactone[54–56]	Feminization	Minimally effective
Oxygen[57–62]	ROP, BPD, free radical–mediated injury	Essential medication, but proper pattern of use is not clearly established

RCA shows the same results: the drugs are perceived as safe and effective. A deeper RCA reveals that several significant changes have happened during this time. NICU census has increased by 20%, resulting in the addition of several new physicians. Nursing turnover during this time has been high, requiring hiring of many new nurses and frequent use of temporary nursing staff. The new physicians and nurses were not part of the previous educational intervention and viewed the drugs as useful. Use of the drugs crept back into routine practice. A repeat educational intervention was planned to again address the knowledge gap regarding these drugs. Ongoing educational refreshers were planned to prevent similar lapses in the future.

SUMMARY

Current medication use and misuse in the NICU may be a significant source of iatrogenesis (**Table 2**). All neonatologists are obligated to critically assess the risks and benefits of any medication they may use in treatment of these fragile infants. The risk/benefit ratio of these drugs must be evaluated and modified in the clinical context of the individual NICU's pattern of morbidity and mortality. The risk/benefit ratio should be further modified as needed in the context of the individual baby's unique clinical status. Ideally, NICU drug usage is compared with national data sets to determine if the NICU is an outlier in usage of the drug. RCA can be used to identify the drivers of the medications use. These drivers can be targeted for modification and changes tested via PDSA cycles. Surveillance of drug use determines if sound systemic changes have been successfully made and maintained.

Thoughtful and effective management of medication use in the NICU can provide enormous benefits to the patient and can avoid repetition of the infamous history of iatrogenesis in neonatal medicine.

REFERENCES

1. Allegaert K. Mechanism based medicine in infancy: complex interplay between developmental pharmacology and pharmacogenetics. Int J Clin Pharm 2011; 33(3):473–4.
2. Allegaert K, Verbesselt R, Naulaers G, et al. Developmental pharmacology: neonates are not just small adults. Acta Clin Belg 2008;63(1):16–24.
3. Leviton LC, Goldenberg RL, Baker CS, et al. Methods to encourage the use of antenatal corticosteroid therapy for fetal maturation: a randomized controlled trial. JAMA 1999;281(1):46–52.
4. Ellsbury DL. Crossing the quality chasm in neonatal-perinatal medicine. Clin Perinatol 2010;37(1):1–10.
5. Robertson AF. Reflections on errors in neonatology: I. The "Hands-Off" years, 1920 to 1950. J Perinatol 2003;23(1):48–55.
6. Robertson AF. Reflections on errors in neonatology: II. The "Heroic" years, 1950 to 1970. J Perinatol 2003;23(2):154–61.
7. Robertson AF. Reflections on errors in neonatology III. The "experienced" years, 1970 to 2000. J Perinatol 2003;23(3):240–9.
8. Ambalavanan N, Walsh M, Bobashev G, et al. Intercenter differences in bronchopulmonary dysplasia or death among very low birth weight infants. Pediatrics 2011;127(1):e106–16.
9. Horbar JD, Badger GJ, Lewit EM, et al. Hospital and patient characteristics associated with variation in 28-day mortality rates for very low birth weight infants. Vermont Oxford Network. Pediatrics 1997;99(2):149–56.

10. Finer NN, Carlo WA, Walsh MC, et al. Early CPAP versus surfactant in extremely preterm infants. N Engl J Med 2010;362(21):1970–9.

11. Morley CJ, Davis PG, Doyle LW, et al. Nasal CPAP or intubation at birth for very preterm infants. N Engl J Med 2008;358(7):700–8.

12. Dunn MS, Kaempf J, de Klerk A, et al. Randomized trial comparing 3 approaches to the initial respiratory management of preterm neonates. Pediatrics 2011; 128(5):e1069–76.

13. Fowlie PW, Davis PG, McGuire W. Prophylactic intravenous indomethacin for preventing mortality and morbidity in preterm infants. Cochrane Database Syst Rev 2010;7:CD000174.

14. Ment LR, Oh W, Ehrenkranz RA, et al. Low-dose indomethacin and prevention of intraventricular hemorrhage: a multicenter randomized trial. Pediatrics 1994; 93(4):543–50.

15. Schmidt B, Davis P, Moddemann D, et al. Long-term effects of indomethacin prophylaxis in extremely-low-birth-weight infants. N Engl J Med 2001;344(26):1966–72.

16. Aher S, Ohlsson A. Late erythropoietin for preventing red blood cell transfusion in preterm and/or low birth weight infants. Cochrane Database Syst Rev 2006; 3:CD004868.

17. Aher SM, Ohlsson A. Early versus late erythropoietin for preventing red blood cell transfusion in preterm and/or low birth weight infants. Cochrane Database Syst Rev 2006;3:CD004865.

18. Ohlsson A, Aher SM. Early erythropoietin for preventing red blood cell transfusion in preterm and/or low birth weight infants. Cochrane Database Syst Rev 2006;3: CD004863.

19. Suk KK, Dunbar JA, Liu A, et al. Human recombinant erythropoietin and the incidence of retinopathy of prematurity: a multiple regression model. J AAPOS 2008; 12(3):233–8.

20. Almirante B, Rodriguez D. Antifungal agents in neonates: issues and recommendations. Paediatr Drugs 2007;9(5):311–21.

21. Avent ML, Kinney JS, Istre GR, et al. Gentamicin and tobramycin in neonates: comparison of a new extended dosing interval regimen with a traditional multiple daily dosing regimen. Am J Perinatol 2002;19(8):413–20.

22. Baley JE, Meyers C, Kliegman RM, et al. Pharmacokinetics, outcome of treatment, and toxic effects of amphotericin B and 5-fluorocytosine in neonates. J Pediatr 1990;116(5):791–7.

23. Bartelink IH, Rademaker CM, Schobben AF, et al. Guidelines on paediatric dosing on the basis of developmental physiology and pharmacokinetic considerations. Clin Pharmacokinet 2006;45(11):1077–97.

24. DiCenzo R, Forrest A, Slish JC, et al. A gentamicin pharmacokinetic population model and once-daily dosing algorithm for neonates. Pharmacotherapy 2003; 23(5):585–91.

25. Fullas F, Padomek MT, Thieman CJ, et al. Comparative evaluation of six extended-interval gentamicin dosing regimens in premature and full-term neonates. Am J Health Syst Pharm 2011;68(1):52–6.

26. Watterberg KL, Papile LA, Adamkin DH. American Academy of Pediatrics. Committee on Fetus and Newborn. Policy statement—postnatal corticosteroids to prevent or treat bronchopulmonary dysplasia. Pediatrics 2010;126(4):800–8.

27. Doyle LW, Halliday HL, Ehrenkranz RA, et al. Impact of postnatal systemic corticosteroids on mortality and cerebral palsy in preterm infants: effect modification by risk for chronic lung disease. Pediatrics 2005;115(3):655–61.

28. Halliday HL, Ehrenkranz RA, Doyle LW. Late (>7 days) postnatal corticosteroids for chronic lung disease in preterm infants. Cochrane Database Syst Rev 2009;1: CD001145.
29. Halliday HL, Ehrenkranz RA, Doyle LW. Early (<8 days) postnatal corticosteroids for preventing chronic lung disease in preterm infants. Cochrane Database Syst Rev 2009;1:CD001146.
30. Clark RH, Bloom BT, Spitzer AR, et al. Reported medication use in the neonatal intensive care unit: data from a large national data set. Pediatrics 2006;117(6):1979–87.
31. Walsh MC, Yao Q, Horbar JD, et al. Changes in the use of postnatal steroids for bronchopulmonary dysplasia in 3 large neonatal networks. Pediatrics 2006; 118(5):e1328–35.
32. Ursprung R, Gray J. Random safety auditing, root cause analysis, failure mode and effects analysis. Clin Perinatol 2010;37(1):141–65.
33. Hibbs AM, Lorch SA. Metoclopramide for the treatment of gastroesophageal reflux disease in infants: a systematic review. Pediatrics 2006;118(2):746–52.
34. Kimball AL, Carlton DP. Gastroesophageal reflux medications in the treatment of apnea in premature infants. J Pediatr 2001;138(3):355–60.
35. Bancalari E. Apnea is not prolonged by acid gastroesophageal reflux in preterm infants. Pediatrics 2005;116(5):1217–8.
36. Clark RH, Spitzer AR. Patience is a virtue in the management of gastroesophageal reflux. J Pediatr 2009;155(4):464–5.
37. Di Fiore JM, Arko M, Whitehouse M, et al. Apnea is not prolonged by acid gastroesophageal reflux in preterm infants. Pediatrics 2005;116(5):1059–63.
38. Wheatley E, Kennedy KA. Cross-over trial of treatment for bradycardia attributed to gastroesophageal reflux in preterm infants. J Pediatr 2009;155(4):516–21.
39. Graham PL 3rd, Begg MD, Larson E, et al. Risk factors for late onset gram-negative sepsis in low birth weight infants hospitalized in the neonatal intensive care unit. Pediatr Infect Dis J 2006;25(2):113–7.
40. Guillet R, Stoll BJ, Cotten CM, et al. Association of H2-blocker therapy and higher incidence of necrotizing enterocolitis in very low birth weight infants. Pediatrics 2006;117(2):e137–42.
41. Saiman L, Ludington E, Pfaller M, et al. Risk factors for candidemia in neonatal intensive care unit patients. The National Epidemiology of Mycosis Survey Study Group. Pediatr Infect Dis J 2000;19(4):319–24.
42. Ellsbury DL, Ursprung R. A primer on quality improvement methodology in neonatology. Clin Perinatol 2010;37(1):87–99.
43. Batalden PB, Nelson EC, Edwards WH, et al. Microsystems in health care: part 9. Developing small clinical units to attain peak performance. Jt Comm J Qual Saf 2003;29(11):575–85.
44. Cole CH. Postnatal glucocorticosteroid therapy for treatment and prevention of neonatal chronic lung disease. Expert Opin Investig Drugs 2000;9(1):53–67.
45. Cotten CM, McDonald S, Stoll B, et al. The association of third-generation cephalosporin use and invasive candidiasis in extremely low birth-weight infants. Pediatrics 2006;118(2):717–22.
46. Clark RH, Bloom BT, Spitzer AR, et al. Empiric use of ampicillin and cefotaxime, compared with ampicillin and gentamicin, for neonates at risk for sepsis is associated with an increased risk of neonatal death. Pediatrics 2006;117(1):67–74.
47. Benjamin DK Jr, Stoll BJ, Fanaroff AA, et al. Neonatal candidiasis among extremely low birth weight infants: risk factors, mortality rates, and neurodevelopmental outcomes at 18 to 22 months. Pediatrics 2006;117(1):84–92.

48. Benjamin DK Jr, Stoll BJ, Gantz MG, et al. Neonatal candidiasis: epidemiology, risk factors, and clinical judgment. Pediatrics 2010;126(4):e865–73.

49. Cantey JB, Sanchez PJ. Prolonged antibiotic therapy for "culture-negative" sepsis in preterm infants: it's time to stop! J Pediatr 2011;159(5):707–8.

50. Cotten CM, Taylor S, Stoll B, et al. Prolonged duration of initial empirical antibiotic treatment is associated with increased rates of necrotizing enterocolitis and death for extremely low birth weight infants. Pediatrics 2009;123(1):58–66.

51. Mejia NI, Jankovic J. Metoclopramide-induced tardive dyskinesia in an infant. Mov Disord 2005;20(1):86–9.

52. Putnam PE, Orenstein SR, Wessel HB, et al. Tardive dyskinesia associated with use of metoclopramide in a child. J Pediatr 1992;121(6):983–5.

53. Rao AS, Camilleri M. Review article: metoclopramide and tardive dyskinesia. Aliment Pharmacol Ther 2010;31(1):11–9.

54. Hoffman DJ, Gerdes JS, Abbasi S. Pulmonary function and electrolyte balance following spironolactone treatment in preterm infants with chronic lung disease: a double-blind, placebo-controlled, randomized trial. J Perinatol 2000;20(1): 41–5.

55. Swiglo BA, Cosma M, Flynn DN, et al. Clinical review: antiandrogens for the treatment of hirsutism: a systematic review and metaanalyses of randomized controlled trials. J Clin Endocrinol Metab 2008;93(4):1153–60.

56. Vachharajani AJ, Shah JK, Paes BA. Ovarian cyst in a premature infant treated with spironolactone. Am J Perinatol 2001;18(6):353–6.

57. Chen ML, Guo L, Smith LE, et al. High or low oxygen saturation and severe retinopathy of prematurity: a meta-analysis. Pediatrics 2010;125(6):e1483–92.

58. Ellsbury DL, Ursprung R. Comprehensive oxygen management for the prevention of retinopathy of prematurity: the pediatrix experience. Clin Perinatol 2010;37(1): 203–15.

59. Johnson K, Scott SD, Fraser KD. Oxygen use for preterm infants: factors that may influence clinical decisions surrounding oxygen titration. Adv Neonatal Care 2011;11(1):8–14 [quiz: 15–6].

60. Carlo WA, Finer NN, Walsh MC, et al. Target ranges of oxygen saturation in extremely preterm infants. N Engl J Med 2010;362(21):1959–69.

61. Saugstad OD. Oxygen and oxidative stress in bronchopulmonary dysplasia. J Perinat Med 2010;38(6):571–7.

62. Saugstad OD, Aune D. In search of the optimal oxygen saturation for extremely low birth weight infants: a systematic review and meta-analysis. Neonatology 2010;100(1):1–8.

Drug Studies in Newborns: A Therapeutic Imperative

George P. Giacoia, MD[a,b,*], Perdita Taylor-Zapata, MD[a,b],
Anne Zajicek, MD[a,b]

KEYWORDS

- Off-patent - Off-label - Drugs - Newborns - Efficacy - Safety

Drug labels frequently include disclaimers stating that safety and efficacy have not been established in children (**Box 1**). This statement is especially true for neonates (birth to 28 postnatal days). As a consequence, pediatric practice frequently involves the use of unlabeled drugs. The percentage of off-label medications used reaches up to 90% in neonatal intensive care units (NICU), particularly in very-low-birth-weight infants (VLBW).[1]

Off-label and unlabeled use of drugs in newborns can be seen as a surrogate for multiple unmet therapeutic needs, although in most cases the choice of a particular drug may not be supported by scientific evidence either. Drugs given to patients in NICUs are frequently affected by conditions not seen later in life. It may, therefore, be more important initially to focus on the indications requiring treatment rather than the drug substances themselves.

The description of the drugs as labeled, not labeled, or used off-label may be subject to different interpretations (eg, extemporaneous drug formulations may be considered either unlabeled or off-label). Off-patent drugs are those whose patent has expired. Off-label uses are those used for different indications than the indication on the label.

The history of neonatology contains numerous examples of drugs introduced in the NICU with little evidence of effectiveness or safety. In 1965, a half-page letter to the editor was published reporting the use of Priscoline (tolazoline) in 5 infants with hyaline membrane disease. That author stated, "No severe gastrointestinal difficulties such as those seen in adults were observed."[2] In the ensuing years, this vasodilator became

The views expressed by the authors in this article do not necessarily reflect those of the NICHD.
[a] Obstetric and Pediatric Pharmacology Branch
[b] Eunice Kennedy Shriver National Institute of Child Health and Human Development (NICHD), Rockville, MD 20852, USA
* Corresponding author. 6100 Executive Boulevard, Room 4AO1C, Bethesda, MD 20852.
E-mail address: giacoiag@mail.nih.gov

Clin Perinatol 39 (2012) 11–23
doi:10.1016/j.clp.2011.12.016
0095-5108/12/$ – see front matter Published by Elsevier Inc.

perinatology.theclinics.com

> **Box 1**
> **Factors responsible for the use of off-label and unlabeled drugs in newborns**
>
> - Developmental characteristics (23–42 weeks) of the population
> - Characterization of newborn conditions and diseases
> - Number of drugs used in the NICU and neonatologist practice standards
> - Limited knowledge of the clinical pharmacology of drugs across viable gestational age span
> - Specific factors that limit or prevent the implementation of drug studies in sick newborns
>   - Limited enrolment and small sample size
>   - Limitations on the amount of blood available
>   - Ethical issues
>   - Lack of pharmacokinetics studies leveraging prior knowledge
>   - Lack of appropriate pharmacodynamic, specific endpoints, and biomarkers
> - Search for evidence: regulatory versus scientific viewpoints
> - Regulatory, academic limitations in relation to economic factors

widely used. Twenty years later, the number and types of complications, including massive gastrointestinal bleeding, resulted in the abandonment of the use of tolazoline in newborns.[3] This experience with the introduction of tolazoline illustrates how off-label, innovative therapies have been sometimes introduced in neonatology for decades in an uncontrolled fashion, without informed consent or institutional review board oversight and not as part of carefully designed protocols. The off-label use of drugs in the newborn requires a systematic approach to detect and identify adverse effects.

It is paradoxic that the legislation and regulations that spurred the performance of labeling studies in children have been largely enacted and promulgated as a result of toxic reactions in newborns, and yet studies of drugs in neonates are wanting. Information about the safety and efficacy of medications in the youngest, and most vulnerable, of the pediatric age groups is especially scarce. Physicians are often asked to practice evidence-based medicine when the evidence is missing.

THE NEWBORN AS A DRUG RECIPIENT

The newborn infant cannot be considered a young child because a child cannot be considered a miniature adult. Developmental characteristics and most of the disease-specific conditions affecting preterm and full-term infants can profoundly affect the efficacy, disposition, and safety of drugs used in this population.

DEVELOPMENTAL CHARACTERISTICS (23–42 WEEKS) OF THE POPULATION

The full impact of developmental immaturity is unknown, particularly at the limits of viability.

Extremely low-birth-weight (ELBW) infants, defined as those with a birth weight less than 1000 g (2 lb, 3 oz), bears little resemblance to the developmental characteristics of a term infant.[4]

Bio-disposition and, subsequently, the effect of drugs are likely to be severely compromised in VLBW infants. The different processes responsible for bio-disposition (absorption, distribution and metabolism, and elimination) change drastically between 23 and 40 weeks of gestation. Gastric pH is higher, gastric emptying prolonged, and intestinal absorption is delayed at low gestational ages. In the newborn, drug-metabolizing enzymes are immature, particularly CYP2D6 and CYP1A1. CYP3A4 increases gradually in preterm infants with increasing gestational age.[5] The role and substrates of CYP3A7, the fetal form of CYP3A4, remain unknown. In general, phase II or conjugation reactions are inefficient in newborns and may play an important role in reducing their ability to eliminate xenobiotics.

Drug distribution is affected by the marked changes in body composition in terms of body water and lipids. The pathways for systemic clearance by the kidney are partially developed, compromising the renal elimination of several compounds. Differences in the developmental expression of metabolic pathways coupled with compromised renal clearance are mostly responsible for the tremendous interindividual differences in drug bio-disposition. The corollary of the developmental changes is the extreme variability of measures of drug disposition in VLBW infants. Given the profound differences at both ends of the gestational age range, the question that remains is can the population be stratified for drug studies according to meaningful gestational age periods?

In addition to developmental immaturity, these infants may have organ dysfunction related to concomitant disease processes that reduce the clearance or elimination of drugs as in cases of hepatic or renal insufficiency. Life-support measures (eg, positive pressure ventilation) may reduce hepatic blood flow, which is particularly important for those drugs that have clearance related to hepatic blood flow (eg, morphine).

A major problem in pediatric pharmacology is the limited availability of validated of pharmacodynamic endpoints. The situation in neonates is even more extreme because immaturity of cellular transporters or receptors is likely to alter the effect of drugs, particularly at the low gestational ages. There is an urgent need for the creation of pharmacodynamic surrogate endpoints. With increasing knowledge, it would be possible to apply novel pharmacometric technologies (eg, in silico simulation of exposure-response relationships and disease-progression modeling) to achieve rational neonatal drug therapy.

NEONATAL DISEASES/INDICATIONS

Many conditions in neonatal medicine are unique to the perinatal period because of the distinctive developmental status of low-birth-weight infants and newborn infants, featuring both immaturity and transitional physiology. Some diseases or conditions vary in severity and frequency with gestational or postnatal age, not only requiring specific longitudinal clinical trial designs but also the study of distinct subgroups.

It is not within the scope of this article to detail the differences in cause, diagnosis, pathophysiology, and response to the therapy for the various conditions affecting newborns in relation to older children and adults. A few examples are described to underscore the problems of studying drugs in the neonatal period.

Shock and Cardiovascular Instability in Preterm Infants

Cardiovascular instability in preterm infants continues to be an elusive therapeutic dilemma. Although about one half of low-birth-weight infants are treated for hypotension or shock, there is a lack of information on normal blood pressure in infants aged between 23 and 26 weeks, particularly when to treat, how to treat, and the effect of treatment on outcome. The immaturity of the myocardium, persistence of fetal shunts, blood loss, and ventilator support may profoundly affect cardiovascular stability in the first week of life. Measurements of cardiac instability (eg, cardiac output, cerebral perfusion, and peripheral perfusion) have not been sufficiently developed or validated in the VLBW infant.[6]

The Neonatal Research Network (NRN), a network sponsored by the National Institute of Child Health and Human Development (NICHD), has undertaken a review of practice standards across their research sites to determine the threshold blood pressure requiring treatment, and a double-blind feasibility study using hydrocortisone or dobutamine was performed by the NRN. Thus far, the results have demonstrated the difficulty in performing such a trial. It remains to be determined to what extent the measurement of blood pressure is a surrogate of shock in VLBW infants.

Neonatal Seizures

Most neonatal seizures are caused by an acute event, such as hypoxic-ischemic encephalopathy, stroke, or infection. Rarely, seizures may caused by genetic conditions (eg, benign familial neonatal seizures) or linked to a syndrome or epilepsy. Neuronal excitability is increased in the immature brain as a consequence of several factors, including the increased number of synapses, transient number of synapses, temporary expression of excitatory receptor subunits, and excitatory expression of γ-aminobutyric acid during early postnatal life.[7]

Because of the characteristics of neonatal brain development, seizures in preterm and term newborns differ in clinical and electroencephalographic (EEG) manifestations from seizures in older children. A classification has been proposed using the terms clonic, tonic, myoclonic, and subtle. Subtle seizures are prevalent in premature infants and may manifest as apnea and, therefore, be confused with apnea of prematurity.[8] Clinical diagnosis of neonatal seizures without EEG documentation is inaccurate, although unfortunately the EEG may not be helpful in confirming a diagnosis of seizures. A phenomenon unique to newborns, called electro-clinical dissociation, refers to generalized tonic seizures without EEG manifestations.[9] Conversely, EEG discharges may occur without clinical seizures, particularly in patients receiving phenobarbital.[10] It is not known if EEG seizures without clinical manifestation can be deleterious and, therefore, require treatment.

Despite its limitations, bedside long-term EEG recording is the gold standard for the diagnosis of neonatal seizures. The incorporation of the amplitude-integrated EEG (aEEG) has been proposed. Recent studies revealed that aEEG cannot replace conventional EEG, but the combination of the 2 techniques increases the detection rate of clinical events.[11]

Despite considerable advances in the pharmacology of antiepileptic drugs (AEDs), continuous EEG monitoring using digital systems with simultaneous video recording, neuroimaging, and basic science research on cellular mechanisms of brain injury, the treatment of neonatal seizures has progressed slowly, lagging behind the therapy offered to older children and adults. Regardless of the pathogenesis of neonatal convulsions, phenobarbital has been a standard therapy for decades despite mounting evidence that the drug may be ineffective in preterm infants[12] and may even be neurotoxic. Phenobarbital, phenytoin, and valproic acid given at therapeutic doses produced marked neuronal apoptotic cells in experimental animal models.[13,14] A rodent study demonstrated phenobarbital induced apoptotic lesions in the striatum, cortex, and limbic regions of the brain.[15] There is a growing body of experimental evidence from rodents to primates, together with epidemiologic studies, that suggests that ketamine and general anesthetics, by producing neuro-apoptotic lesions in early life, may impair future cognitive development.[16] Currently, a large international epidemiologic study is seeking to ascertain if the experimental evidence can be linked to human outcome data. Newborn infants receiving chronic administration of phenobarbital should also be included in this type of long-term outcome study. In view of toxic and efficacy concerns, other AEDs should be studied in newborn patients.

Neonatal Encephalopathy

Neonatal encephalopathy is a heterogeneous syndrome resulting from different conditions affecting newborns born at term or late preterm ($\geq$36 weeks' gestation). Birth asphyxia and hypoxic-ischemic (anoxic) encephalopathy are responsible for many cases. In many others, however, the cause remains unexplained. The term neonatal encephalopathy has largely replaced hypoxic-ischemic encephalopathy to avoid implying a specific pathophysiology.

There is a need to adopt a consensus as to definition and degree of severity of neonatal encephalopathy. Some investigators adopt stringent criteria (ie, 2 or more symptoms of brain dysfunction, abnormal level of consciousness, seizures, tone and reflex abnormalities, apnea, and feeding difficulties) at 24 hours,[17] whereas others include infants born with a low 5-minute Apgar score.[18] The Sarnat classification or other scoring systems have also been used to predict outcome.[19,20]

Over the last 10 years, specific neuroprotective therapies have been tested in animal and clinical studies. There are encouraging reports on the effect of hypothermia in increasing survival and reducing neurodevelopmental sequelae in newborns with moderate neonatal encephalopathy. The persistence of clinical symptoms at 72 hours of age has a high risk of death or disability, however.[21] There are several potential candidate therapies that could be tested in conjunction with hypothermia (eg, antioxidants, anticonvulsants, and erythropoietin), with additional novel treatments under consideration.[22] The effect of induced hypothermia on the disposition and effect of drugs remains understudied.

As with other neonatal conditions, outcome endpoints other than clinical evaluations will be needed to define neonatal encephalopathy and to gauge progression, regression, and recovery of patients with neonatal encephalopathy. There is an urgent need to identify biomarkers for disease stratification, toxicity evaluation, and outcome prediction. Considerable progress has been made on the use of imaging technology, although quantification and standardization across institutions are still lacking.

Apnea of Prematurity

Apnea of prematurity is defined as a sudden cessation of breathing that lasts for at least 20 seconds or that is accompanied by bradycardia or oxygen desaturation in an infant younger than 37 weeks' gestational age.[23]

In practice, the definition of apnea of prematurity varies in relationship to symptoms, and the duration of apnea considered to be abnormal while the degree of change in oxygen saturation varies by NICU practice. As with other neonatal conditions, the definition, diagnosis, and treatment have not been harmonized. The influence of confounding conditions (eg, sedation, oxygen therapy, and the presence of a patent ductus arteriosus [PDA]) has not been characterized. For decades, the treatment of apnea of prematurity has consisted of methylxanthines (caffeine or theophylline) and doxapram. Doxapram was abandoned because of toxicity concerns (gastrointestinal disturbances and hypertension), as well as the lack of an oral preparation and the lack of evidence of superiority over methylxanthines.[24]

Over the years, caffeine has prevailed as the standard of care. The long-term effects of apnea or its treatment on neurodevelopment has not been sufficiently characterized. Experimental studies in animal models have raised concerns that caffeine acting as a nonspecific adenosine receptor antagonist could lead to neurologic damage. Studies of adenosine receptors in caffeine-treated animal models have yielded conflicting results.[25,26] A recent large trial of caffeine versus placebo in infants with birth weight less than 1250 g found a reduced incidence of cerebral palsy and cognitive deficits,[27] demonstrating the difficulty in interpreting and animal data. The standard dosage of caffeine has been a loading dose of 20 mg/kg followed by a maintenance dose of 5 to 10 mg/kg/d. Higher doses, however, were found to be more effective in the treatment of apnea of prematurity.[28] A recent randomized trial of 2 dosages (standard- and high-dose regimes using a loading dose of 80 mg/kg and maintenance of 20 mg/kg/d) did not demonstrate adverse outcomes for development, and behavior.[29]

The results of these studies have lead to the widespread use of high doses of caffeine in the NICUs across the United States. Despite the beneficial effects, toxicity concerns remain. The results of a brain magnetic resonance imaging study in a placebo-controlled trial of preterm infants (<1250 g birth weight) are consistent with an enhancement in white matter microstructural development in infants treated with standard doses of caffeine.[30] This finding provides evidence of a beneficial effect in preterm infants. The routine use of large doses of caffeine may require further epidemiologic and experimental toxicity studies before their wide implementation.

The Food and Drug Administration (FDA) labeled caffeine citrate (CAFCIT) for short-term use in preterm infants (between 28 and <33 weeks of gestational age) in April 2000. Efficacy was established from a multi-institutional, double-blind, placebo-controlled trial in which apnea was defined as an infant having at least 6 apneic episodes of greater than 20 seconds in a 24-hour period. Altogether, 82 preterm infants were studied. The 45 treated infants received CAFCIT at the standard loading dose of 20 mg/kg and a maintenance dose of 5 mg/Kg/d for a treatment period limited to 10 to 12 days.

A Cochrane review analyzed 5 randomized trials comparing caffeine and theophylline and did not find differences in efficacy; however, toxicity was lower in those patients treated with caffeine.[31]

Bronchopulmonary Dysplasia

Bronchopulmonary dysplasia (BPD) exemplifies the difficulties of demonstrating the efficacy of drugs used in newborns, including (1) evolving definitions of the disease, (2) disease heterogeneity, (3) the need to develop an approach to stratify affected newborns according to pathophysiological changes and postnatal age, and (4) matching therapeutic strategies to the stage of the disease.

Northway and colleagues[32] first described the disease in 1967. Over the ensuing 44 years, the definition of BPD has been extensively revised. Bancalari and colleagues[33] developed a definition based on the ventilation criteria and oxygen requirement at 28 days to maintain arterial oxygen tension more than 50 mm Hg. A modification was proposed by Shennan[34] to add the need for supplemental oxygen at 36 weeks of postmenstrual age.

In 2001, the NICHD consensus conference on bronchopulmonary dysplasia developed a severity scoring system based on oxygen requirements and the need for ventilator support. Walsh and colleagues[35] proposed a physiology definition at 35 to 37 weeks' postmenstrual age (PMA) who received mechanical ventilation, continuous airway pressure, or supplemental oxygen of 30%. This physiologic definition reduced the rate of BPD by eliminating those patients that were misdiagnosed.

Models have been developed recently for estimating the probability of BPD at specific postnatal age using available clinical data.[36] This approach is important because BPD is an evolving process of lung injury, and the pathophysiology is likely to differ at various times. In the initial stage, pathophysiologic changes are self-limited or can be reversed (up to age 7 days). Stage 2 is an evolving disease, and stage 3 is established chronic disease beginning at 28 ± 7 days. Therapeutic interventions should be targeted to either prevent the development of the disease or arrest/reverse the pathophysiologic alterations. In addition to minimizing barotraumas and oxygen exposure, treatment of BPD has included steroids, diuretics, and antiinflammatory agents. The cause of chronic lung disease (CLD) is multifactorial. The inflammation of pulmonary parenchyma plays a pivotal role in evolution of CLD. During inflammation, there is a massive influx of neutrophils into the alveoli, with liberation of proinflammatory mediators, such as cytokines and the release of oxygen free radicals and proteinases in the alveoli. Therapeutic approaches to arrest and reverse the process with the use of antioxidants (eg, superoxide dismutase) and antiproteases (alpha 1 proteinase inhibitor) have not been impressive. A new approach being considered is the use of recombinant Clara cell protein to prevent or ameliorate the disease.[37] A number of studies have tested the efficacy of early (<8 days) postnatal administration of corticosteroids for preventing CLD in preterm infants. A Neonatal Cochrane review included 28 randomized controlled trials (RCTs) enrolling a total of 3740 participants.[38] A meta-analysis of these trials demonstrated significant benefits, such as earlier extubation and decreased risk of CLD at 28 days and 36 weeks' PMA, death or CLD at 28 days and 36 weeks PMA, and rates of PDA and retinopathy of prematurity (ROP), including severe ROP. Steroids (most commonly dexamethasone) were given orally or intravenously. Safety was not established. Steroids have also been administered by aerosol delivery in the first 2 weeks of life. A Cochrane review analyzing 5 trials enrolling 429 neonates reported on the incidence of CLD at 36 weeks' PMA. There was no statistically significant difference in the incidence of CLD at 36 weeks' PMA in the inhaled steroid group versus the placebo group.[39]

A serious concern is the significant suppression of the pituitary-adrenal axis exhibited by some infants treated with inhaled corticosteroids for the prevention of CLD. Thus, the use of inhaled steroids in this population is not indicated. A major concern with studies of inhalation therapy in neonates is the uncertainty regarding drug delivery and deposition in the peripheral airways. Because of their submicrometer size, aerosolized nanoparticles can potentially overcome many of the problems associated with traditional inhalation therapy if their lung deposition can be significantly increased. To make the many next-generation inhaled medications effective, viable drug delivery alternatives and neonatal-specific delivery devices need to be developed.

RARE DISEASES OF THE NEWBORN

There is a group of diseases/conditions that have low prevalence in the newborn population (eg, stroke, neonatal hypertension, transient diabetes, severe cardiac arrhythmias) in which multiple drugs have been used for treatment. This group of conditions could be grouped as orphan neonatal diseases for which RCTs likely could not be used but could be studied using models of orphan drug development.

NUMBER OF DRUGS USED IN THE NICU AND STANDARDS OF PRACTICE

The large number of off-label drugs used in the NICU has been widely recognized.[40,41] The extent of the overuse was not recognized until 2006 with the publication of data collected from a large national database of practicing neonatologists. From January 1996 to April 2005, 409 different drugs were prescribed.[42] The drugs recorded included the following number of different drugs within therapeutic classes: antibiotics (53); steroids (10); diuretics (6); antihypertensives, beta-blockers, bronchodilators, and neuromuscular blocking agents (7 each); and calcium channel blocking drugs (3).

During the last 2 years (2010–2011), the number of drugs used decreased to 288 (Clark RH, personal communication, 2011).

Because an overwhelming amount of drugs are not labeled nor are there sufficient data in the literature to provide adequate guidance, there are large variations in treatment practices. Although tools and resources for the practice of evidence-based neonatology have been developed, there remains a significant tendency to prescribe different drugs within therapeutic classes for which there is a paucity of safety and efficacy information. The solution to the problem of unlabeled drugs in newborns will require a combined approach of decreasing the number and variety of drugs prescribed while acquiring the needed information in high-priority drugs thus potentially augmenting the knowledge base and the labeling.

FACTORS THAT LIMIT AND PREVENT THE DEVELOPMENT AND IMPLEMENTATION OF NEWBORN DRUG STUDIES
Sample Size and Heterogeneity of Study Population

Small sample size, heterogeneity of study population, and reliance on a single efficacy study are major factors leading to failed trials in neonates. Several means allow for the reduction of the number of children required for an RCT without decreasing its statistical power; this consideration may include a homogeneous subpopulation within a single cause that is likely to decrease the interindividual variability as well as potentially facilitating the demonstration of a clinically significant treatment effect size. Unfortunately, many studies are based on stratification of birth weight rather than gestational age. The later is associated with a more homogeneous population in terms of developmental state of maturation and allows one to better predict changes in neonatal drug elimination in relation to maturational changes.[43]

Availability and Limitations on Amount and Frequency of Blood Sampling

The relative small blood volume of VLBW infants imposes severe limitations to the amount of blood available for pharmacokinetics (PK) studies. This limitation can be circumvented by using scavenged blood samples and the use of dried blood spots in filter paper, coupled with the development of very small blood volume assays technology. Samples may also be collected from other sources (urine, saliva, expired air).

Ethical Issues

There are important limitations in performing studies in particularly vulnerable, medically fragile populations. Clinical trials in sick preterm infants may involve more than minimal risks. Studies seeking to demonstrate evidence for dosing, safety, or efficacy for drugs that have been and are currently widely used must be ethically justified and in compliance with FDA regulations. The inclusion of a placebo group in patients receiving intensive care may prove to be a major challenge requiring special study designs.

Obtaining consent from a parent or guardian faced with a sick newborn remains problematic. It has been suggested that informed consent could be obtained from mothers in premature labor at high risk to deliver sick newborns. It is postulated that when prematurity and illness are only a possibility, mothers will be able to exercise their judgment before facing the emotional stress of an unexpected critical event that requires intensive care. Considering the tremendous differences in the physiologic characteristics of the VLBW infant and the possibility of overtreatment or undertreatment, a case may be made to consider it unethical not to perform dosing studies when a new drug is introduced in the NICU. Academicians and regulators should strive to perform adequate dosing studies when there is no available information in this population, particularly in life-threatening conditions.

LACK OF PHARMACOKINETIC STUDIES AND ABILITY TO LEVERAGE PRIOR KNOWLEDGE IN OLDER CHILDREN AND ADULTS

Information on PK of the numerous drugs used in the NICU is either not available or may be the result of flawed studies using adult parameters. Differences between adults, older children, and newborns need to be taken into account. Dosing information may only be available in adults. Prior information may be assembled to build an information system that will allow the use of modeling techniques to determine the initial dose selection that can be used in clinical trial simulations to determine appropriate dosing recommendations.[44]

LACK OF APPROPRIATE PHARMACODYNAMIC MEASUREMENTS, SPECIFIC ENDPOINTS, AND BIOMARKERS

Although advanced technological support remains the backbone of NICUs, much of the equipment, instruments, and devices used are miniaturized versions of those used for older patients. With few exceptions, it is rare to find instruments and devices that have been developed and rigorously evaluated specifically for newborn infants and small children.

Biomarkers have been sparingly used in neonatology, more for patient management rather than drug development. Limitations of their use include lack of specificity, high cost, nonautomated, labor intensive, lack of real-time accessibility, and lack of normative data.

An important role of biomarkers in neonatology is to define potential subject cohorts and as potential surrogate endpoints, to define molecular endpoints, or to measure desired effects. A considerable body of literature exists on the use of biomarkers for the diagnosis of sepsis.[45,46] Despite the large number of biomarkers studied to date, including acute phase reactants, chemokines and cytokines, cell-surface antigens, and the application of genomics and proteomics, no single biomarker fulfills the requirements for application in clinical trials. The investigation of prognostic biomarkers and of disease progression is an area that deserves further consideration.

SEARCH FOR EVIDENCE: REGULATORY VERSUS SCIENTIFIC VIEWPOINTS

Practicing and academic neonatologists may be aware of the labeling requirements of new drugs specifically developed for the treatment of neonatal conditions (eg, surfactant for the treatment of respiratory distress syndrome) but are largely unaware that hundreds of the off-label drugs that they prescribe daily have never been studied in this population. The problem is compounded because many of these drugs have been used for many years, and there is a lack of a readily available reference on the labeling status of pediatric drugs.

FDA regulators have done a remarkable job in increasing the number of drugs labeled in pediatrics. Faced with the large number of unlabeled drugs in pediatrics, the FDA developed an approach based on extrapolation of efficacy in adults to the pediatric population under which no efficacy trials are needed if the pathophysiology of the disease, response to therapy, and disease characteristics are sufficiently similar in children and adults.[47] PK and safety cannot be extrapolated and therefore additional neonatal trials will be required. In addition, labeling is based on the evidence available for different pediatric age groups. As a consequence, drugs are more likely to be labeled and used in older children before in infants. Due to the above difficulties in performing studies in neonates, neonatal labeling is frequently inadequate even if efficacy extrapolation is possible, PK and safety cannot be extrapolated and, therefore, additional neonatal trials will be required.

SAFETY ISSUES

There is a lack of adequate data systems to detect adverse drug effects despite the multiplicity of drugs used concomitantly in the NICU setting and the potential toxicity of the excipients used in drug formulations. The identification of biomarkers of toxicity is greatly needed. Consideration must also be given to the possible effect of xenobiotics in organ development. For example, angiotensin-converting enzyme inhibitors may influence on-going renal development in neonates aged less than 36 weeks of life.

CHANGE OF PARADIGM: PROMOTE RATIONAL THERAPEUTICS FOR THE MOST VULNERABLE POPULATION

The most pressing need is to develop a knowledge base by which regulatory compliant neonatal studies can be designed and performed.

Because most drugs in need of study are off-patent in addition to being off-label, the major priority is to cover gaps that prevent the study of drugs in newborns. Here are a few suggestions:

1. Develop a consensus on the diagnostic criteria of the most common neonatal conditions (eg, BPD, neonatal seizures, Hypoxic-ischemic encephalopathy [HIE]) including common data elements.
2. Involve the leadership and encourage the participation of the major US and international neonatal collaborative networks in off-label studies in the newborn population.
3. An incremental approach for developing dosing recommendations and demonstration of efficacy and safety should be adopted. It should be recognized that although the RCTs are the gold standard for the establishment of efficacy, this may not be possible in this patient population, and other clinical trial designs may be needed. Data gathering using pharmacoepidemiologic approaches may be required. The use of modeling and simulation could be hight valuable in this population.
4. Large-scale efficacy trials should be undertaken following the analysis of preliminary dosing and safety data, evaluation of trial feasibility, and use of modeling and simulation to insure proper clinical trial design, potentially incorporating novel clinical endpoints and biomarkers of efficacy and safety.
5. A partnership between academia and industry could result in the development of new diagnostic and clinically relevant neonatal biomarkers to be validated in clinical trials. Another benefit of this partnership could be the prompt application in neonatology of new, specific biomarkers that could replace the nonspecific biomarkers currently in use.

Commercially available neonatal-specific formulations are needed for oral as well as parenteral drugs.

SUMMARY

The prevalent use of off-label drugs in the NICU clearly illustrates the need to reevaluate the current approach to the study of drugs in this special population.

Despite attempts to increase the number of FDA-compliant studies we remain unenlightened about the proper dosing, safety and efficacy of most drugs used in newborns, particularly preterm infants. Most drugs are off-patent, although they have been in use for many years.

Labeling in pediatrics is most prevalent in the older age groups (more than 6 years of age), and is the exception in infants unless a condition is judged to be an exclusive neonatal condition (respiratory distress syndrome, persistence of the PDA of pulmonary fetal circulation).

Lack of appropriate outcome measures, pharmacodynamic markers, biomarkers, and outcome measures are major obstacles to performing FDA-compliant trials.

REFERENCES

1. Choonara I, Conroy S. Unlicensed and off-label drug use in children: implications for safety. Drug Saf 2002;25:1–5.
2. Cotton EK. The use of Priscoline in the treatment of the hypoperfusion syndrome. Pediatrics 1965;36:149.
3. Ward RM. Pharmacology of tolazoline. Clin Perinatol 1984;11(3):703–13.
4. Reiter PD. Neonatal pharmacology and pharmacokinetics. NeoReviews 2002; 3(11):e229.
5. Ilegaert K, van den Anker JN, Naulaers G. Determinants of drug metabolism in early neonatal life. Curr Clin Pharmacol 2007;2(1):23–9.
6. Summary in proceedings from the cardiovascular group on cardiovascular instability in preterm infants. Pediatrics 2006;117:S34.
7. Holmes GL, Ben Ari Y. The neurobiology and consequences of epilepsy in the developing brain. Pediatr Res 2002;49:320–5.
8. Mizrahi EM, Kellaway P. Characterization and classification of neonatal seizures. Neurology 1987;37:1837–44.
9. Weinder SP, Painter MJ, Geva D, et al. Neonatal seizures: electro-clinical dissociation. Pediatr Neurol 1991;5:363–8.
10. Zhang L, Zhou YX, Chang XP. Diagnostic value of amplitude-integrated electroencephalogram in neonatal seizures. Neurosci Bull 2011;27:251–7.
11. Volpe JJ. Neonatal seizures. In: Volpe JJ, editor. Neurology of the newborn. Philadelphia (PA): Saunders, Elisivier; 2008. p. 203–44. Chapter 5.
12. Boylean BG, Rennie JM, Wilson G, et al. Phenobarbitone, neonatal seizures and video EEG. Arch Dis Child Fetal Neonatal Ed 2002;86:F165–70.
13. Uckermann O, Luksch H, Stefovska V, et al. Matrix metalloproteinases 2 and 9 fail to influence drug-induced neuroapoptosis in developing rat brain. Neurotox Res 2011;19(4):638.
14. Katz I, Kim J, Gale K, et al. Effects of lamotrigine alone and in combination with MK-801, phenobarbital, or phenytoin on cell death in the neonatal rat brain. J Pharmacol Exp Ther 2007;322(2):494–500.
15. Forcelli PA, Kim J, Kondratyev A, et al. Pattern of antiepileptic drug-induced cell death in limbic regions of the neonatal rat brain. Epilepsia 2011;52(12):e207–11.
16. Vutskits L. Anesthetic-related neurotoxicity and the developing brain: shall we change practice? Paediatr Drugs 2011;14(1):13–21.
17. Badawi N, Kurinczuk JJ. Antepartum risk factors for newborn encephalopathy: the Western Australian case-control study. BMJ 1998;317:1549–53.
18. Bartha AI, Foster-Barber A, Miller SP, et al. Neonatal encephalopathy: association of cytokines with MR spectroscopy and outcome. Pediatr Res 2004;56:960.
19. Thompson CM, Puterman AS, Linley LL, et al. The value of a scoring system for hypoxic ischemic encephalopathy, in predicting neurodevelopmental outcome. Acta Pediatr 1997;86:757–61.

20. Miller SP, Latal B, Clark H, et al. Clinical signs predict 30 month neurodevelopmental outcome after neonatal encephalopathy. Am J Obstet Gynecol 2004; 190:93–9.
21. Shankaran S, Laptook AR, Tyson JE, et al. Evolution of encephalopathy during whole body hypothermia for neonatal hypoxic-ischemic encephalopathy. J Pediatr 2011, in press.
22. Rees S, Harding R, Walker D. The biologic basis of injury and neuroprotection in the fetal and neonatal brain. Int J Dev Neurosci 2011;29(6):551–63.
23. American Academy of Pediatrics, Committee on Fetus and Newborn. Apnea, sudden infant death syndrome, and home monitoring. Pediatrics 2003;111(4): 914–7. Available at: http://pediatrics.aappublications.org/content/111/4/914.full.
24. Henderson-Smart DJ, Steer PA. Doxapram treatment for apnea in preterm infants. Cochrane Database Syst Rev 2004;4:CD000074.
25. Black AM, Pandya S, Clark D, et al. Effect of caffeine and morphine on the developing pre-mature brain. Brain Res 2008;1219:136–42.
26. Desfrere L, Olivier P, Schwendimann L, et al. Transient inhibition of astrocytogenesis in developing mouse brain following postnatal caffeine exposure. Pediatr Res 2007;62(950):604–9.
27. Schimidt B, Roberts RS, Davis P, et al. Long term effects of caffeine therapy for apnea of prematurity. N Engl J Med 2007;357:1893–902.
28. Gray PH, Flenady VJ, Charles BG, et al. Caffeine citrate for very preterm infants: effects on development, temperament and behavior. J Paediatr Child Health 2011;47:167–72.
29. Steer PA, Fienady VJ, Lee TC, et al. Periextubation caffeine in preterm neonates: a randomized dose response trial. J Paediatr Child Health 2003;39:511–5.
30. Doyle LW, Cheong J, Hunt RW, et al. Caffeine and brain development in very preterm infants. Ann Neurol 2010;68:734–42.
31. Henderson-Smart DJ, Steer PA. Caffeine versus theophylline for apnea in preterm infants. Cochrane Database Syst Rev 1998;2:CD000273.
32. Norhway WH Jr, Rosan RC, Porter DY. Pulmonary disease following respirator therapy of hyaline membrane disease. Bronchopulmonary dysplasia. N Engl J Med 1967;276:357–68.
33. Bancalari E, Abdenour GE, Feller R, et al. Bronchopulmonary dysplasia: clinical presentation. J Pediatr 1979;95(5 Pt 2):819–23.
34. Shennan AT, Dunn MS, Ohlsson A, et al. Abnormal pulmonary outcomes in premature infants: prediction from oxygen requirement in the neonatal period. Pediatrics 1988;82(4):527–32.
35. Walsh MC, Yao Q, Gettner P, et al. Impact of a physiologic definition on bronchopulmonary dysplasia rates. Pediatrics 2004;114:1305–11.
36. Laughon MM, Langer JC, Bose CL, et al. Prediction of bronchopulmonary dysplasia by postnatal age in extremely premature infants. Am J Respir Crit Care Med 2011;183(12):1715–22.
37. Abel-Latik ME, Osborn DA. Intratracheal Clara cell secretory protein (CCSP) administration in preterm infants with or at risk of respiratory distress syndrome. Cochrane Database Syst Rev 2011;5:CD00830.
38. Halliday HL, Ehrenkranz RA, Doyle LW. Early (<8 days) postnatal corticosteroids for preventing chronic lung disease in preterm infants. Cochrane Database Syst Rev 2003;1:CD001146.
39. Shah V, Ohlsson A, Halliday HL, et al. Early administration of inhaled corticosteroids for preventing chronic lung disease in ventilated very low birth weight preterm neonates. Cochrane Database Syst Rev 2000;1. Updated search August 2007.

40. Prandstetter C, Tamesberger M, Wagner O, et al. [Medical prescriptions to premature and newborn infants in an Austrian neonatal intensive care unit]. Klin Padiatr 2009;221:312–7 [in German].
41. Neubert A, Lukas K, Leis T, et al. Drug utilisation on a preterm and neonatal intensive care unit in Germany: a prospective, cohort-based analysis. Eur J Clin Pharmacol 2010;66:87–95.
42. Clark RH, Bloom BT, Spitzer AR, et al. Reported medication use in the neonatal intensive care unit: data from a large national data set. Pediatrics 2006;117: 1979–87.
43. Anderson BJ, Holford NH. Mechanistic basis for using body size and maturation to predict clearance in humans. Drug Metab Pharmacokinet 2009;24:25–36.
44. Jadhau PR, Zhang J, Gobburu VS. Leveraging prior quantitative knowledge in pediatric drug development: a case study. Pharm Stat 2009;8:216–24.
45. Polin RA, Randis L. Biomarker for late-onset sepsis. Genome Med 2010;6(2):58.
46. Ng PC, Lam HS. Biomarkers for late onset neonatal sepsis: cytokines and beyond. Clin Perinatol 2010;37:599–610.
47. Dunne J, Rodriguez WJ, Murphy MD, et al. Extrapolation of adult data and other data in pediatric drug-development programs. Pediatrics 2011;128(5):e1242–9.

Therapeutic Drug Monitoring–the Appropriate Use of Drug Level Measurement in the Care of the Neonate

Thomas E. Young, MD[a,b,*]

KEYWORDS

- Theraputic drug monitoring • Aminoglycosides • Vancomycin
- Caffeine • Digoxin • Hypothermia

The goal of therapeutic drug monitoring (TDM) is to tailor drug dosage to maximize therapeutic benefits while minimizing toxicity. Traditionally, this approach has been performed by measuring serum drug concentrations, applying pharmacokinetic and pharmacodynamic principles, and then adjusting the dose to keep the drug concentration in the therapeutic range. By its very nature, TDM is primarily applicable for medications that possess narrow therapeutic indices (ie, the drug concentration required for therapeutic effect is close to the toxic concentration) and for agents that demonstrate a good correlation between serum concentrations and pharmacologic effect. In clinical situations with a wide therapeutic index for the medication in question, it is less important for the clinician to closely follow drug levels.

NEONATAL PHARMACOKINETIC CONSIDERATIONS

Neonates and young infants are in a unique and dynamic pharmacokinetic (PK) state, where they undergo relatively rapid maturational changes in drug absorption, distribution, metabolism, and excretion.[1] These PK variables are strongly influenced both by gestational age, being most pronounced in the extremely premature infants, and postnatal age, when the changes are greatest in the first few weeks after birth. Body composition also significantly affects the distribution of drugs in the body. Neonates,

---

[a] WakeMed Faculty Physicians-Neonatology, 3000 New Bern Avenue, Raleigh, NC 27610, USA
[b] University of North Carolina, Chapel Hill, NC, USA
* WakeMed Faculty Physicians-Neonatology, 3000 New Bern Avenue, Raleigh, NC 27610.
E-mail address: tyoung@wakemed.org

Clin Perinatol 39 (2012) 25–31
doi:10.1016/j.clp.2011.12.009
0095-5108/12/$ – see front matter © 2012 Elsevier Inc. All rights reserved.

especially premature infants, have a relatively high proportion of total body water and a low proportion of fat; this increases the apparent volume of distribution (V_d) for water-soluble compounds, and decreases the V_d for fat-soluble compounds. In addition, because the brain-to-body mass ratio is high, and body fat content is low, lipid-soluble drugs tend to concentrate in the central nervous system. Protein binding in neonates is diminished, so that free drug concentrations are higher even if total serum drug concentrations are the same as in older patients. Clearance of drugs is prolonged, due to both immature hepatic metabolism and immature renal excretion. This physiology leads to both higher drug concentrations and higher metabolite concentrations. Clearance is even more prolonged in infants with intrauterine growth restriction because of altered renal morphogenesis.[2] In addition to these maturational factors, most drug PK studies in neonates show wide interindividual variability despite similar gestational and postnatal ages. In some neonates, a portion of this variability may be explained by the presence of a patent ductus arteriosus or its treatment with indomethacin or ibuprofen. For most infants, however, this variability remains unexplained; hence TDM is a necessary tool in the neonatal intensive care unit (NICU).

SPECIFIC MEDICATIONS
Aminoglycosides

The bactericidal effect of aminoglycosides (gentamicin, tobramycin, amikacin) is strongly associated with the peak serum concentration (C_{max}) drawn 30 minutes after a 30-minute infusion. Studies in adults have demonstrated that a C_{max}/minimum inhibitory concentration (MIC) ratio of at least 8 to 10 is associated with improved outcomes.[3] Studies in neonates have been underpowered to assess clinical outcomes because of the infrequency of documented neonatal infections.[4] Nonetheless, current recommendations suggest that when treating serious infections with gentamicin, where the bacterial MIC = 0.5 μg/mL, the target C_{max} is at least 4 to 5 mg/dL; if MIC = 1, the target C_{max} is at least 8–10 μg/mL.

Ototoxicity and nephrotoxicity are the most concerning adverse effects of aminoglycosides. Neonates may be less susceptible to these toxicities than adults.[5] Nonetheless, measuring trough serum concentrations continues to be recommended, both to minimize the risk of toxicity, and as a surrogate assessment of renal function. In the past, the target trough concentration to lessen the risk of toxicity was less than 2 μg/mL. With the recognition of the postantibiotic effect of aminoglycosides, the in vitro demonstration of adaptive resistance with high trough levels, and the efficacy of prolonged ($\geq$24 hours) dosing intervals, the target trough concentration has been revised and is now considered to be less than 1 μg/mL.

Aminoglycosides are small hydrophilic molecules with a volume of distribution similar to extracellular fluid volume and clearance directly proportional to glomerular filtration rate. During the first week of life, V_d is higher and clearance prolonged, especially in the most premature neonates. Neonatal dosage nomograms with extended dosing intervals take these factors into account. Interindividual variability is wide, however, and the large number of dosing schedules reported in the literature indicates that the optimal schedule has yet to be determined.[6]

Most neonates treated for suspected sepsis have antibiotic therapy discontinued within 48 hours of initiation, negating the need to measure serum drug concentrations in these patients. For those being treated for more than 5 days due to positive blood cultures or clinical suspicion of true sepsis, or for those with disease states or therapies discussed in the sections that follow, TDM is indicated. For treating mild-to-moderate infections in clinically stable patients in whom the aminoglycoside is being used primarily for its synergistic effect, measuring peak concentrations is usually not necessary, and trough concentrations would be sufficient.

Vancomycin

Vancomycin is a glycopeptide used primarily to treat infections caused by methicillin-resistant *Staphylococcus aureus* and *S epidermidis*. Unlike aminoglycosides, vancomycin activity against staphylococci is primarily a time-dependent process. Pharmacodynamic efficacy, on the basis of in vitro, animal, and limited human data, is best predicted by the 24-hour area under the concentration curve (AUC) divided by the MIC (AUC/MIC). Vancomycin dosing and monitoring remain sources of controversy. Recent Infectious Diseases Society of America (IDSA) recommendations suggest a target AUC/MIC value of 400 to adequately treat serious staphylococcal infections (bacteremia, infective endocarditis, osteomyelitis, meningitis, pneumonia, and necrotizing fasciitis) if the MIC is no more than 1 μg/mL; if the MIC is 2 μg/mL or greater, an alternative drug should be used.[7] For adults with normal renal function, a serum trough concentration of 15 to 20 μg/mL reliably predicts that the AUC/MIC will be greater than 400 and has been shown to modestly improve patient outcomes.[8] Whether these PK targets are associated with an increased risk of nephrotoxicity or ototoxicity remains a point of controversy, although toxicity appears to be related more to the underlying disease state and concurrent use of medications such as furosemide and gentamicin. If these PK targets are desired when treating serious infections in neonates, then higher and more frequent dosing than most current nomograms will be required. There are no studies of outcomes in neonates treated using these recommendations. Monitoring of peak serum concentrations is not recommended, as they do not correlate with efficacy or toxicity. The uncertainties mentioned have resulted in a wide range of practice methods, from very infrequent to excessive monitoring of concentrations.

Caffeine

Caffeine has been one of the most frequently prescribed drugs in the NICU for many years. Usage has increased recently since publication of the caffeine for apnea of prematurity (CAP) trial results showing improvement in both short- and long-term outcomes.[9] The traditional therapeutic concentration range to treat apnea of prematurity is wide—5 to 20 μg/mL—and traditional standard dosages (20 mg/kg loading dose and 5 mg/kg/d maintenance) attain these concentrations independent of low gestational age, elevated liver enzymes, or renal dysfunction.[10] In the CAP trial, which used these dosages and enrolled over 900 neonates in the treatment arm, serum concentrations were not measured, and no significant toxicity was observed.[9] In studies using doses fourfold higher than standard doses, efficacy is improved in some patients without any increase in adverse events.[11] Monitoring of plasma caffeine concentrations is therefore not necessary.[12] The usual clinical sign of mild toxicity in neonates is tachycardia, which is treated by holding doses or stopping the drug without the need for measuring serum concentrations.

Anticonvulsants

The pharmacodynamic target of anticonvulsants is the cessation of seizures, but it remains controversial as to whether complete cessation of both clinical and electrographic seizures leads to improved outcomes in neonates with hypoxic–ischemic encephalopathy.[13,14] Treating all electrical seizures may require higher dosages of anticonvulsants and potentially increase the risk of toxicity. Many clinicians now use continuous electroencephalogram (EEG) monitoring to assess efficacy, yielding an individualized patient therapeutic level.

Phenobarbital remains the first-line drug for most neonatal seizures. The dosage predicts the serum concentration fairly well in the newborn period; a loading dose of 20 mg/kg yields a serum concentration of 17 to 23 μg/mL in the great majority of neonates. The serum concentration necessary to control clinical seizures in approximately 70% of neonates is 17 to 40 μg/mL, and additional loading doses of 5 to 10 mg/kg are often used.[15,16] The success rate for cessation of all electrographic seizures is somewhat less. Somnolence is common if the serum concentration is greater than 50 μg/mL. The half-life of phenobarbital in the first few days of life is greater than 100 hours, and drug accumulation may occur. A trough concentration measured several days after the loading dose therefore does not assess steady state, which may not occur for 2 weeks.

Fosphenytoin has replaced phenytoin as a commonly used second drug in the treatment of neonatal seizures because of its improved water solubility and reduced infusion-related toxicity. It is completely and rapidly converted to phenytoin in neonates. Dosing is expressed in phenytoin equivalents, and TDM continues to be measurement of serum phenytoin concentrations. Pharmacokinetics are dose-dependent, nonlinear, and change significantly over the first few weeks of life, so TDM is especially important. Trough levels should be measured 48 hours after the loading dose, and obtained at least 2 hours after an intravenous dose and 4 hours after an intramuscular dose to avoid fosphenytoin interaction with immunoanalytic methods. The therapeutic range for total phenytoin concentrations in children and adults is 10 to 20 μg/mL[17]; in neonates it is approximately 8 to 15 μg/mL due to less protein binding. Measuring free phenytoin concentrations may be preferred in neonates, and this is especially important in patients with hypoalbuminemia or hyperbilirubinemia.[18] The therapeutic range for serum free phenytoin concentrations is 1 to 2 μg/mL.

Serum concentrations for the other anticonvulsants frequently used in neonates—levetiracetam, lorazepam, and lidocaine—are not routinely monitored, as there is no clear relationship between serum concentration and either effect or toxicity.

Digoxin

The pharmacologic mechanisms of action of digoxin are complex and beyond the scope of this article. The pharmacodynamic target in neonates is resolution of supraventricular tachycardia or improvement in congestive heart failure. Digoxin is an example where TDM consists of a combination of measuring serum drug concentrations and monitoring other clinical parameters—in this case serial electrocardiograms (EKGs)—to assess for both therapeutic and toxic effects on heart rate and rhythm.[19] In addition, it is important to maintain normal serum potassium, calcium, and magnesium levels.

Pharmacokinetic studies indicate that infants require a larger weight-adjusted dose of digoxin than adults to attain comparable serum levels, principally because of higher body clearance and larger volume of distribution. Yet, with similar serum levels in infants and adults, the myocardium of infants and children contains more digoxin than adult myocardium. Therapeutic serum levels are approximately 1 to 2 ng/mL, with the lower end of the range more desirable. Serum levels obtained during digitalization and for the first few days of therapy are usually higher than when the steady state is reached. Serum digoxin levels must be interpreted in the context of the total clinical picture, including EKG changes and serum electrolyte values.

Serum digoxin levels may bear a relationship to digoxin content in the myocardium, but digitalis toxicity is a manifestation of dysfunction at the pacemaker site or in the conduction tissue. EKG changes reflective of therapeutic effect (shortening of QT interval, sagging of ST segment, diminished T wave amplitude, lower heart rate) are related to ventricular repolarization, whereas signs of toxicity (prolongation of PR interval, sinus bradycardia, atrial or ectopic beats, ventricular arrhythmias) reflect disturbances in the formation and conduction of the impulse. Electrolyte disturbances such as hypokalemia and hypercalcemia can predispose to digitalis toxicity, even in the presence of low serum digoxin levels.

SPECIAL CIRCUMSTANCES THAT MAY REQUIRE TDM
Therapeutic Hypothermia

The effects of hypothermia on pharmacodynamics and PK in neonates are incompletely understood due to limited data.[20] Most research has been done in animals and in adults, without the effects of perinatal asphyxia. Some of these studies were done under conditions of severe hypothermia (28° C), rather than moderate hypothermia (33–34° C) as used to treat neonatal asphyxia.

Hypothermia causes redistribution of regional blood flow, which may significantly alter drug distribution and clearance.[21] Volume of distribution is increased for phenobarbital and midazolam, while V_d is decreased for gentamicin, fentanyl, morphine, and pancuronium. The drug metabolizing activity of hepatic enzymes is impaired at lower temperatures.[22] This phenomenon likely explains the prolonged clearance of morphine[23] and phenobarbital[24] observed in asphyxiated neonates treated with hypothermia compared with a normothermic control group. Decreased drug clearance may also occur due to diminished renal blood flow. A recent study in neonates, however, showed that the effects of asphyxia on renal function overwhelm any changes in gentamicin clearance related to hypothermia.[25]

Extracorporeal Membrane Oxygenation

The apparent volume of distribution is increased during extracorporeal membrane oxygenation (ECMO) due to increased circulating blood volume. There is also drug lost in the ECMO circuit, the amount depending on the type of circuit used, the age of the circuit, and the characteristics of the drug.[26] The largest number of PK studies has been conducted with gentamicin and vancomycin. Both drugs have been found to have an increased V_d and prolonged elimination half-lives during ECMO, with several studies demonstrating a return to expected values after decannulation.[27]

SUMMARY

The known wide variability in neonatal PK makes the concept of therapeutic drug monitoring very attractive. The value of routine TDM for most drugs used in neonates remains uncertain, however, due to the paucity of neonatal-specific outcome data. Prevention of toxicity continues to be a primary goal of TDM, as neonatal drug clearance is often unpredictable, and drug accumulation may occur.

Therapeutic drug monitoring is evolving toward a new era of personalized therapeutics. There is increasing recognition that many adverse drug reactions or treatment failures, initially characterized as idiosyncratic, find their origin in genetic or genomic variation. As more is learned about pharmacogenomics, it is likely that the overall approach to TDM and PK testing will evolve into more than just measuring serum drug concentrations.

REFERENCES

1. Alcorn J, McNamara PJ. Pharmacokinetics in the newborn. Adv Drug Deliv Rev 2003;55:667–86.
2. Allegaert K, Anderson BJ, van den Anker JN, et al. Renal drug clearance in preterm neonates: relation to prenatal growth. Ther Drug Monit 2007;29:284–91.
3. Moore RD, Lietman PS, Smith CR. Clinical response to aminoglycoside therapy: importance of the ratio of peak concentration to minimal inhibitory concentration. J Infect Dis 1987;155:93–9.
4. Rao SC, Srinivasjois R, Hagan R, et al. One dose per day compared to multiple doses per day of gentamicin for treatment of suspected or proven sepsis in neonates. Cochrane Database Syst Rev 2011;11:CD005091.
5. deHoog M, vanZanten BA, Hop WC, et al. Newborn hearing screening: tobramycin and vancomycin are not risk factors for hearing loss. J Pediatr 2003;142:41–6.
6. Pacifici GM. Clinical pharmacokinetics of aminoglycosides in the neonate: a review. Eur J Clin Pharmacol 2009;65:419–27.
7. Rybak M, Lomaestro B, Rotschafer JC, et al. Therapeutic monitoring of vancomycin in adult patients: a consensus review of the American Society of Health-System Pharmacists, the Infectious Diseases Society of America, and the Society of Infectious Diseases Pharmacists. Am J Health Syst Pharm 2009;66:82–98.
8. Kullar R, Davis SL, Levine DP, et al. Impact of vancomycin exposure on outcomes in patients with methicillin-resistant *Staphylococcus aureus* bacteremia: support for consensus guidelines suggested targets. Clin Infect Dis 2011;52:975–81.
9. Schmidt B, Roberts RS, Davis P, et al. Caffeine for apnea of prematurity. N Engl J Med 2006;354:2112–21.
10. Natarajan G, Botica ML, Thomas R, et al. Therapeutic drug monitoring for caffeine in preterm neonates: an unnecessary exercise? Pediatrics 2007;119:936–40.
11. Steer P, Flenady V, Shearman A, et al. High dose caffeine for extubation of preterm infants: a randomised controlled trial. Arch Dis Child Fetal Neonatal Ed 2004;89:F499–503.
12. Charles BG, Townsend SR, Steer PA, et al. Caffeine citrate treatment for extremely premature infants with apnea: population pharmacokinetics, absolute bioavailability, and implications for therapeutic drug monitoring. Ther Drug Monit 2008;30:709–16.
13. Kwon JM, Guillet R, Shankaran S, et al. Clinical seizures in neonatal hypoxic-ischemic encephalopathy have no independent impact on neurodevelopmental outcome: secondary analyses of data from the Neonatal Research Network hypothermia trial. J Child Neurol 2011;26:322–8.
14. Glass HC, Glidden D, Jeremy RJ, et al. Clinical neonatal seizures are independently associated with outcome in infants at risk for hypoxic–ischemic brain injury. J Pediatr 2009;155:318–23.
15. Lockman LA, Kriel R, Zaske D, et al. Phenobarbital dosage for control of neonatal seizures. Neurology 1979;29:1445–9.
16. Gilman JT, Gal P, Duchowny MS, et al. Rapid sequential phenobarbital treatment of neonatal seizures. Pediatrics 1989;83:674–8.
17. Patsalos PN, Berry DJ, Bourgeois BF, et al. Antiepileptic drugs—best practice guidelines for therapeutic drug monitoring: a position paper by the subcommission on therapeutic drug monitoring, ILAE Commission on Therapeutic Strategies. Epilepsia 2008;49:1239–76.

18. Wolf GK, McClain CD, Zurakowski D. Total phenytoin concentrations do not accurately predict free phenytoin concentrations in critically ill children. Pediatr Crit Care Med 2006;7:434–9.
19. Park MK. Use of digoxin in infants and children, with specific emphasis on dosage. J Pediatr 1986;108:871–7.
20. Zanelli S, Buck M, Fairchild K. Physiologic and pharmacologic considerations for hypothermia therapy in neonates. J Perinatol 2011;31:377–86.
21. van den Broek MP, Groenendaal F, Egberts AC, et al. Effects of hypothermia on pharmacokinetics and pharmacodynamics. Clin Pharmacokinet 2010;49:277–94.
22. Tortorici MA, Kochanek PM, Poloyac SM. Effects of hypothermia on drug disposition, metabolism, and response: a focus of hypothermia-mediated alterations on the cytochrome P450 enzyme system. Crit Care Med 2007;35:2196–204.
23. Roka A, Melinda KT, Vasarhelyi B, et al. Elevated morphine concentrations in neonates treated with morphine and prolonged hypothermia for hypoxic ischemic encephalopathy. Pediatrics 2008;121:e844–9.
24. Thoresen M, Stone J, Hoem NO, et al. Hypothermia after perinatal asphyxia more than doubles the plasma half life of phenobarbitone [abstract]. In: Pediatric Academic Societies 2003 annual meeting. Seattle (WA), May 3–6, 2003. E-PAS2003–137.
25. Liu X, Borooah M, Stone J, et al. Serum gentamicin concentrations in encephalopathic infants are not affected by therapeutic hypothermia. Pediatrics 2009;124: 310–5.
26. Wildschut ED, Ahsman MJ, Allegaert K, et al. Determinants of drug absorption in different ECMO circuits. Intensive Care Med 2010;36:2109–16.
27. Buck ML. Pharmacokinetic changes during extracorporeal membrane oxygenation. Clin Pharmacokinet 2003;42:403–17.

Obstetric Interventions Beneficial to Prematurely Delivering Newborn Babies: Antenatal Corticostetroids, Progesterone, Magnesium Sulfate

Thomas J. Garite, MD[a,b,c],*, C. Andrew Combs, MD, PhD[b,d]

KEYWORDS

- Prematurity • Antenatal corticosteroids • Magnesium sulfate
- Progesterone

Although improvements in neonatal care have continued to result in reduced mortality and morbidity of prematurely delivering newborns for decades, the results of a myriad of obstetric efforts and interventions have failed to reduce the overall rate of prematurity or prolong pregnancy at any gestational age. Efforts to prolong pregnancy, including tocolysis, cervical cerclage, bed rest, antibiotics, and comprehensive prematurity prevention programs, have proved to be failures. Thus, the prematurity rate since the time data began to be collected on the subject has not declined whatsoever and, in recent years, has actually been on the rise, increasing by 36% since the 1980s reaching a high of 12.7% of all births in 2007.[1] This recent increase has largely been caused by the increase in multiple gestations associated with assisted

[a] Department of Obstetrics and Gynecology, University of California Irvine, College of Medicine, Irvine, CA, USA
[b] Pediatrix Medical Group, Sunrise, FL, USA
[c] American Journal of Obstetrics and Gynecology, USA
[d] Obstetrix Medical Group, San Jose, CA, USA
* Corresponding author. Department of Obstetrics and Gynecology, University of California Irvine, College of Medicine, Irvine, CA.
E-mail address: tjgarite@uci.edu

Clin Perinatol 39 (2012) 33–45
doi:10.1016/j.clp.2011.12.012   **perinatology.theclinics.com**
0095-5108/12/$ – see front matter © 2012 Elsevier Inc. All rights reserved.

reproduction technologies, such as in vitro fertilization, and iatrogenic prematurity caused by early labor inductions and cesarean sections; however, these two factors do not account for the entire increase. It is estimated that at least 50% of all sponta-neous deliveries (not indicated for maternal or fetal concerns) are caused by an infec-tious process, but no real inroads beyond increased understanding, have been made into altering prematurity rates and associated complications caused by infection. Despite this dismal record, a few new developments or refinements of established interventions give increased hope for an improved obstetric contribution to the problem of prematurity. These include a better understanding of how best to use ante-natal corticosteroids (ACSs) and the newer options of magnesium sulfate to ameliorate or avoid cerebral palsy (CP) associated with prematurity and maternal progesterone administration to selected at-risk populations to decrease the likelihood of premature delivery.

ANTENATAL CORTICOSTEROIDS

Since Liggins and Howie[2] while investigating the mechanisms of the onset of labor serendipitously discovered that maternally administered corticosteroids improved lung compliance in prematurely delivered lambs, a large number of randomized controlled trials (RCT) have consistently substantiated the beneficial effects of ACSs.[3] Although this approach was, for some time, the only clearly beneficial obstetric intervention for prematurely delivering babies, only a minority of patients at risk actu-ally received ACS before delivering prematurely. Leviton and colleagues,[4] fully 25 years after Liggins' initial RCT and many confirming RCT's,[3] found that only 15% of babies who delivered at less than 34 weeks had actually received ACS before delivery. This finding compelled the National Institute of Child Health and Human Development (NICHD) to hold its first consensus conference on ACS in 1994.[5] This conference concluded the following:

- The benefits of ACS vastly outweigh the potential risks
- The benefits include a reduction in respiratory distress syndrome (RDS), intraven-tricular hemorrhage (IVH), and neonatal death
- All fetuses from 24 to 34 weeks should be considered candidates for ACS
- The decision for ACS should not be altered by fetal gender, race, or availability of surfactant therapy
- Treatment should be either:
  - Betamethasone, 12 mg intramuscularly, two doses 24 hours apart, or
  - Dexamethasone, 6 mg intramuscularly, four doses 12 hours apart
- Optimal benefit begins 24 hours after the first dose and lasts 7 days
- Because there is benefit within even less than 24 hours, ACS should still be given unless delivery is immediate
- In premature rupture of membranes (PROM) less than 30 to 32 weeks, ACS is recommended because of the high risk of IVH
- In complicated pregnancies less than 34 weeks, ACS should be given unless corticosteroids will have an adverse effect or delivery is imminent.

The most important question that remained after this conference was what to do with the patient who received a course of ACS but did not deliver and still remained at risk for premature delivery. The dramatic 50% reduction in RDS in babies who receive ACS at least 24 hours before delivery seems to disappear in patients who remain undelivered for a week or more but still deliver before 34 weeks.[2,6–11] Further-more, most patients who do actually receive ACS do not deliver within 1 week because of the inaccuracy of the diagnosis of premature labor or prediction of immi-nent preterm delivery in other clinical settings, such as placenta previa, preeclampsia, or preterm PROM (PPROM). A survey of perinatologists dealing with this problem in the ensuing years revealed that 91% would repeat treatment after 1 week if premature labor recurred and 58% would be willing to give more than six courses.[12] Thus, weekly repeat courses of ACS in patients at risk seemed to be the prevailing approach. However, a large body of evidence emerged regarding the potential harmful effects of repeat courses of ACS. Animal studies consistently showed decreased body weight and decreased growth of various organs including brain, thymus, and liver; glucose intolerance; adrenal suppression; and subtle changes in neurobehavioral develop-ment.[13] Retrospective studies in humans also raised similar concerns. In 1999, Banks and colleagues[14] did an analysis of a randomized thyrotropin releasing hormone (TRH) trial in which all of the mothers had also received ACS in one or more courses. This study found a decrease in birth weight in those who had received two or more courses and an increase in neonatal deaths in those who had received three or more courses. French and coworkers[15] found decreasing birth weight with increasing number of courses and a reduction in head circumference and increased long-term behavioral problems (3 years) with multiple doses of ACS. Because of these concerns, issues over questionable efficacy, and the NICHD's conclusion that this question needed further study, four large RCTs were concluded and published.

Guinn and colleagues[16] performed a multicenter RCT comparing a single course of ACS with weekly courses. Although there was no difference in RDS or other compli-cations of prematurity between the groups, the study was discontinued early because of findings of lower birth weights and increased rates of severe IVH in the babies who had received multiple courses. Wapner and the Maternal Fetal Medicine Network of the NICHD[17] performed a large multicenter RCT. Although they did not find a difference in the primary outcome of composite morbidity, they did observe some benefit with weekly courses that included less need for mechanical ventilation, lower surfactant requirement, and fewer pneumothoraces. There was no difference in head circumfer-ences between the groups but there was a significant reduction in birth weight in those receiving four or more courses of ACS. Crowther and colleagues[18] performed a similar study in Australia and did find a modest 10% reduction in RDS and severe lung disease; but they also showed a reduction in birth weights and head circumference in the repeat ACS group and did find a relationship between the number of courses and these adverse outcomes. Finally, the Canadian multicenter trial by Murphy and colleagues[19] showed no difference in morbidity, but found that babies in the multiple course group had birth weights that were smaller, infants were shorter, and they had smaller head circumferences. Two of these studies reported the long-term follow-up of babies in these studies.[20,21] In the Wapner study,[20] there were no significant differ-ences in Bayley results or anthropometric measurements. However, six children (2.9% of pregnancies) in the repeat-corticosteroid group had CP compared with one child (0.5% of pregnancies) in the placebo group. These infants were restricted to those whose mothers had received four or more courses. In the Crowther study,[21] the rate of survival free of major disability was similar in the repeat-corticosteroid and placebo groups. There were no significant differences between the groups in body size, blood pressure, use of health services, respiratory morbidity, or child behavior scores, although children exposed to repeat doses of corticosteroids were more likely than those exposed to placebo to warrant assessment for attention-deficit problems. Given the inconsistency in reported benefit and the concerns about adverse effects raised by all these studies, the NICHD convened a second consensus conference. This confer-ence concluded that: "because of insufficient scientific data regarding the efficacy and safety of repeated courses of corticosteroids, such therapy should not be used routinely… …should be reserved for patients enrolled in randomized trials."[13] They further recommended that one course of ACS is safe and effective and should be used whenever appropriate, that routine repeat courses of ACS should not be used, and that there is still an open question on at least one "rescue course" of ACS.

The issue of a rescue course of ACS therefore was raised. A rescue course as opposed to routine weekly courses of ACS relies on the accurate prediction of the likelihood that a patient who had received a course of ACS more than 1 week previously again has a high likelihood of delivering in the upcoming week because of the recurrence of a problem, such as premature labor, worsening preeclampsia, bleeding with placenta previa, and so forth. These patients would then be retreated with an additional single course. One retrospective study was encouraging. Vermillion and coworkers[22] performed a retrospective study and found a reduction in RDS in the rescue group compared with a single course of ACS with no difference in birth weight or other outcomes. Mercer,[23] in a study of 189 patients presented only in abstract, compared weekly ACS with a single rescue course and found that although the weekly course group had more optimal exposure (delivery within a week of treatment), the rates of RDS were similar between the two groups. In addition, the weekly treated group had a linear correlation between the number of courses and reduced newborn birth weight, length, and head circumference. Garite and the Obstetrix Collaborative Research Network[24] in a multicenter RCT of more than 400 patients comparing a single rescue course with placebo found that 55% of treated patients actually delivered in the ensuing week, and that there was a 40% reduction in RDS compared with placebo, but no differences in birth weight, length, or head circumference. McEvoy and colleagues[25] in a smaller RCT of a single rescue course versus placebo found a nonstatistically significant reduction in RDS but significant improvement in respiratory compliance and need for O_2 greater than 30% and greater than 40%.

The American Congress of Obstetricians and Gynecologists (ACOG) recently recommended in a Committee Opinion[26]:

A single course of corticosteroids is recommended for pregnant women between 24 weeks and 34 weeks of gestation who are at risk of preterm delivery within 7 days. A single course of antenatal corticosteroids should be administered to women with premature rupture of membranes before 32 weeks of gestation to reduce the risks of respiratory distress syndrome, perinatal mortality, and other morbidities. The efficacy of corticosteroid use at 32–33 completed weeks of gestation for preterm premature rupture of membranes is unclear, but treatment may be beneficial, particularly if pulmonary immaturity is documented. Sparse data exist on the efficacy of corticosteroid use before fetal age of viability, and such use is not recommended. A single rescue course of antenatal corticosteroids may be considered if the antecedent treatment was given more than 2 weeks prior, the gestational age is less than 32 6/7 weeks, and the women are judged by the clinician to be likely to give birth within the next week. However, regularly scheduled repeat courses or multiple courses (more than two) are not recommended. Further research regarding the risks and benefits, optimal dose, and timing of a single rescue course of steroid treatment is needed.

There are two remaining important issues to be resolved regarding ACS. One is the issue of use of ACS in the setting of PPROM. Clearly, if one compiles all the RCTs of ACS with PPROM, the benefits in terms of reduction of RDS and other morbidities are not as uniformly seen as with intact membranes and preterm delivery. After these RCTs began to couple the use of ACS with the use of antibiotics, the benefits of ACS were more uniformly reported. Broad-spectrum antibiotics clearly prolong the latency period (interval between rupture and delivery) in the setting of PPROM and, in all probability, the unmasking of the benefits of ACS in this setting with antibiotics relates to a reduction in neonatal pneumonia. The current recommendation is that ACS be used in patients with PPROM before 32 weeks.[13] Two studies[27,28] have looked at one or more additional courses of ACS with PPROM and both showed an increase in infectious complications including neonatal sepsis and chorioamnionitis in the repeated course group, even with only one additional course. Thus, even a single rescue course of ACS cannot be recommended at this time with PPROM.

The other issue is the question of whether betamethasone or dexamethasone is the better choice for ACS benefit or risk. Data on this question are confusing and conflicting and at present no clear recommendation can be made for one over the other. ACOG in its committee opinion comments[13]: "Of the 10 trials included in a Cochrane review on this issue, there were no differences in perinatal death or alterations in biophysical activity, but there was a decreased incidence of IVH with dexamethasone treatment. Alternatively, an observational study reported less frequent adverse neurologic outcome at 18–22 months after betamethasone exposure. These inconsistent and limited data are not considered sufficient to recommend one steroid regimen over the other," and both options remain recommended by ACOG and the NICHD consensus conference. Thus, ACS remain one of the most well-proved obstetric interventions to reduce neonatal death and morbidity in prematurely delivering newborns, has stood the test of time, and must be used in appropriate patients less than 34 weeks who are threatening to deliver prematurely.

MAGNESIUM SULFATE TO REDUCE CP

Magnesium sulfate has been used for decades, initially as an antiseizure medication in preeclampsia, and subsequently as the most widely used tocolytic drug in the United States. Controversy regarding its efficacy as a tocolytic, and even possible dangers to the newborn, emerged and extensive pro and con discussions saturated the obstetric literature. Although the controversy continued regarding $MgSO_4$ as a tocolytic agent, a new application for this drug emerged. Nelson and Grether,[29] in an observational study, showed that in babies less than 1500 g, 7% of 42 babies with CP and 36% of 75 non-CP controls were exposed to $MgSO_4$ (odds ratio, 0.14; 95% confidence interval [CI], 0.05–0.41). This sparked interest in performing studies to see if $MgSO_4$ could be used specifically for the purpose of preventing CP. The idea of performing such a study was daunting because of the very large number of subjects it would take to do a large RCT, and this delayed the performance of these trials. The study was further complicated by not knowing the optimal dose and what the best timing for drug administration before delivery was, and the optimal gestational age. Ultimately, however, four larger multicenter prospective RCTs were performed.

Conde-Agudelo and Romero[30] reviewed 331 studies on the subject and included six in a meta-analysis of the issue, including the four multicenter trials with creative acronyms: the ACTOMagSulfate trial,[31] the PreMag trial,[32] the BEAM trial,[33] and MAGPIE trial.[34] Among more than 5000 randomized subjects, there was a 39% reduction in the overall incidence of CP of prematurity. The primary benefit was seen in reducing moderate and severe CP but not mild CP and there was no difference in neonatal death. The optimal gestational age and dosing differed in these trials ranged from upper limits of 30 to 36 weeks and doses of 4 to 6 g loads and 1 to 2 g per hour for 12 to 24 hours before delivery. A potentially important observation in the Beam trial[33] was that the benefit of $MgSO_4$ was restricted to those treated at less than 28 weeks of gestation.

In those cases, the rate of moderate or severe CP with magnesium treatment (2.7%) was less than half the rate in the placebo group (6%; relative risk, 0.45; 95% CI, 0.23–0.87). Among cases treated at 28 weeks or more, there was no difference in rates of CP between the groups. However, the frequency of CP is lower as gestational age advances, so this lack of difference in the babies beyond 28 weeks could be caused by an inadequate sample size. The authors of this review[30] concluded that only 52 mothers would be needed to treat to prevent one case of CP at a cost of $10,291 per case prevented. Compared with the cost of taking care of a child with CP this is a modest investment.

The mechanism whereby $MgSO_4$ may prevent neuronal injury in the fetus or newborn is unclear and there are certainly some diverse biochemical reasons that it might work. Perhaps the most convincing argument favors that the drug prevents CP by preventing inflammatory injury to the brain, common in very prematurely delivering babies and associated with periventricular leukomalacia. Because there is a strong association between CP in prematures and intrauterine infection, and because there is no reduction in IVH in $MgSO_4$ studies yet there is reduction in CP, and because most of the prospective RCTs of $MgSO_4$ for CP were dominated by PPROM where infection is more common than in premature labor with intact membranes, the evidence is certainly suggestive. In a mouse model of lipopolysaccharide-induced neuronal injury, the injury to the brain cells was prevented by the intraperitoneal injection of $MgSO_4$ without altering the proinflammatory response, thereby providing a good animal model for how this drug might work.[35]

Based on this evidence should clinicians then be using $MgSO_4$ to prevent CP in prematurely delivering newborns? ACOG stops short of recommending the use of $MgSO_4$ for neuroprotection concluding: "Physicians electing to use magnesium sulfate for fetal neuroprotection should develop specific guidelines regarding inclusion criteria, treatment regimens, concurrent tocolysis, and monitoring in accordance with one of the larger trials."[36] However, Rouse[37] poses the following arguments in favor of use: current studies are unanimous in efficacy; safety is not questioned; there probably will not be any more large studies done; and $MgSO_4$ (as a tocolytic) can buy time for corticosteroids.

PROGESTERONE TO PROLONG PREGNANCY

The goal of reducing prematurity and its consequences can be accomplished in theory in one or more of three basic approaches. Tocolytics can be considered a tertiary approach, and because this is done at the last minute, and its other limitations, this approach is least likely to result in any great impact. Primary prevention relies on encompassing interventions, such as smoking prevention or work reduction, which would be ideal, but again because of the multifactorial nature of premature delivery, it has had limited success. Secondary prevention relies on identification of patients at risk and applying interventions specifically aimed at their most likely causes of premature delivery (**Table 1**). Until recently, such options as cervical cerclage for patients with "incompetent cervix" have had limited impact because of the minority of patients who have such a specific problem. Broader programs, such as aggressive prematurity-prevention programs in patients at risk, have been largely unsuccessful. In the last decade hope has emerged because of the reintroduction of prophylactic progesterone administration in specific at-risk groups. Although this hormone has been know for decades to be critical in the control of the onset of labor and previously used (albeit unsuccessfully) for many years for the prevention of miscarriage, the careful and critical evaluation of this agent for the prevention of prematurity has surprisingly only recently occurred.

Table 1
Interventions intended to reduce morbidity and mortality of preterm birth

		Examples
Primary	Preventive measures for all women	Public education (eg, risk factor reduction, risks of repeated dilation and curettage) Professional policies (eg, avoidance of multiple-embryo in vitro fertilization, standardized ovulation induction protocols) Societal policies (eg, paid pregnancy leave, time off from work for prenatal visits, protection from workplace hazards) Nutritional supplementation Smoking cessation Prenatal care Periodontal care Risk factor screening Sonographic cervical length screening Fetal fibronectin screening
Secondary	Preventive measures for women with risk factors	Prophylactic interventions for women with history of prior preterm birth (eg, progesterone, cerclage, cervical length screening, antibiotic therapy) Prophylactic interventions for women with history of preeclampsia (eg, low-dose aspirin, dietary modifications, antihypertensive medications) Activity restrictions Nutritional supplementation Antibiotic therapy of bacterial vaginosis
Tertiary	Treatments designed to reduce neonatal complications when given to women with anticipated preterm delivery	Early diagnosis of preterm labor (eg, home uterine monitoring, education about symptoms) Tocolysis for acute preterm labor or PPROM Maintenance tocolysis after acute episode Antenatal corticosteroids for impending preterm birth Magnesium sulfate for neuroprotection with impending early preterm birth Antibiotic treatment after preterm labor or PPROM Cesarean delivery of preterm neonate

Some of these interventions have been proved not effective, others are under investigation, and a few are believed to be effective in some circumstances.

Adapted from Iams JD, Romero R, Culhane JF, et al. Primary, secondary, and tertiary interventions to reduce the morbidity and mortality of preterm birth. Lancet 2008;371:164–75; with permission.

It is well know that in many mammalian animal species progesterone concentration drops in the hours or days before the onset of spontaneous labor.[38] It has been shown in animals that the removal of progesterone early in pregnancy, when it is produced primarily by the corpus luteum, results in the onset of labor and the resulting miscarriage. In the classic experiments by Csapo,[39] replacement of exogenous progesterone prevents this loss even when the corpus luteum is removed. However, human parturition is different from other mammalian species in that there is no apparent drop in progesterone concentration before the onset of labor; rather, it is thought that either receptor deactivation or a relative change in the estrogen/progesterone ratio is more likely responsible for the trigger that starts the cascade leading to the onset of labor. For decades, largely without good evidence, progesterone was given to patients with recurrent miscarriage, with first-trimester vaginal bleeding, known as "threatened abortion," and with such conditions as appendicitis to prevent premature contractions and delivery as a complication. In 1975, Johnson and colleagues[40] performed a RCT demonstrating efficacy of 17-hydroxyprogesterone caproate given weekly in lowering the rate of prematurity in treated patients. Although there was initial enthusiasm for this approach, several small studies failed to confirm this finding and the use of progesterone to prevent premature delivery fell out of favor. In 1990, Keirse[41] performed a meta-analysis restricted to five trials using the specific agent 17-hydroxyprogesterone caproate in women at high risk of preterm birth. In this group, this drug substantially reduced the risk of preterm birth (odds ratio, 0.50; 95% CI, 0.30–0.85). Subsequently, two recent large randomized trials of Meis and the NICHD MFMU network[42] in the United States and de Fonseca and colleagues[43] in Brazil in patients with a history of premature delivery caused by premature labor or PROM, renewed interest in progesterone. In the Meis study, 463 patients were randomized to receive 250 mg of 17-hydroxyprogesterone caproate imtramuscularly or placebo weekly from randomization at 15 to 20 weeks until 36 weeks. The results were that there was a reduction in the rate of premature delivery from 55% in the placebo group to 36% in the treatment group. They also found a nearly statistically significant reduction in neonatal death, need for ventilator support, and IVH. Da Fonseca and colleagues[43] randomized 142 patients with previous preterm deliveries to 100 mg of progesterone vaginal suppositories versus placebo nightly from 24 to 34 weeks. They also found a significant reduction in premature delivery from 29% to 14%. However, a large RCT by O'Brien and colleagues,[44] using a vaginal gel form of progesterone, failed to demonstrate any benefit in prolonging pregnancy. This failure, along with the previous meta-analysis[41] that suggested that benefit was restricted to 17-hydroxyprogesterone caproate, raises the question of whether benefit for women with a previous preterm birth is restricted to 17-hydroxyprogesterone caproate rather than vaginal progesterone.

Thus, the door was opened to investigate the question of benefit in other at-risk groups. The most obvious risk factor occurs in patients with multiple gestations where there is 50% or greater risk of premature delivery. To date, there have been published results from five RCTs of prophylactic 17-hydroxyprogesterone[45–49] and three trials of vaginal progesterone[50–52] in twin pregnancies. None of these showed any benefit of progestin treatment, or even a suggestive trend toward reducing the rate of early preterm birth or reducing neonatal complications. Subanalyses have not yet demonstrated benefit in twins with short cervices or with a history of prior preterm birth, although the number of patients with these risk factors is small. In triplet pregnancy, where risk of preterm birth is nearly 100%, there have been two trials of 17-hydroxyprogesterone caproate.[53,54] Neither showed a reduction in either preterm birth or neonatal morbidity.

Most recently, the use of endovaginal ultrasound for cervical length has been exploited to find another at-risk group on which to test the efficacy of progesterone.

For the last 15 years, multiple studies have demonstrated that patients whose cervices shortened early in pregnancy were at much greater risk for early delivery. For example, with a cervical length in the second trimester of less than 25 mm the risk is increased by 6-fold, at less than 22 mm by 10-fold, and at less than 12 cm by 14-fold.[55] Because these patients represent a very-high-risk group, and because they present with this finding in the second trimester, well before the actual delivery occurs and where starting progesterone has been shown to be most effective, this represents a potentially excellent group for hope of outcome improvement with progesterone. Indeed, several recent trials have confirmed the value of progesterone in patients with a short cervix. DeFranco and colleagues[56] performed a subanalysis of the negative trial of vaginal progesterone[44] in patients with previous preterm delivery and found that in those with a cervical length of less than 28 mm the rate of preterm birth less than 32 weeks was zero among those treated with progesterone versus 29.5% in the placebo group. Two RCTs in patients with short cervices have now been concluded. Fonseca and colleagues[57] found that in patients with a cervical length of 15 mm or less, delivery before 34 weeks was less frequent with nightly vaginal progesterone (19%) than with placebo (34%). Hassan and colleagues[58] (the PREGNANT trial) randomized 465 patients with a short cervix of between 10 and 20 mm to vaginal progesterone compared with placebo and found a reduction in delivery before 33 weeks (8.9% vs 16.1%). Reductions in the rates of RDS and any neonatal morbidity were also observed. Studies using endovaginal ultrasound for cervical length and treatment with progesterone in multiple pregnancies have not yet been performed, but subanalyses of larger studies of cervical length suggest this approach may hold promise for success.

The safety of progesterone has been well established. Progesterone has been extensively studied in many mammalian species and no virilizing or teratogenic effects have been found.[59] This statement is true for progesterone and 17α-hydoxyprogesterone. There are also numerous studies in humans, including some with long-term follow-up, that show no virilizing or teratogenic effects or any deleterious effects on neurodevelopment. Nothen and colleagues[59] reported on the follow-up of children exposed to 17α-hydroxyprogesterone caproate in the initial NICHD trial. They followed 278 of the 348 originally randomized children with a mean age of 48 months at evaluation. There were no differences in genital anomalies, health status, physical examination, or indices of neurodevelopment. Similarly, 2-year follow-up of children exposed to vaginal progesterone in the twins trial of Klein and colleagues[60] showed no adverse effect on neurodevelopment. Thus, it is reasonable to conclude that treatment with progestational agents, including those used for prevention of preterm delivery, is safe.

What then are the best recommendations for use of progestesterone? ACOG developed a Committee Opinion in 2008 and reaffirmed it in 2011.[61] They state:

> ...progesterone supplementation reduces preterm birth in a select group of women. Despite the apparent benefits of progesterone, the ideal progesterone formulation is unknown. The American College of Obstetricians and Gynecologists' Committee on Obstetric Practice and the Society for Maternal Fetal Medicine believe that further studies are needed to evaluate the optimal preparation, dosage, route of administration, and other indications for the use of progesterone for the prevention of preterm delivery. Based on current knowledge, it is important to offer progesterone for pregnancy prolongation to only women with a documented history of a previous spontaneous birth at less than 37 weeks of gestation.

We would amend and add to this statement to state specifically that 17-hydroxyprogesterone caproate is the agent with demonstrated benefit for women with a history of prior spontaneous preterm birth. Studies of vaginal or oral progesterone have been inconsistent in women with this history. And with women with a short cervix the current literature restricts benefit to vaginally administered progesterone. It is likely that this discrepancy will be sorted out with future studies. There is strong evidence that progestins are not beneficial for unselected twin or triplet pregnancies. The data are inconclusive regarding use of progestins for other indications, such as PPROM, arrested preterm labor, or twin pregnancy with added risk factors, such as short cervix or a history of prior preterm birth. Additional clinical trials are needed to evaluate the role of progestins in these settings.

Only a minority of women actually delivering prematurely has a history of previous preterm delivery, however, and the approach so far endorsed by ACOG will have limited impact on the overall prematurity rate. Routine screening of all pregnant women with endovaginal ultrasound is one option that holds great promise. Although only 1% to 2% of women screened have a very short cervix ($\leq$20 mm), the benefit of reduced neonatal complications with progesterone treatment for such women may actually justify the costs of a universal screening program. In a recent article by Cahill and colleagues,[62] the potential cost effectiveness of various approaches for the use of progesterone to prevent preterm delivery was analyzed. The authors concluded that "universal sonographic screening for short cervical length and treatment with vaginal progesterone appears to be cost effective and yields the greatest reduction in preterm birth <34 wks." They calculated that this approach would result in a reduction of more than 95,000 preterm births and more than 13,000 cases of severe morbidity in the United States annually with a cost savings of almost $13 billion per year.

Although this approach has not yet been endorsed by any group, it is certainly appealing and promising and, of all the approaches yet to be proposed to actually impact the rate of preterm delivery and its consequences, this is by far the most promising single approach that has come along in the history of studying this problem.

REFERENCES

1. Prematurity: March of dimes web site. Available at: http://www.marchofdimes.com/mission/prematurity_indepth.html. Accessed December 20, 2011.
2. Liggins GC, Howie RN. A controlled trial of antepartum glucocorticoid treatment for prevention of the respiratory distress syndrome in premature infants. Pediatrics 1972;50:515–25.
3. Crowley P. Antenatal corticosteroid therapy: a metaanalysis of the randomized trials 1972-1994. Am J Obstet Gynecol 1995;173:322–35.
4. Leviton LL, Baker S, Hassol A, et al. An exploration of opinion and practice patterns affecting low use of antenatal corticosteroids. Am J Obstet Gynecol 1995;173:312–6.
5. NIH Consensus Conference Panel on the Effect of Corticosteroids for Fetal Maturation on Perinatal Outcomes. JAMA 1995;273:413–8.
6. Doran TA, Swyer P, MacMurray B, et al. Results of a double-blind controlled study on the use of betamethasone in the prevention of respiratory distress syndrome. Am J Obstet Gynecol 1980;136:313–20.
7. Shutte MF, Treffers PE, Koppe JG, et al. The influence of betamethasone and orciprenaline on the incidence of respiratory distress syndrome in the newborn after premature labor. Br J Obstet Gynaecol 1980;87:127–31.
8. Terramo K, Hallman M, Raivio KO. Maternal glucocorticoid in unplanned premature labor. Pediatr Res 1980;14:326–9.

9. Collaborative Group on Antenatal Steroid Therapy. Effect of antenatal steroid administration on prevention of respiratory distress syndrome. Am J Obstet Gynecol 1981;141:276–87.

10. Morales WJ, Diebel ND, Lazar AJ, et al. The effect of antenatal dexamethasone of the prevention of respiratory distress syndrome in preterm gestation with premature of membranes. Am J Obstet Gynecol 1986;154:591–5.

11. Garite TJ, Rumney PJ, Briggs GG, et al. A randomized placebo controlled trial of betamethasone for the prevention of respiratory distress syndrome at 24–18 weeks gestation. Am J Obstet Gynecol 1992;166:646–51.

12. Planer BC,, Ballard RA,, Ballard P. Antenatal corticosteroid use in preterm labor in the USA. Pediatr Res 1996;39:110.

13. Antenatal corticosteroids revisited: repeat courses. NIH Consens Statement 2000;17:1–18.

14. Banks BA, Cnaan A, Morgan MA, et al. Multiple courses of antenatal corticosteroids and outcome of premature neonates. Am J Obstet Gynecol 1999;181:709–17.

15. French NP, Hagan R, Evans SF, et al. Repeated antenatal corticosteroids: size at birth and subsequent development. Am J Obstet Gynecol 1999;180:114–21.

16. Guinn DA, Atkinson MW, Sullivan L, et al. Single vs. weekly courses of antenatal for corticosteroids for women at risk of preterm delivery: a randomized controlled trial. JAMA 2001;286:1581–7.

17. Wapner RJ, Sorokin Y, Thom EA, et al, National Institute of Child Health and Human Development Maternal Fetal Medicine Units Network. Single vs. weekly courses of antenatal corticosteroids: evaluation of safety and efficacy. Am J Obstet Gynecol 2006;195:633–42.

18. Crowther CA, Haslam RR, Hiller JE, et al, Australian Collaborative Trial of Repeat Doses of Steroids (ACTORDS) Study Group. Neonatal respiratory distress after repeat exposure to antenatal corticosteroids: a randomised controlled trail. Lancet 2006;367:1913–9.

19. Murphy KE, Hannah ME, Willan AR, et al. MACS Collaborative Group Multiple courses of antenatal corticosteroids for preterm birth (MACS): a randomised controlled trial. Lancet 2008;372:2143–251.

20. Wapner RJ, Sorokin Y, Mele L, et al. Long-term outcomes after repeat doses of antenatal corticosteroids. N Engl J Med 2007;357:1190–8.

21. Crowther CA, Doyle LW, Haslam RR, et al. Outcomes at 2 years after repeat doses of antenatal corticosteroids. N Engl J Med 2007;357:1179–89.

22. Vermillion ST, Bland ML, Soper DE. Effectiveness of a rescue dose of antenatal betamethasone after an initial single dose. Am J Obstet Gynecol 2001;185:1086–9.

23. Mercer B. Randomized controlled trial of weekly vs. rescue antenatal corticosteroids [abstract]. Presented at the Annual Meeting of the Society of Maternal Fetal Medicine. Reno, February 1–3, 2001.

24. Garite TJ, Kurtzman J, Maurel K, et al, Obstetrix Collaborative Research Network. Impact of a rescue course of antenatal corticosteroids: a multicenter randomized placebo-controlled trial. Am J Obstet Gynecol 2009;200:248.e1–9.

25. McEvoy C, Schilling D, Peters D, et al. Respiratory compliance in preterm infants after a single rescue course of antenatal steroids: a randomized controlled trial. Am J Obstet Gynecol 2010;202:544.

26. American Congress of Obstetricians and Gynecologists. Antenatal corticosteroid therapy for fetal maturation. ACOG Committee Opinion #475, February, 2011.

27. Vermillion ST, Soper DE, Chasedunn-Roark J. Neonatal sepsis after betamethasone to patients with preterm premature rupture of membranes. Am J Obstet Gynecol 1999;181:320–7.

28. Lee M, Davies J, Guinn D, et al. Single vs. weekly course of antenatal corticosteroids in preterm premature rupture of membranes. Obstet Gynecol 2004;103:274–81.

29. Nelson KB, Grether JK. Can magnesium sulfate reduce the risk of cerebral palsy in very low birthweight infants? Pediatrics 1995;95:263–9.

30. Conde-Agudelo A, Romero R. Antenatal magnesium sulfate for the prevention of cerebral palsy in preterm infants less than 34 weeks' gestation: a systematic review and metaanalysis. Am J Obstet Gynecol 2009;200:595–609.

31. Crowther CA, Hiller JE, Doyle LW, et al. Australasian Collaborative Trial of Magnesium Sulphate (ACTOMg SO4) Collaborative Group Effect of magnesium sulfate given for neuroprotection before preterm birth: a randomized controlled trial. JAMA 2003;290:2669.

32. Marret S, Marpeau L, Zupan-Simunek V, et al. PREMAG trial group Magnesium sulphate given before very-preterm birth to protect infant brain: the randomised controlled PREMAG trial. Br J Obstet Gynaecol 2007;114:310–8.

33. Rouse DJ, Hirtz DG, Thom E, et al. A randomized, controlled trial of magnesium sulfate for the prevention of cerebral palsy. N Engl J Med 2008;359:895–905.

34. Magpie Trial Follow-Up Study Collaborative Group. The Magpie Trial: a randomised trial comparing magnesium sulphate with placebo for pre-eclampsia: outcome for children at 18 months. Br J Obstet Gynaecol 2007;114:289–99.

35. Burd I, Breen K, Friedman A, et al. Magnesium sulfate reduces inflammation-associated brain injury in fetal mice. Am J Obstet Gynecol 2010;202:292.e1–9.

36. American Congress of Obstetricians and Gynecologists. Magnesium Sulfate Before Anticipated Preterm Birth for Neuroprotection. ACOG Committee Opinion #455, March 2010.

37. Rouse D. Magnesium sulfate for the prevention of cerebral palsy. Am J Obstet Gynecol 2009;200:610–2.

38. Romero R. Prevention of spontaneous preterm birth: the role of sonographic cervical length in identifying patients who may benefit from progesterone treatment. Ultrasound Obstet Gynecol 2007;30:675–86.

39. Csapo AI. The "see-saw" theory of parturition. In: Knight J, O'Connor M, editors. The fetus and birth. Amsterdam: Elsevier/Excerpta Medica; 1977. p. 159.

40. Johnson JW, Austin KL, Jones GS, et al. Efficacy of 17 alpha-hydroxyprogesterone caproate in the prevention of premature labor. N Engl J Med 1975;293:675–80.

41. Keirse MJ. Progestogen administration in pregnancy may prevent preterm delivery. Br J Obstet Gynaecol 1990;97:149–54.

42. Meis PJ, Klebanoff M, Thom E, et al. Prevention of recurrent preterm delivery by 17 alpha-hydroxyprogesterone caproate. N Engl J Med 2003;348:2379–85.

43. da Fonseca EB, Bittar RE, Carvalho MH, et al. Prophylactic administration of progesterone by vaginal suppository to reduce the incidence of spontaneous preterm birth in women at increased risk: a randomized placebo-controlled double-blind study. Am J Obstet Gynecol 2003;188:2419–24.

44. O'Brien JM, Adair CD, Lewis DF, et al. Progesterone vaginal gel for the reduction of recurrent preterm birth: primary results from a randomized, double-blind, placebo-controlled trial. Ultrasound Obstet Gynecol 2007;30:687–96.

45. Hartikainen-Sorri AL, Kauppila A, Tuimala R. Inefficacy of 17 alpha-hydroxyprogesterone caproate in the prevention of prematurity in twin pregnancy. Obstet Gynecol 1980;56:692–5.

46. Rouse DJ, Caritis SN, Peaceman AM, et al. A trial of 17 alpha-hydroxyprogesterone caproate to prevent prematurity in twins. N Engl J Med 2007;357:454–61.

47. Briery CM, Veillon EW, Klauser CK, et al. Progesterone does not prevent preterm births in women with twins. South Med J 2009;102:900–4.

48. Combs CA, Garite T, Maurel K, et al. 17-hydroxyprogesterone caproate for twin pregnancy: a double-blind, randomized clinical trial. Am J Obstet Gynecol 2011;204, e1–8.
49. Lim AC, Schuit E, Bloemenkamp K, et al. 17alpha-hydroxyprogesterone caproate for the prevention of adverse neonatal outcome in multiple pregnancies: a randomized controlled trial. Obstet Gynecol 2011;118:513–20.
50. Rode L, Klein K, Nicolaides KH, et al. Prevention of preterm delivery in twin gestations (PREDICT): a multicenter, randomized, placebo-controlled trial on the effect of vaginal micronized progesterone. Ultrasound Obstet Gynecol 2011;38:272–80.
51. Cetingtoz E, Cam C, Sakalli M, et al. Progesterone effects on preterm birth in high-risk pregnancies: a randomized placebo-controlled trial. Arch Gynecol Obstet 2011;283:423–9.
52. Norman JE, Mackenzie F, Owen P, et al. Progesterone for the prevention of preterm birth in twin pregnancy (STOPPIT): a randomized, double-blind, placebo-controlled study and meat-analysis. Lancet 2009;372:2034–240.
53. Caritis SN, Rouse DJ, Peaceman AM, et al. Prevention of preterm birth in triplets using 17 alpha-hydroxyprogesterone caproate: a randomized controlled trail. Obstet Gynecol 2009;113(2 Pt 1):285–92.
54. Combs CA, Garite T, Maurel K, et al. Failure of 17-hydroxyprogesterone to reduce neonatal morbidity or prolong triplet pregnancy: a doubleblind, randomized clinical trial. Am J Obstet Gynecol 2010;203:248.e1–9.
55. Iams JD, Goldenberg RL, Meis PJ, et al. NICHD MFM Network. The length of the cervix and the risk of spontaneous premature delivery. N Engl J Med 1996;334:567–72.
56. DeFranco EA, O'Brien JM, Adair CD, et al. Vaginal progesterone is associated with a decrease in risk for early preterm birth and improved neonatal outcome in women with a short cervix: a secondary analysis from a randomized, double-blind, placebo-controlled trial. Ultrasound Obstet Gynecol 2007;30:697–705.
57. Fonseca EB, Celik E, Parra M, et al. Progesterone and the risk of preterm birth among women with a short cervix. N Engl J Med 2007;357:462–9.
58. Hassan SS, Romero R, Vidyadhari D, et al. Vaginal progesterone reduces the rate of preterm birth in women with a sonographic short cervix: a milticenter, randomized, double-blind, placebo-controlled trial. Ultrasound Obstet Gynecol 2011;38(1):18–31.
59. Nothen AT, Norman GS, Anderson K, et al. follow up of children exposed in utero to 17 alpha-hydroxyprogesterone caproate compared with placebo. Obstet Gynecol 2007;110:865–72.
60. Klein K, Rode L, Nicolaides KH, et al. Vaginal micronized progesterone and risk of preterm delivery in high-risk twin pregnancies: secondary analysis of a placebo-controlled randomized trial and meta-analysis. Ultrasound Obstet Gynecol 2011;38(3):281–7.
61. American Congress of Obstericians and Gynecologists. Use of Progesterone to Reduce Preterm Birth. ACOG Committee Opinion #419, October, 2008.
62. Cahill AG, Odibo AO, Caughey AB, et al. Universal cervical length screening and treatment with vaginal progesterone to prevent preterm birth: a decision and economic analysis. Am J Obstet Gynecol 2010;202:548, e1–8.

Evidence-Based Neonatal Pharmacotherapy: Postnatal Corticosteroids

Kristi Watterberg, MD

KEYWORDS

- Dexamethasone • Hydrocortisone
- Bronchopulmonary dysplasia • Cardiovascular insufficiency
- Hypotension • Preterm infant • Newborn infant

ACTIONS OF CORTICOSTEROIDS

Corticosteroids are hormones produced by the adrenal cortex and the synthetic compounds that mimic the actions of those natural hormones. Corticosteroids affect almost all body functions and are therefore among the most powerful agents used in clinical practice. The actions of these hormones can be divided into mineralocorticoid and glucocorticoid actions; however, cortisol, the primary glucocorticoid produced by the adrenal cortex, also has mineralocorticoid actions, as shown in **Box 1**. Cortisol regulates protein, carbohydrate, lipid, and nucleic acid metabolism; maintains cardiac and vascular response to vasoconstrictors; regulates extracellular water and promotes free water excretion; suppresses the inflammatory response and decreases capillary permeability during inflammation; and modulates central nervous system processing and behavior.[1,2] Aldosterone, the primary mineralocorticoid produced in the adrenal cortex, is rarely used as its synthetic equivalent, fludrocortisone, in the neonatal intensive care unit (NICU), and is not discussed in this article.

Synthetic corticosteroids, such as dexamethasone, betamethasone, and prednisone, have variable effects on these multiple functions, differing degrees of mineralocorticoid activity, and widely varying half-lives.[3,4] Thus, determining the relative potency of these different agents can be difficult. Nevertheless, those differences are highly relevant to the actions and effects of the synthetic steroids in clinical practice. For example, dexamethasone has a much longer biologic half-life than cortisol, which may amplify its nominal potency from 25 to 40 times greater than that of hydrocortisone to as much as 150 times higher for some actions.[1,5]

Department of Pediatrics, University of New Mexico School of Medicine, Albuquerque, NM 87131-0001, USA
E-mail address: kwatterberg@salud.unm.edu

Clin Perinatol 39 (2012) 47–59
doi:10.1016/j.clp.2011.12.017
0095-5108/12/$ – see front matter © 2012 Elsevier Inc. All rights reserved.

Box 1
Cortisol actions

Glucocorticoid effects

Regulation of protein, carbohydrate, lipid, and nucleic acid metabolism

Maintenance of cardiac and vascular response to vasoconstrictors

Regulation of extracellular water and promotion of free water excretion

Suppression of the inflammatory response

Lowering of capillary permeability

Modulation of central nervous system processing and behavior

Mineralocorticoid effects

Sodium reabsorption

Potassium excretion

Dexamethasone, the most widely used synthetic steroid in neonatology, has essentially no mineralocorticoid activity but suppresses endogenous cortisol secretion, creating what is sometimes referred to as a *chemical adrenalectomy*.[2,3] This effect, in conjunction with its high potency and long half-life, may help explain the observed adverse effects of dexamethasone on the neurodevelopmental outcomes of preterm infants. The brain contains both mineralocorticoid and glucocorticoid receptors, which are present in particularly high density in the hippocampus, an area of the brain critical to learning and memory.[2,3] At usual physiologic concentrations, cortisol binds primarily to the mineralocorticoid receptors in the brain; only at higher, stress-induced concentrations does it bind substantially to glucocorticoid receptors.[2,3] Because dexamethasone suppresses cortisol secretion, the mineralocorticoid receptors are left unoccupied, leading to neuronal apoptosis in the hippocampus both in vitro and in animal models.[6,7] Administration of corticosterone (the rodent equivalent of cortisol) or aldosterone protects against this apoptosis.[6,7]

Observational human studies have associated impaired learning and memory with smaller hippocampal volumes in children and adolescents born preterm.[8–10] In turn, other observational studies have associated dexamethasone therapy in the preterm infant with smaller brain or hippocampal volumes at term gestation and with adverse neurodevelopmental outcomes.[11–13] Because these observations have not been studied in randomized trials, they may only reflect increased severity of illness in infants who received dexamethasone. However, neither published observational studies nor a preliminary report from a randomized controlled trial (RCT) of hydrocortisone has shown an association between hydrocortisone therapy and decreased hippocampal volume.[14–16] One observational study of approximately 20 infants who were treated with hydrocortisone and had no dexamethasone exposure reported an association between hydrocortisone therapy and decreased cerebellar volume (another area of the brain with high density of corticosteroid receptors). However, the preliminary report from an RCT of hydrocortisone (23 patients treated with hydrocortisone) found no such effect.[16,17]

In addition to differences related to variable mineralocorticoid and glucocorticoid actions and relative potency, corticosteroids have both genomic and nongenomic effects. Genomic actions are those traditionally associated with glucocorticoids, requiring transport to the cell nucleus, transcription, and translation to new protein, with significant time delay to achieve effect (eg, prenatal administration to stimulate lung maturation). Nongenomic effects, however, occur as soon as the molecule binds to the cell surface, and directly affect multiple cellular events, including calcium and sodium transmembrane cycling[18,19]; these effects are seen clinically within a few hours of administration (eg, hydrocortisone given to treat hypotension). Synthetic glucocorticoids have effect profiles that differ in their nongenomic versus genomic actions, adding even more complexity to estimations of equivalence.[18]

Postnatal corticosteroids have been primarily administered to treat two conditions in the NICU: bronchopulmonary dysplasia (BPD) and hypotension (cardiovascular insufficiency); this article focuses on those two therapeutic indications.

BPD
A Brief History of Dexamethasone for BPD: A Cautionary Tale

The story of dexamethasone for treatment or prevention of BPD in preterm infants has become a quintessential cautionary tale in neonatology, illustrating the hazards of adopting a therapy based on minimal human evidence and ignoring previously existing neonatal animal data documenting adverse effects of high-dose corticosteroids on brain and somatic growth.[20–22] Dexamethasone therapy was adopted based on a few small studies published in the late 1980s that showed positive short-term respiratory effects.[23–25] High dosages (0.5–1.0 mg/kg/d), effectively equivalent to well over 20 times the basal cortisol secretion rate,[1,4,26] were administered to thousands of very preterm infants and tapered over as long as 42 days[25,27,28] before follow-up of RCTs began to document adverse effects on neurodevelopment.[29–32]

During those years, dexamethasone studies often documented a decrease in weight gain and/or head circumference during therapy and frequent occurrence of other short-term side effects, such as hyperglycemia and hypertension.[23,27,33] Over time, a wide variety of other serious adverse effects became evident, including increased protein catabolism[34] and cardiac hypertrophy,[35] and gastrointestinal perforation when therapy was initiated in the first postnatal week.[36,37] With documentation of these numerous short- and long-term adverse effects of high-dose dexamethasone, initial enthusiasm waned, fewer infants received dexamethasone,[38] and investigators began to study the effects of lower doses.

In summary, the approach to the use of dexamethasone for BPD was the opposite of the model used for testing of a novel therapeutic agent: begin with a low dose and increase in increments while monitoring efficacy and toxicity. In addition, the wrong primary outcome measure—short-term respiratory benefit—was chosen. On a positive note, an important result of the dexamethasone story has been the recognition that assessment of long-term outcomes is an essential part of the evaluation of any drug administered to neonates.

Dexamethasone for BPD: Current Evidence

After publication of studies documenting adverse neurodevelopmental effects of high-dose dexamethasone treatment, the American Academy of Pediatrics and Canadian Paediatric Society jointly recommended in 2002 that routine dexamethasone therapy for the prevention or treatment of BPD be limited to RCTs with long-term follow-up, that alternative corticosteroids undergo further study, and that infants currently enrolled in RCTs undergo long-term neurodevelopmental follow-up.[39] Outside the context of RCTs, "the use of corticosteroids should be limited to exceptional clinical circumstances (eg, an infant on maximal ventilatory and oxygen support). In those circumstances, parents should be fully informed about the known short- and long-term risks and agree to treatment."[39]

Unfortunately for the recommendation for further RCTs, the results of previous high-dose studies dampened enthusiasm for further study of dexamethasone at any dose. This resulted in early closure of several clinical trials of lower-dose dexamethasone, including one specifically designed to evaluate neurodevelopmental outcomes.[40,41] This trial, designed to enroll 800 patients, was closed after only 80 patients were enrolled, severely limiting its power to detect important differences. The authors found that a dexamethasone dosage of 0.15 mg/kg/d tapered over 10 days facilitated extubation, did not significantly lower mortality or BPD, and had no significant adverse effect on neurodevelopmental outcomes at 2 years.[40,41] Another group of investigators performed two small RCTs comparing starting dosages of 0.5 mg/kg versus 0.2 mg/kg tapered over 7 days and found similar pulmonary effects and outcomes using either dosage.[42,43] Two recently reported small observational studies showed significant effects on pulmonary mechanics with a starting dosage of only 0.05 mg/kg/d tapered over 9 or 16 days ("minidex").[44,45] The effects of this very low dose have not yet been reported in a randomized trial. In summary, although a much lower daily dose of dexamethasone may have equal efficacy with fewer adverse effects, data are currently insufficient for an evidence-based dosing recommendation.[46]

In seeming contradiction to the data described earlier, a recent meta-analysis found that a higher cumulative dose of dexamethasone was associated with decreased death or neurodevelopmental impairment (NDI)[47]; however, only one of the included RCTs used a starting daily dose of less than 0.5 mg/kg; therefore, this meta-analysis primarily evaluated the effect of shorter versus longer courses of high-dose therapy, and found a benefit to longer courses of therapy. In a separate analysis, these authors highlight the effect of open-label glucocorticoid use on the results of these RCTs.[48] They found that moderately early dexamethasone therapy (initiated between 7 and 14 days' postnatal age) reduced mortality in trials with less than 30% open-label contamination of the placebo arm, a benefit that was not seen in trials with greater than 30% contamination.[48] Later therapy (>3 weeks' postnatal age) showed no such benefit, but instead an increase in cerebral palsy in the treated patients. However, their analysis of trials with less than 30% contamination included only 35 dexamethasone-treated infants. This meta-analysis highlights the difficulty of evaluating drug effect in RCTs with significant open-label medication use; fewer than one-fourth of the patients were enrolled in trials with less than 30% open-label use of dexamethasone.

Another difficulty in comparing RCTs in a meta-analysis is variation in patient populations. In an attempt to address this issue, Doyle and colleagues[49] performed a "risk-weighted" meta-analysis to evaluate the effect of the baseline risk of BPD on study outcomes. They found that studies enrolling infants with a low risk of BPD (<35%) showed an increased incidence of death or cerebral palsy among dexamethasone-treated infants compared with placebo-treated infants. In contrast, studies enrolling infants at high risk for BPD (>50%) showed that dexamethasone treatment decreased the risk for death or cerebral palsy in treated infants. Thus, for infants at highest risk of BPD, the beneficial effect of dexamethasone in reducing lung disease seemed to outweigh its adverse effect in terms of cerebral palsy.

This risk-weighted meta-analysis illustrates several important issues, including the difficulty of comparing RCTs with different patient populations and treatment regimens. In addition, it indicates the importance of trying to balance the risks of a therapeutic agent against the risks of the disease itself. BPD consistently has been shown to be a risk factor for impaired growth and adverse neurodevelopment in preterm infants[50,51]; therefore, for infants at very high risk of BPD, such as those who remain intubated after the first or second week of life, a trial of lower-dose dexamethasone may be a reasonable choice.[46,52,53]

Hydrocortisone for BPD: Current Evidence

Four RCTs of hydrocortisone therapy in the first week of life to prevent BPD have been published (N = 501).[54–57] These studies were similar in design, dosing, and duration of therapy (approximately 2 weeks), and were based on the premise that many extremely preterm infants have immature adrenal gland function, leaving them vulnerable to inflammatory lung injury during the first several weeks of life.[58–62] Two of the smaller studies showed a significant increase in survival without BPD in the hydrocortisone-treated infants, and the direction of effect favored hydrocortisone in all studies. The largest trial (N = 360) did not show a significant benefit of hydrocortisone treatment in the overall study group; however, for infants exposed to histologic chorioamnionitis (n = 149), hydrocortisone-treated infants had a significant decrease in mortality and increase in survival without BPD.[55] Patient enrollment was stopped early in three of these studies because of a significant increase in spontaneous gastrointestinal perforations in hydrocortisone-treated infants, possibly caused by an interaction between hydrocortisone and indomethacin therapy.[55] A recent meta-analysis of the effect of early hydrocortisone on BPD included an additional four RCTs of hydrocortisone therapy in the first postnatal week and found "few beneficial or harmful effects"; however, the additional four studies had different primary aims and shorter treatment courses, limiting their comparability.[63]

Neurodevelopmental outcomes at 18 to 22 months' corrected age have been published for children enrolled in three of these trials, with no reported adverse effects of hydrocortisone treatment.[64,65] In the largest trial, which evaluated 87% of 291 survivors, the incidence of death or major NDI, NDI alone, and cerebral palsy were similar between groups. The only significant differences favored the hydrocortisone-treated group, including fewer infants with a Bayley Scales of Infant Development (2nd edition) Mental Developmental Index less than 70, and increased attainment of object permanence, which is an early test of working memory.[64]

Currently, no RCTs of later hydrocortisone therapy for BPD have been published, although one small RCT has been presented in abstract form[16] and several trials are currently enrolling patients. Peer-reviewed data are limited to cohort studies of infants treated with a 3-week course of hydrocortisone beginning with 5 mg/kg/d, which may be roughly equivalent to 0.15 mg/kg/d of dexamethasone.[1] Structural and functional assessments have been performed at school age (8–10 years) for 62 hydrocortisone-treated infants and a comparison group of 164 infants.[14] Hydrocortisone-treated infants were smaller, less mature, and sicker than their counterparts. After adjustment for differences in neonatal variables (eg, gestational age, birth weight), their cognitive, motor, and MRI outcomes were similar.[14] Although these results are reassuring, data are insufficient to make an evidence-based recommendation for using hydrocortisone to treat BPD.

Inhaled Steroids for BPD: Current Evidence

The option of using inhaled rather than systemic glucocorticoids to prevent or treat BPD is clearly attractive, because it would provide a direct topical application and limit systemic exposure. Unfortunately, a variety of factors limit drug delivery and deposition in intubated babies, including particle size; type of nebulizer and its placement in the ventilator circuit; flow rate; small endotracheal tube diameter; and short inspiratory times.[66] Studies using sodium cromoglycate as a marker of lung deposition have shown that effective drug delivery is low in intubated and spontaneously breathing infants.[67,68] In addition, nonintubated infants may have greatly increased steroid exposure from deposition of drug in the oropharynx.[66] RCTs thus far have not shown a benefit of inhaled steroids in preventing or treating BPD.[69,70]

SUMMARY OF CURRENT EVIDENCE-BASED RECOMMENDATIONS FOR BPD

- Glucocorticoid therapy in the first week of life has been associated with spontaneous gastrointestinal perforation. Although this may be from concurrent indomethacin or ibuprofen administration, steroid therapy currently cannot be recommended in the first postnatal week to prevent BPD.
- High dosages of dexamethasone (eg, ≥ 0.5 mg/kg/d) may decrease the incidence of BPD, but have been associated with numerous short- and long-term adverse effects. Based on existing evidence, this therapy cannot be recommended.
- Lower doses of dexamethasone (≤ 0.2 mg/kg/d) may be equally efficacious, facilitate extubation, and result in fewer adverse effects; however, data from RCTs are currently insufficient to allow an evidence-based recommendation for this therapy.
- Low-dose hydrocortisone (1 mg/kg/d) given during the first 2 weeks of life may decrease BPD in specific patient populations, such as infants exposed to prenatal inflammation; however, because of the risk of spontaneous gastrointestinal perforation, this therapy cannot currently be recommended.
- Hydrocortisone therapy in antiinflammatory doses (3–5 mg/kg/d) after the first week of life has not been reported to decrease BPD in an RCT; therefore, an evidence-based recommendation currently cannot be made.
- Inhaled glucocorticoids have not been shown to decrease BPD in an RCT; therefore, this therapy currently cannot be recommended.
- Because data are insufficient to form a clear evidence-based recommendation for the use of glucocorticoid therapy for BPD, clinicians must weigh the risks of glucocorticoid therapy against the risks of BPD in an individual patient. For example, infants who remain on mechanical ventilation through an endotracheal tube after the first postnatal week are at very high risk of developing BPD. For these infants, clinicians, together with the family, may decide that a short tapering course of lower-dose glucocorticoid therapy (eg, a starting dosage of approximately 0.15 mg/kg/d of dexamethasone or approximately 5 mg/kg/d of hydrocortisone) is warranted.

Cardiovascular Insufficiency (Shock)

Treatment aimed at improving cardiac output and systemic circulation is highly prevalent and variable in the NICU. A cohort study of 1387 extremely low-gestational-age newborns (<28 weeks' gestational age) found that more than 80% received some form of this treatment, and a third of the population received vasopressors.[71] In the 14 participating centers, the proportion of infants treated with vasopressors ranged from 6% to 64%, with no apparent relationship to blood pressure. Similarly, a 16-center cohort study of 830 term and late-preterm infants undergoing mechanical ventilation showed that 61% of infants underwent therapy for hypotension.[72] Of the treated infants, 97% received a fluid bolus, 44% received vasopressors, and 21% received corticosteroids.

Data regarding the relationship of early cardiovascular insufficiency to outcome are variable and conflicting, probably at least partly due to differing definitions and a multitude of possible causes. The most commonly used measure, blood pressure, is a poor reflector of cardiac function[73]; some hypotensive infants may have otherwise normal indicators of cardiovascular function and benefit from watchful waiting, or "permissive hypotension."[74] Others may have poor perfusion, decreased urine output, and metabolic acidosis, indicating inadequate cardiovascular function that may benefit from supportive measures. Monitoring of more direct measures of blood flow, oxygen delivery, and oxygen consumption could provide a better evaluation of the link between cardiac insufficiency and outcomes[75]; however, these techniques are not easily applied. In the meantime, clinicians need to exercise clinical judgment regarding treatment of cardiovascular insufficiency, or shock, in the absence of good evidence.

The use of glucocorticoids, primarily hydrocortisone, to support cardiovascular function in acutely ill preterm infants was first described in a series of six hypotensive patients with very low cortisol values who responded to hydrocortisone.[76] Further studies documented that infants with higher illness severity scores or those receiving dopamine had lower cortisol values or response to adrenocorticotropic hormone stimulation,[59,77,78] suggesting the presence of a relative adrenal insufficiency in these infants similar to that described in critically ill adults.[79] Furthermore, cohort studies, RCTs, and meta-analyses have consistently shown that hydrocortisone results in an increase in blood pressure and cardiac output, and a decrease in vasopressor requirements in preterm infants (**Fig. 1**).[19,55,80,81] Hydrocortisone may produce these effects through treating relative adrenal insufficiency, counteracting the inflammation-mediated down-regulation of cardiovascular adrenergic receptors, or other nongenomic effects on cell membranes.[19,82]

Although hydrocortisone results in an increase in blood pressure and cardiac output, RCTs of hydrocortisone for hypotension are small,[80,83] and do not include vital evaluation of long-term outcomes. A cohort study of 1401 very low-birth-weight infants reported that administration of hydrocortisone for hypotension was associated with a significantly higher incidence of intraventricular hemorrhage, periventricular leukomalacia, and death.[84] As the authors of the study pointed out, this increased morbidity was most likely secondary to the hypotension itself, but they urged caution regarding the possible contributing role of hydrocortisone.

The difference in apparent drug effect between a cohort study such as described above and a randomized trial is shown by the multicenter RCT of early hydrocortisone for preventing BPD.[55] In that study of 360 infants, 21 (6%) were receiving open-label

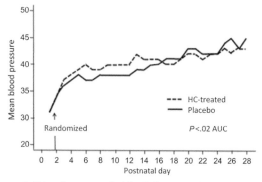

Fig. 1. Daily mean arterial blood pressure (pr) for infants randomized to hydrocortisone (HC; 1 mg/kg/d) versus placebo in the study of 360 infants by Watterberg and colleagues.[55] Hypotension was neither an inclusion nor an exclusion criterion; 37% of the infants were receiving vasopressor therapy on their first postnatal day. AUC, area under the curve. (*Data from* Kristi Watterberg, unpublished data, 2004; and Watterberg KL, Gerdes JS, Cole CH, et al. Prophylaxis of early adrenal insufficiency to prevent bronchopulmonary dysplasia: a multicenter trial. Pediatrics 2004;114:1649–57.)

hydrocortisone at the time of randomization. Of those, 33% died (Kristi Watterberg, unpublished data, 2004), a significantly higher mortality rate than that of the overall study population (16%). However, in the randomized groups, the mortality rates were similar (16% vs 17% for placebo), as were the incidence of intraventricular hemorrhage, periventricular leukomalacia, and outcomes at 18 to 22 months' corrected age.[64] As this example shows, RCTs often lead to different conclusions than do cohort studies.

As with BPD, therefore, insufficient data are available for clinicians to make an evidence-based decision regarding whether and how to treat cardiovascular insufficiency in preterm or term infants. The evidence described earlier shows that, statistically, these infants have lower cortisol values than those with stable cardiovascular status, and that hydrocortisone will result in an increase in blood pressure in most infants. If the patient's cardiac insufficiency is from a relative adrenal insufficiency or down-regulation of cardiovascular adrenergic receptors, then hydrocortisone may be a more appropriate treatment than vasopressors; however, no data from RCTs are available regarding long-term outcomes after use of hydrocortisone to treat these infants, or after any treatment for hypotension. Thus, clinicians must exercise clinical judgment when treating an infant exhibiting systemic signs of cardiovascular insufficiency.

If hydrocortisone treatment is chosen, consideration must be given to its prolonged half-life in newborns, particularly in preterm infants. Studies of hydrocortisone pharmacokinetics are difficult, because of the inability to distinguish exogenous hydrocortisone from endogenous cortisol. The only study published in term babies involved eight infants and found the half-life of hydrocortisone to be approximately 4 hours, more than twice that of adults.[85] Results for preterm infants are only available in abstract form, and report the half-life in extremely preterm infants to be prolonged and highly variable, likely 8 to 12 hours.[86,87] Although several studies have used higher doses of hydrocortisone in preterm infants (eg, 1 mg/kg every 8 hours[80]), these doses may result in very high serum concentrations.[86] The large RCT of hydrocortisone to prevent BPD in extremely preterm infants showed that a dose of 0.5 mg/kg every 12 hours resulted in a statistically significant increase in both blood cortisol concentrations and blood pressure (see **Fig. 1**).[55,87] In the absence of better data, and in keeping with the goal of minimizing drug exposure, a reasonable strategy might be to administer a test dose of 1 mg/kg and observe the patient for response over the next 2 to 6 hours. If cardiovascular status improves, therapy can be continued at a dose of 0.5 mg/kg given every 12 hours for the extremely preterm infant and every 6 to 8 hours for the late preterm or term infant, weaning quickly when clinical improvement is seen.

This article clearly illustrates that many more questions than answers exist regarding treatment with glucocorticoids in the NICU. RCTs are urgently needed to answer these questions and improve care for patients; however, the practical difficulties of performing some of these trials (eg, early hydrocortisone for cardiovascular insufficiency) are enormous and may preclude generating the evidence so badly needed.

REFERENCES

1. Williams HW, Dluhy RG. Diseases of the adrenal cortex. In: Fauci AS, Braunwald E, Isselbacher KJ, et al, editors. Harrison's principles of internal medicine. 14th edition. New York: McGraw-Hill Companies; 1998. p. 2035–57.
2. De Kloet RE, Vreugdenhil E, Oitzl MS, et al. Brain corticosteroid receptor balance in health and disease. Endocr Rev 1998;19:269–301.

3. McEwen BS. The brain is an important target of adrenal steroid actions: a comparison of synthetic and natural steroids. Ann N Y Acad Sci 1997;823: 201–13.

4. Schimmer BP, Parker KL. Adrenocorticotropic hormone; adrenocortical steroids and their synthetic analogs; inhibitors of the synthesis and actions of adrenocortical hormones. In: Hardman JG, Limbird LE, editors. Goodman & Gilman's the pharmacologic basis of therapeutics. 10th edition. New York: McGraw-Hill; 2001. p. 1649–77.

5. Meikle AW, Tyler FH. Potency and duration of action of glucocorticoids: effects of hydrocortisone, prednisone and dexamethasone on human pituitary-adrenal function. Am J Med 1977;63:200–7.

6. Crochemore C, Lu J, Wu Y, et al. Direct targeting of hippocampal neurons for apoptosis by glucocorticoids is reversible by mineralocorticoid receptor activation. Mol Psychiatry 2005;10:790–8.

7. Hassan AH, von Rosenstiel P, Patchev VK, et al. Exacerbation of apoptosis in the dentate gyrus of the aged rat by dexamethasone and the protective role of corticosterone. Exp Neurol 1996;140:43–52.

8. Isaacs EB, Lucas A, Chong WK, et al. Hippocampal volume and everyday memory in children of very low birth weight. Pediatr Res 2000;47:713–20.

9. Giménez M, Junqué C, Narberhaus A, et al. Hippocampal gray matter reduction associates with memory deficits in adolescents with history of prematurity. Neuroimage 2004;23:869–77.

10. Nosarti C, Al-Asady MH, Frangou S, et al. Adolescents who were born very preterm have decreased brain volumes. Brain 2002;125:1616–23.

11. Murphy BP, Inder TE, Huppi PS, et al. Impaired cerebral cortical gray matter growth after treatment with dexamethasone for neonatal chronic lung disease. Pediatrics 2001;107:217–21.

12. Parikh NA, Lasky RE, Kennedy KA, et al. Postnatal dexamethasone therapy and cerebral tissue volumes in extremely low birth weight infants. Pediatrics 2007; 119:265–72.

13. Thompson DK, Wood SJ, Doyle LW, et al. Neonate hippocampal volumes: prematurity, perinatal predictors, and 2-year outcome. Ann Neurol 2008;63:642–51.

14. Rademaker KJ, Uiterwaal CS, Groenendaal F, et al. Neonatal hydrocortisone treatment: neurodevelopmental outcome and MRI at school age in preterm-born children. J Pediatr 2007;150:351–7.

15. Rademaker KJ, Rijpert M, Uiterwaal CS, et al. Neonatal hydrocortisone treatment related to 1H-MRS of the hippocampus and short-term memory at school age in preterm born children. Pediatr Res 2006;59:309–13.

16. Parikh NA, Lasky R, Tyson J, et al. Does low dose hydrocortisone improve volumetric MRI measures of cerebral growth in extremely low birth weight infants at high risk for bronchopulmonary dysplasia?: a randomized trial [abstract]. Presented at the annual meeting of Pediatric Academic Societies. E-PAS 2009:3212.2.

17. Tam EW, Chau V, Ferriero DM, et al. Preterm cerebellar growth impairment after postnatal exposure to glucocorticoids. Sci Transl Med 2011;3:105ra105.

18. Buttgereit F, Brand MD, Burmester GR. Equivalent doses and relative drug potencies for non-genomic glucocorticoid effects: a novel glucocorticoid hierarchy. Biochem Pharmacol 1999;58:363–8.

19. Noori S, Friedlich P, Wong P, et al. Hemodynamic changes after low-dosage hydrocortisone administration in vasopressor-treated preterm and term neonates. Pediatrics 2006;118:1456–66.

20. Howard E. Reductions in size and total DNA of cerebrum and cerebellum in adult mice after corticosterone treatment in infancy. Exp Neurol 1968;22:191–208.

21. Howard E, Benjamin JA. DNA, ganglioside and sulfatide in brains of rats given corticosterone in infancy, with an estimate of cell loss during development. Brain Res 1975;92:73–87.

22. De Souza SW, Adlard BP. Growth of suckling rats after treatment with dexamethasone or cortisol. Implications for steroid therapy in human infants. Arch Dis Child 1973;48:519–22.

23. Mammel MC, Green TP, Johnson DE, et al. Controlled trial of dexamethasone therapy in infants with bronchopulmonary dysplasia. Lancet 1983;1(8338): 1356–8.

24. Avery GB, Fletcher AB, Kaplan M, et al. Controlled trial of dexamethasone in respirator-dependent infants with bronchopulmonary dysplasia. Pediatrics 1985;75:106–11.

25. Cummings JJ, D'Eugenio DB, Gross SJ. A controlled trial of dexamethasone in preterm infants at high risk for bronchopulmonary dysplasia. N Engl J Med 1989;320:1505–10.

26. Metzger DL, Wright NM, Veldhuis JD, et al. Characterization of pulsatile secretion and clearance of plasma cortisol in premature and term neonates using deconvolution analysis. J Clin Endocrinol Metab 1993;77:458–63.

27. Yeh TF, Torre JA, Rastogi A, et al. Early postnatal dexamethasone therapy in premature infants with severe respiratory distress syndrome: a double-blind, controlled study. J Pediatr 1990;117:273–82.

28. Kothadia JM, O'Shea TM, Roberts D, et al. Randomized placebo-controlled trial of a 42-Day tapering course of dexamethasone to reduce the duration of ventilator dependency in very low birth weight infants [erratum appears in Pediatrics 2004;114:1746]. Pediatrics 1999;104:22–7.

29. Yeh TF, Lin YJ, Huang CC, et al. Early dexamethasone therapy in preterm infants: a follow-up study. Pediatrics 1998;101:E7.

30. O'Shea TM, Kothadia JM, Klinepeter KL, et al. Randomized placebo-controlled trial of a 42-day tapering course of dexamethasone to reduce the duration of ventilator dependency in very low birth weight infants: outcome of study participants at 1-year adjusted age. Pediatrics 1999;104:15–21.

31. Barrington KJ. The adverse neuro-developmental effects of postnatal steroids in the preterm infant: a systematic review of RCTs. BMC Pediatr 2001;1:1.

32. Yeh TF, Lin YJ, Lin HC, et al. Outcomes at school age after postnatal dexamethasone therapy for lung disease of prematurity. N Engl J Med 2004;350:1304–13.

33. Papile LA, Tyson JE, Stoll BJ, et al. A multicenter trial of two dexamethasone regimens in ventilator-dependent premature infants. N Engl J Med 1998;338: 1112–8.

34. Tsai FJ, Tsai CH, Wu SF, et al. Catabolic effect in premature infants with early dexamethasone treatment. Acta Paediatr 1996;85:1487–90.

35. Zecca E, Papacci P, Maggio L, et al. Cardiac adverse effects of early dexamethasone treatment in preterm infants: a randomized clinical trial. J Clin Pharmacol 2001;41:1075–81.

36. Garland JS, Alex CP, Pauly TH, et al. A three-day course of dexamethasone therapy to prevent chronic lung disease in ventilated neonates: a randomized trial. Pediatrics 1999;104:91–9.

37. Stark AR, Carlo WA, Tyson JE, et al. National Institute of Child Health and Human Development Neonatal Research Network. Adverse effects of early dexamethasone in extremely-low-birth-weight infants. National Institute of Child Health and

Human Development Neonatal Research Network. N Engl J Med 2001;344: 95–101.

38. Walsh MC, Yao Q, Horbar JD, et al. Changes in the use of postnatal steroids for bronchopulmonary dysplasia in 3 large neonatal networks. Pediatrics 2006;118: e1328–35.

39. Committee on Fetus and Newborn. Postnatal corticosteroids to treat or prevent chronic lung disease in preterm infants. Pediatrics 2002;109:330–8.

40. Doyle LW, Davis PG, Morley CJ, et al. DART Study Investigators. Low-dose dexamethasone facilitates extubation among chronically ventilator-dependent infants: a multicenter, international, randomized, controlled trial. Pediatrics 2006;117: 75–83.

41. Doyle LW, Davis PG, Morley CJ, et al. DART Study Investigators. Outcome at 2 years of age of infants from the DART study: a multicenter, international, randomized, controlled trial of low-dose dexamethasone. Pediatrics 2007; 119:716–21.

42. Durand M, Mendoza ME, Tantivit P, et al. A randomized trial of moderately early low-dose dexamethasone therapy in very low birth weight infants: dynamic pulmonary mechanics, oxygenation, and ventilation. Pediatrics 2002;109:262–8.

43. McEvoy C, Bowling S, Williamson K, et al. Randomized, double-blinded trial of low-dose dexamethasone: II. Functional residual capacity and pulmonary outcome in very low birth weight infants at risk for bronchopulmonary dysplasia. Pediatr Pulmonol 2004;38:55–63.

44. Yates HL, Newell SJ. Minidex: very low dose dexamethasone (0.05 mg/kg/day) in chronic lung disease. Arch Dis Child Fetal Neonatal Ed 2011;96:F190–4.

45. Tanney K, Davis J, Halliday HL, et al. Extremely low-dose dexamethasone to facilitate extubation in mechanically ventilated preterm babies. Neonatology 2011; 100:285–9.

46. Watterberg KL, American Academy of Pediatrics. Committee on Fetus and Newborn. Policy statement–postnatal corticosteroids to prevent or treat bronchopulmonary dysplasia. Pediatrics 2010;126:800–8.

47. Onland W, Offringa M, De Jaegere AP, et al. Finding the optimal postnatal dexamethasone regimen for preterm infants at risk of bronchopulmonary dysplasia: a systematic review of placebo-controlled trials. Pediatrics 2009;123:367–77.

48. Onland W, van Kaam AH, De Jaegere AP, et al. Open-label glucocorticoids modulate dexamethasone trial results in preterm infants. Pediatrics 2010;126: e954–64.

49. Doyle LW, Halliday HL, Ehrenkranz RA, et al. Impact of postnatal systemic corticosteroids on mortality and cerebral palsy in preterm infants: effect modification by risk for chronic lung disease. Pediatrics 2005;115:655–61.

50. Ehrenkranz RA, Walsh MC, Vohr BR, et al. National Institutes of Child Health and Human Development Neonatal Research Network. Validation of the National Institutes of Health consensus definition of bronchopulmonary dysplasia. Pediatrics 2005;116:1353–60.

51. Gargus RA, Vohr BR, Tyson JE, et al. Unimpaired outcomes for extremely low birth weight infants at 18 to 22 months. Pediatrics 2009;124:112–21.

52. Halliday HL, Ehrenkranz RA, Doyle LW. Early (<8 days) corticosteroids for preventing chronic lung disease in preterm infants. Cochrane Database Syst Rev 2009;1:CD001146.

53. Halliday HL, Ehrenkranz RA, Doyle LW. Late (>7 days) postnatal corticosteroids for chronic lung disease in preterm infants. Cochrane Database Syst Rev 2009;1: CD001145.

54. Watterberg KL, Gerdes JS, Gifford KL, et al. Prophylaxis against early adrenal insufficiency to prevent chronic lung disease in premature infants. Pediatrics 1999;104:1258–63.

55. Watterberg KL, Gerdes JS, Cole CH, et al. Prophylaxis of early adrenal insufficiency to prevent bronchopulmonary dysplasia: a multicenter trial. Pediatrics 2004;114:1649–57.

56. Peltoniemi O, Kari MA, Heinonen K, et al. Pretreatment cortisol values may predict responses to hydrocortisone administration for the prevention of bronchopulmonary dysplasia in high-risk infants. J Pediatr 2005;146:632–7.

57. Bonsante F, Latorre G, Iacobelli S, et al. Early low-dose hydrocortisone in very preterm infants: a randomized, placebo-controlled trial. Neonatology 2007;91:217–21.

58. Watterberg KL, Scott SM. Evidence of early adrenal insufficiency in babies who develop bronchopulmonary dysplasia. Pediatrics 1995;85:120–5.

59. Huysman MW, Hokken-Koelega AC, De Ridder MA, et al. Adrenal function in sick very preterm infants. Pediatr Res 2000;48:629–33.

60. Watterberg KL, Scott SM, Backstrom C, et al. Links between early adrenal function and respiratory outcome in preterm infants: airway inflammation and patent ductus arteriosus. Pediatrics 2000;105:320–4.

61. Watterberg KL, Gerdes JS, Cook KL. Impaired glucocorticoid synthesis in premature infants developing chronic lung disease. Pediatr Res 2001;50:190–5.

62. Nykänen P, Anttila E, Heinonen K, et al. Early hypoadrenalism in premature infants at risk for bronchopulmonary dysplasia or death. Acta Paediatr 2007; 96:1600–5.

63. Doyle LW, Ehrenkranz RA, Halliday HL. Postnatal hydrocortisone for preventing or treating bronchopulmonary dysplasia in preterm infants: a systematic review. Neonatology 2010;98:111–7.

64. Watterberg KL, Shaffer ML, Mishefske MJ, et al. Growth and neurodevelopmental outcomes after early low-dose hydrocortisone treatment in extremely low birth weight infants. Pediatrics 2007;120:40–8.

65. Peltoniemi OM, Lano A, Puosi R, et al. Trial of early neonatal hydrocortisone: two-year follow-up. Neonatology 2009;95:240–7.

66. Mazela J, Polin RA. Aerosol delivery to ventilated newborn infants: historical challenges and new directions. Eur J Pediatr 2011;170:433–44.

67. Watterberg KL, Clark AR, Kelly HW, et al. Delivery of aerosolized medication to intubated babies. Pediatr Pulmonol 1991;10:136–41.

68. Köhler E, Jilg G, Avenarius S, et al. Lung deposition after inhalation with various nebulisers in preterm infants. Arch Dis Child Fetal Neonatal Ed 2008; 93:F275–9.

69. Shah SS, Ohlsson A, Halliday H, et al. Inhaled versus systemic corticosteroids for the treatment of chronic lung disease in ventilated very low birth weight preterm infants. Cochrane Database Syst Rev 2007;4:CD002057.

70. Shah V, Ohlsson A, Halliday HL, et al. Early administration of inhaled corticosteroids for preventing chronic lung disease in ventilated very low birth weight preterm neonates. Cochrane Database Syst Rev 2007;4:CD001969.

71. Laughon M, Bose C, Allred E, et al. Factors associated with treatment for hypotension in extremely low gestational age newborns during the first postnatal week. Pediatrics 2007;119:273–80.

72. Fernandez EF, Watterberg KL, Kendrick D, et al. Incidence, management and short term outcomes of hypotension in the critically ill term and late preterm newborn [abstract]. Presented at the annual meeting of Pediatric Academic Societies. E-PAS 2011:3832.305.

73. Logan JW, O'Shea TM, Allred EN, et al. Early postnatal hypotension and developmental delay at 24 months of age among extremely low gestational age newborns. Arch Dis Child Fetal Neonatal Ed 2011;96:F321–8.
74. Dempsey EM, Al Hazzani F, Barrington KJ. Permissive hypotension in the extremely low birthweight infant with signs of good perfusion. Arch Dis Child Fetal Neonatal Ed 2009;94:F241–4.
75. Soleymani S, Borzage M, Seri I. Hemodynamic monitoring in neonates: advances and challenges. J Perinatol 2010;30(Suppl):S38–45.
76. Helbock HJ, Insoft RM, Conte FA. Glucocorticoid-responsive hypotension in extremely low birth weight newborns. Pediatrics 1993;92:715–7.
77. Scott SM, Watterberg KL. Effect of gestational age, postnatal age, and illness on plasma cortisol concentrations in premature infants. Pediatr Res 1995;37:112–6.
78. Ng PC, Lee CH, Lam CW, et al. Transient adrenocortical insufficiency of prematurity and systemic hypotension in very low birthweight infants. Arch Dis Child Fetal Neonatal Ed 2004;89:F119–26.
79. Cooper MS, Stewart PM. Adrenal insufficiency in critical illness. J Intensive Care Med 2007;22:348–62.
80. Ng PC, Lee CH, Bnur FL, et al. A double-blind, randomized, controlled study of a "stress dose" of hydrocortisone for rescue treatment of refractory hypotension in preterm infants. Pediatrics 2006;117:367–75.
81. Higgins S, Friedlich P, Seri I. Hydrocortisone for hypotension and vasopressor dependence in preterm neonates: a meta-analysis. J Perinatol 2010;30:373–8.
82. Yoder B, Martin H, McCurnin DC, et al. Impaired urinary cortisol excretion and early cardiopulmonary dysfunction in immature baboons. Pediatr Res 2002;51: 426–32.
83. Bourchier D, Weston PJ. Randomised trial of dopamine compared with hydrocortisone for the treatment of hypotensive very low birthweight infants. Arch Dis Child Fetal Neonatal Ed 1997;76:F174–8.
84. Finer NN, Powers RJ, Ou CH, et al. California Perinatal Quality Care Collaborative Executive Committee. Prospective evaluation of postnatal steroid administration: a 1-year experience from the California Perinatal Quality Care Collaborative. Pediatrics 2006;117:704–13.
85. Reynolds JW, Colle E, Ulstrom RA. Adrenocortical steroid metabolism in newborn infants. V. Physiologic disposition of exogenous cortisol loads in the early neonatal period. J Clin Endocrinol Metab 1962;22:245–54.
86. Watterberg KL, Cook K, Gifford KL. Pharmacokinetics of hydrocortisone in extremely low birth weight infants in the first week of life. Pediatr Res 1996;39: 251A.
87. Watterberg KL, Shaffer ML, for the PROPHET study group. Cortisol concentrations and apparent serum half-life during hydrocortisone therapy in extremely low birth weight infants. PAS 2005;57:1501.

Antibiotic Use and Misuse in the Neonatal Intensive Care Unit

Nidhi Tripathi, BS[a,b], C. Michael Cotten, MD, MHS[c],
P. Brian Smith, MD, MPH, MHS[b,d],*

KEYWORDS

- Neonatal intensive care unit • Empiric • Antibiotic • Sepsis
- Infection

Antibiotics are the most commonly used therapeutics in neonatal intensive care units (NICUs).[1] Neonatal sepsis often has a subtle, nonspecific presentation and results in serious consequences ranging from neurodevelopmental deficits to death.[2–5] As a result, clinicians frequently administer empiric antibiotics to symptomatic infants or infants at high risk of sepsis while awaiting culture results.[1] However, antibiotic treatment in the setting of negative cultures may not be benign. Broad-spectrum antibiotics (eg, third-generation cephalosporins) are associated with an increased risk of invasive candidiasis and death,[6,7] and prolonged duration of antibiotic therapy is associated with increased risks of necrotizing enterocolitis (NEC), death, and late-onset sepsis (LOS).[8–10]

The cumulative incidence of early-onset sepsis (EOS; infection within 72 hours of birth) is 0.98 per 1000 live births.[11] However, the burden of disease increases with decreasing birth weight. Very low birth weight (VLBW; <1500 g birth weight) infants have a cumulative incidence of EOS of 11 per 1000 live births.[11] Of those who survive longer than 3 days, 21% have an episode of LOS (infection occurring after 3 days of life).[11,12]

A cohort study of VLBW infants in Israel from 1995 to 1998 revealed an increased risk of death with LOS (17% vs 9%; $P<.001$).[13] In a more recent cohort of 400,000 live births from 2006 to 2009, 389 infants were diagnosed with EOS or early-onset

---

Competing interests: Dr Smith received support from NICHD 1K23HD060040-01, DHHS-1R18AE000028-01, and from industry for neonatal and pediatric drug development (http://www.dcri.duke.edu/research/coi.jsp). Ms Tripathi was supported in part by Duke University's CTSA grant TL1RR024126 from NCRR/NIH. Dr Cotten has no conflicts to report.

[a] Duke University Medical Center, DUMC 3710, Durham, NC 27710, USA
[b] Duke Clinical Research Institute, Duke University Medical Center, 2400 Pratt Street, Durham, NC 27705, USA
[c] Division of Neonatal-Perinatal Medicine, Department of Pediatrics, Duke University, Durham, NC, USA
[d] Department of Pediatrics, Duke University Medical Center, Duke University, Box 3352, DUMC, Durham, NC 27710, USA
* Corresponding author. Duke Clinical Research Institute, Box 17969, Durham, NC 27715.
E-mail address: brian.smith@duke.edu

Clin Perinatol 39 (2012) 61–68
doi:10.1016/j.clp.2011.12.003
0095-5108/12/$ – see front matter © 2012 Elsevier Inc. All rights reserved.

meningitis.[11] Overall, 16% died, and mortality was inversely related to gestational age (22–24 weeks, 54%; 25–28 weeks, 30%; 29–33 weeks, 12%; 34–36 weeks, 0%; ≥37 weeks, 3%).[11] In an National Institute of Child Health and Human Development Neonatal Research Network study, VLBW infants with LOS were also significantly more likely to die than unaffected infants (18% vs 7%; P<.001).[12] Survivors of neonatal sepsis are at a high risk of adverse outcomes. VLBW infants with a history of EOS have a significantly higher risk of severe intraventricular hemorrhage or periventricular leukomalacia (odds ratio [OR] 3.2, 95% confidence interval [CI] 1.9, 5.5) and bronchopulmonary dysplasia (OR 2.4, 95% CI 1.2–4.7) than uninfected infants.[14] A prospective cohort study of 6093 extremely low birth weight (ELBW; <1000 g birth weight) infants revealed that 65% of survivors had a history of at least 1 infection.[2] Survivors were at increased risk of impaired neurodevelopmental outcomes at 18 to 22 weeks corrected gestational age including cerebral palsy (OR 1.4, 95% CI 1.1–1.8), vision impairments (OR 1.7, 95% CI 1.3–2.2), and low Bayley Scales of Infant Development II scores on the mental development index (OR 1.3, 95% CI 1.1–1.6) and psychomotor development index (OR 1.5, 95% CI 1.2–1.9).[2] In addition, they were more likely to have a head circumference less than the 10th percentile (OR 1.5, 95% CI 1.2–1.7), a finding associated with poor cognitive function, academic achievement, and behavior at school age.[2,15]

BACTERIOLOGY

EOS is most often caused by group B Streptococcus (GBS; 43%) followed by Escherichia coli (29%).[11] Among VLBW infants, rates of E coli infection exceed those of GBS (5.1 vs 2.1 per 1000 live births).[11] LOS in the NICU is predominantly caused by gram-positive organisms (70%), primarily coagulase-negative Staphylococcus (CoNS, 48%) and Staphylococcus aureus (8%).[12] Gram-negative LOS is less common but is associated with greater mortality (19%–36%).[4,12] Fungal infections account for roughly 12% of LOS in VLBW infants,[12] although the incidence among centers varies widely.[7]

COMMONLY USED ANTIBIOTICS: BACTERIAL SUSCEPTIBILITY AND RISKS

Investigators examined reports of neonatal bacteremia received by the Health Protection Agency's voluntary surveillance scheme from 90% of microbiological laboratories in England and Wales between January 2006 and March 2008.[16] Most of the 1516 EOS episodes were caused by gram-positive organisms (82%), with GBS (31%) and CoNS (22%) being the most common. LOS was similarly dominated by gram-positive organisms (81%), with CoNS (45%) and S aureus (13%) comprising most of the 3482 episodes, followed by Enterobacteriaceae other than E coli (9%), E coli (7%), and GBS (7%).

In the UK study, 94% of the EOS isolates were susceptible to penicillin or gentamicin, 100% to amoxicillin or cefotaxime, and 96% to cefotaxime alone.[16] The LOS isolates had a 96% susceptibility to amoxicillin or gentamicin, 93% to amoxicillin or cefotaxime, and 78% to cefotaxime alone. These susceptibilities were the same or higher when CoNS isolates were excluded from the analysis. The investigators concluded that, despite an overall susceptibility of 93% or more for the amoxicillin and cefotaxime combination, cefotaxime should not be included in the empiric regimen. Virulent late-onset pathogens, such as Enterobacteriaceae other than E coli (75%) and Pseudomonas spp (46%), are often not susceptible to cefotaxime, and cefotaxime is not considered to be effective against other common pathogens including Enterococcus spp, Acinetobacter spp, and Listeria monocytogenes.

Use of cefotaxime in empiric regimens may also promote bacterial resistance.[16–18] To study the effects of empiric antibiotics on the emergence of resistant bacterial strains, investigators examined 436 infants admitted to 2 NICUs within the same hospital who were assigned to either a narrow-spectrum antibiotic regimen (penicillin plus tobramycin or flucloxacillin plus tobramycin) or a broad-spectrum regimen (amoxicillin plus cefotaxime).[18] Bacterial screening of respiratory and rectal cultures were performed on admission and then weekly for the presence of resistant bacteria. After 6 months of study, the units exchanged regimens. The rates of colonization with bacteria resistant to the empiric regimen of the unit was 18-fold higher in the cefotaxime plus amoxicillin group than in the penicillin/flucloxacillin plus tobramycin group.[18] Infants treated with penicillin plus tobramycin were better protected against nosocomial infection because they were more likely to be infected with pathogens susceptible to empiric therapy than those in the amoxicillin plus cefotaxime group.

Neonatal sepsis often presents with subtle and nonspecific signs such as lethargy, feeding intolerance, apnea, and hypotonia.[5,19,20] Because of the devastating consequences of untreated sepsis, clinicians have a low threshold for initiating empiric antibiotic therapy in high-risk or symptomatic newborns. Empiric therapy is begun once an infant exhibits signs of sepsis, and continues while awaiting culture results. Ampicillin (#1), gentamicin (#2), and cefotaxime (#3) are the most commonly used therapeutics in infants.[1] Although more than 95% of infants admitted to the NICU receive empiric antibiotics in the first postnatal days, only 1% to 5% have positive initial blood cultures.[6,8,21]

RISKS ASSOCIATED WITH EMPIRIC BROAD-SPECTRUM ANTIBIOTIC TREATMENT

In addition to the potential for promoting bacterial antibiotic resistance,[16] broad-spectrum antibiotics have been associated with altered gut colonization,[22] increased risk of *Candida* colonization and subsequent invasive candidiasis,[7,23] and increased risk of death.[6] In a cohort of 3702 preterm ELBW infants who survived for 72 hours or longer, previous broad-spectrum antibiotic (third-generation cephalosporin or carbapenem) use was associated with an increased risk of invasive candidiasis (OR 2.2, 95% CI 1.4–3.3).[7] The incidence of candidiasis between centers ranged from 2.4% to 20.2% and correlated with the average number of days of broad-spectrum antibiotic use per infant with sterile cultures throughout hospitalization. A multicenter retrospective cohort study of 128,914 infants found an increased risk of death when infants were treated with ampicillin plus cefotaxime versus ampicillin plus gentamicin in the first 3 postnatal days (OR 1.5, 95% CI 1.4–1.7).[6] This risk persisted despite adjustment for potential confounding factors such as gestational age, degree of respiratory support, and perinatal or neonatal depression. There was significant site variation in the use of ampicillin plus cefotaxime versus ampicillin plus gentamicin. From the wide variation in center use of ampicillin plus cefotaxime versus ampicillin plus gentamicin, it seems that the empiric antibiotic choice was often made programmatically rather than from the patient's level of apparent illness.

ADVERSE EFFECTS WITH PROLONGED DURATION OF ANTIBIOTIC THERAPY

Culture-proven neonatal sepsis is treated with a full course of antibiotics informed by antimicrobial susceptibility results. A more difficult consideration is determining the appropriate length of antibiotic treatment in the setting of suspected sepsis in an infant with negative cultures. Modern automated blood culture systems are able to detect bacteremia caused by common neonatal pathogens within 48 hours.[24] However, obtaining blood cultures from preterm infants is technically difficult, with small total blood volumes (often <1 mL) measuring less than the 2 mL needed for reliable culture results.[25] Low blood volume decreases the sensitivity of the blood culture, leading to frequent prolonged antibiotic treatment in infants with sterile cultures that may have simply missed collecting the offending organism.

A multicenter retrospective cohort study examined the duration of empiric antibiotic therapy in 790 ELBW infants with suspected or confirmed EOS.[9] Investigators compared infants who received 3 days or less of empiric therapy with those who received 7 days or more. Six-hundred and ninety-five infants had negative cultures, and, of these, 40% received 3 days or less of therapy, whereas 34% received 7 days or more. The duration of therapy was unrelated to perinatal risk factors for EOS or measures of illness severity including birth weight, gestational age, sex, preeclampsia, chorioamnionitis, prolonged premature rupture of membranes, premature labor, cesarean section, Clinical Risk Index for Babies scores, ventilator use, or survival.[9] Half of the 30 centers administered antibiotics beyond 3 days in 50% or more of the infants with sterile cultures, suggesting that the duration of empiric antibiotic therapy in infants with sterile cultures is an institutional decision and not dictated by clinical indicators of illness. Infants less than or equal to 26 weeks' gestational age at the time of initial empiric therapy who received 7 days or more of antibiotics had a longer average length of hospitalization (75 days vs 59 days, $P = .01$) and more ventilator days (31 days vs 26 days, $P = .05$) compared with infants who received 3 days or less.

A 19-center study of 5693 ELBW infants with sterile cultures who began initial empiric antibiotic treatment within the first 3 postnatal days found that the initial median duration of empiric antibiotic treatment was 5 days.[8] However, there was a large degree of center variability in antibiotic prescribing practice, and the median duration by center ranged from 3 to 9.5 days. The proportion of infants receiving prolonged treatment (defined as ≥ 5 days) ranged from 27% to 85% by center. In risk-adjusted multivariable analyses, prolonged duration of antibiotic therapy was associated with NEC or death (OR 1.30, 95% CI 1.10–1.54) or death alone (OR 1.46, 95% CI 1.19–1.78).[8] Each additional day of antibiotic therapy was associated with a 4% increase in the odds of NEC or death, a 7% increase in the odds of NEC alone, and a 16% increase in the odds of death alone. This analysis was repeated in infants who were intubated for the first 7 postnatal days as an indicator of illness severity. The association between prolonged antibiotic therapy and NEC or death, NEC alone, and death alone remained.

A case-control study examined the association between antibiotic use and the risk of NEC in a single center.[26] One-hundred and twenty-four cases of NEC were matched with 248 controls by gestational age, birth weight, and year of admission. Potential risk factors for NEC were collected, including antenatal corticosteroid exposure, 5-minute Apgar score, small for gestational age, respiratory distress syndrome, the presence of a patent ductus arteriosus, laboratory-confirmed bloodstream infection, feeding practices (day of first enteral feeding, type of feeding, maximum enteral volume achieved, and day of full enteral feedings), antibiotic exposure, and umbilical catheter use. The duration of antibiotics was calculated as the cumulative number of days of antibiotic therapy before the day of an NEC diagnosis in case subjects. In subjects without a history of bloodstream infection, each day of antibiotic exposure was associated with a 20% increase in the risk of NEC. After 1 to 2 days of antibiotic therapy, the OR for the development of NEC was 1.19 and continued to increase to 1.43 at 3 to 4 days, 1.71 at 5 to 6 days, 2.05 at 7 to 8 days, 2.45 at 9 to 10 days, and 2.94 at more than 10 days of exposure.

Prolonged antibiotic therapy has also been associated with LOS. In the study of 5693 subjects discussed earlier, both 4 and 5 days of initial empiric antibiotic treatment were associated with increased risk of the combined outcome of LOS caused by organisms other than CoNS or death (4 days, OR 1.32 [95% CI 1.11–1.58]; 5 days, OR 1.24 [95% CI 1.06–1.44]).[8] A study of 365 infants less than or equal to 32 weeks' gestation and less than or equal to 1500 g birth weight found that prolonged antibiotic therapy (≥5 days) initiated on the day of birth was associated with LOS alone (OR 2.45, 95% 1.28, 4.67) and the composite outcome of LOS, NEC, or death (OR 2.66, 95% CI 1.12, 6.30) after 7 days of life.[10] The regression models controlled for birth weight, gestational age, race, prolonged premature rupture of membranes, number of days on high-frequency ventilation in the first week of life, and the amount of breast milk received in the first 14 days of life. Each additional day of antibiotics was associated with increased risk of these outcomes (LOS: OR 1.27, 95% CI 1.09–1.49. LOS, NEC, or death: OR 1.24, 95% 1.07–1.44).

PERINATAL GBS PREVENTION: OPPORTUNITIES MISSED

In 1996, the Centers for Disease Control and Prevention (CDC) and the American College of Obstetricians and Gynecologists released guidelines for intrapartum antibiotic prophylaxis (IAP) to prevent perinatal GBS infections, the leading cause of early neonatal infectious morbidity and mortality in the United States. Candidates for IAP were identified by either a risk-based or screening-based approach under the initial guidelines, but the revised 2002 guidelines recommended a universal screening-based approach to better identify appropriate IAP candidates.[27] Since the initiation of IAP, the cumulative incidence of early-onset GBS disease has fallen from 1.7 cases per 1000 live births in the early 1990s to 0.41 cases per 1000 live births from 2006 to 2009.[11,14] However, the potential for improvement in the implementation of guidelines still exists.

In 2002, the IAP guidelines recommended culture-based screening at 35 to 37 weeks for all pregnant women.[27] The guidelines stipulated that women who presented with threatened preterm labor and no culture results within 4 weeks should undergo rectovaginal cultures and receive IAP if delivery seemed imminent.[27] However, only 50% of the mothers who delivered preterm were screened before delivery, and only 18% were screened at admission.[28] Women were more likely to be screened with longer intervals between admission and delivery. Among those for whom the interval between admission and delivery was 48 hours or longer, 59% were screened at admission.

Proper implementation of IAP was also lacking during preterm births.[28] Mothers who delivered preterm were less likely to receive IAP when indicated than mothers who delivered at term (relative risk 0.81, 95% CI 0.75–0.87). Of the women who delivered preterm and had positive cultures, 84% received IAP; however, only 63% of women who delivered preterm with unknown GBS colonization status were given IAP. Those with unknown status were less likely to receive IAP when the interval between admission and delivery was less than 4 hours compared with 4 hours or longer.

Guidelines regarding proper antibiotic choice in the setting of a penicillin allergy also were rarely followed.[28] The 2002 guidelines recommended the use of cefazolin in women with penicillin allergies at low risk for anaphylaxis, a recommendation that was reiterated in the 2010 guidelines.[27] However, 70% of allergic women at low risk for anaphylaxis received clindamycin for prophylaxis, and only 14% received cefazolin.[28] There is limited evidence that clindamycin crosses the placenta and concentrates in fetal tissues and amniotic fluid at bacteriocidal concentrations, and the available data suggest that it does not do so adequately.[29,30] Furthermore, GBS resistance to clindamycin has increased in the last 20 years to 13% to 20%.[31–33] Only 1% of GBS-positive women who were allergic to penicillin had documented susceptibilities to clindamycin.[28] Because the effectiveness of clindamycin, erythromycin, or vancomycin (their alternative in the case of resistance) has not been studied, no duration of these therapies is considered adequate prophylaxis.[27]

The result of these failures of screening and treatment is that well-appearing preterm newborns undergo a limited evaluation for sepsis including a complete blood count with differential and blood culture under both the 2002 and 2010 CDC guidelines.[27] Lack of screening or proper administration of IAP leads to increased sepsis evaluations of infants and subsequent increased administration of empiric antibiotic therapy to these infants.

SUMMARY

Neonatal sepsis causes significant morbidity and mortality, especially in preterm infants. Consequently, clinicians are compelled to empirically administer antibiotics to infants with risk factors and infants with signs of suspected sepsis. However, both broad-spectrum antibiotics and prolonged treatment with empiric antibiotics are associated with adverse outcomes including invasive candidiasis, increased antimicrobial resistance, NEC, LOS, and death. Most common neonatal pathogens are susceptible to narrow-spectrum antibiotics. As a result, clinicians should treat with short courses of narrow-spectrum antibiotics whenever possible. The choice of antibiotic or duration of empiric treatment is often not associated with risk factors for sepsis or indicators of illness severity but rather with center. Antibiotic exposure in infants could be minimized through conscientious monitoring of culture results, antibiotic choice, and duration. Improving adherence to guidelines for GBS IAP provides another opportunity to potentially reduce unnecessary antibiotic exposure in hospitalized infants.

REFERENCES

1. Clark RH, Bloom BT, Spitzer AR, et al. Reported medication use in the neonatal intensive care unit: data from a large national data set. Pediatrics 2006;117(6): 1979–87.
2. Stoll BJ, Hansen NI, Adams-Chapman I, et al. Neurodevelopmental and growth impairment among extremely low-birth-weight infants with neonatal infection. JAMA 2004;292(19):2357–65.
3. Klinger G, Levy I, Sirota L, et al. Outcome of early-onset sepsis in a national cohort of very-low-birth-weight infants. Pediatrics 2010;125(4):e736–40.
4. Benjamin DK, DeLong E, Cotten CM, et al. Mortality following blood culture in premature infants: increased with Gram-negative bacteremia and candidemia, but not Gram-positive bacteremia. J Perinatol 2004;24(3):175–80.
5. Fanaroff AA, Korones SB, Wright LL, et al. Incidence, presenting features, risk factors and significance of late onset septicemia in very-low-birth-weight infants. Pediatr Infect Dis J 1998;17(7):593–8.
6. Clark RH, Bloom BT, Spitzer AR, et al. Empiric use of ampicillin and cefotaxime, compared with ampicillin and gentamicin, for neonates at risk for sepsis is associated with an increased risk of neonatal death. Pediatrics 2006;117(1): 67–74.

7. Cotten CM, McDonald S, Stoll B, et al. The association of third-generation ceph-alosporin use and invasive candidiasis in extremely-low-birth-weight infants. Pediatrics 2006;118(2):717–22.
8. Cotten CM, Taylor S, Stoll B, et al. Prolonged duration of initial empirical antibiotic treatment is associated with increased rates of necrotizing enterocolitis and death for extremely-low-birth-weight infants. Pediatrics 2009;123(1): 58–66.
9. Cordero LM, Ayers LW. Duration of empiric antibiotics for suspected early-onset sepsis in extremely-low-birth-weight infants. Infect Control Hosp Epidemiol 2003; 24(9):662–6.
10. Kuppala VS, Meinzen-Derr J, Morrow AL, et al. Prolonged initial empirical antibiotic treatment is associated with adverse outcomes in premature infants. J Pediatr 2011;159(5):720–5.
11. Stoll BJ, Hansen NI, Sánchez PJ, et al. Early-onset neonatal sepsis: the burden of group B streptococcal and E. coli disease continues. Pediatrics 2011;127(5): 817–26.
12. Stoll BJ, Hansen N, Fanaroff AA, et al. Late-onset sepsis in very-low-birth-weight neonates: the experience of the NICHD Neonatal Research Network. Pediatrics 2002;110(2):285–91.
13. Makhoul IR, Sujov P, Smolkin T, et al. Epidemiological, clinical, and microbiological characteristics of late-onset sepsis among very-low-birth-weight infants in Israel: a national survey. Pediatrics 2002;109(1):34–9.
14. Stoll BJ, Hansen N, Fanaroff AA, et al. Changes in pathogens causing early-onset sepsis in very-low-birth-weight infants. N Engl J Med 2002;347(4):240–7.
15. Hack M, Breslau N, Weissman B, et al. Effect of very low birth weight and subnormal head size on cognitive abilities at school age. N Engl J Med 1991; 325(4):231–7.
16. Muller-Pebody B, Johnson AP, Heath PT, et al. Empirical treatment of neonatal sepsis: are the current guidelines adequate? Arch Dis Child Fetal Neonatal Ed 2011;96(1):F4–8.
17. Gupta A, Ampofo K, Rubenstein D, et al. Extended-spectrum lactamase-producing Klebsiella pneumoniae infections: a review of the literature. J Perinatol 2003;23(6):439–43.
18. de Man P, Verhoeven B, Verbrugh H, et al. An antibiotic policy to prevent emergence of resistant bacilli. Lancet 2000;355(9208):973–8.
19. Bonadio WA, Hennes H, Smith D, et al. Reliability of observation variables in distinguishing infectious outcome of febrile young infants. Pediatr Infect Dis J 1993; 12(2):111–4.
20. Ottolini MC, Lundgren K, Mirkinson LJ, et al. Utility of complete blood count and blood culture screening to diagnose neonatal sepsis in the asymptomatic at risk newborn. Pediatr Infect Dis J 2003;22(5):430–4.
21. Stoll BJ, Hansen NI, Higgins RD, et al. Very-low-birth-weight preterm infants with early-onset neonatal sepsis: the predominance of Gram-negative infections continues in the National Institute of Child Health and Human Development Neonatal Research Network, 2002–2003. Pediatr Infect Dis J 2005; 24(7):635–9.
22. Gewolb I, Schwalbe R, Taciak V, et al. Stool microflora in extremely-low-birthweight infants. Arch Dis Child Fetal Neonatal Ed 1999;80(3):F167.
23. Saiman L, Ludington E, Dawson JD, et al. Risk factors for Candida species colonization of neonatal intensive care unit patients. Pediatr Infect Dis J 2001;20(12): 1119–24.

24. Garcia-Prats JA, Cooper TR, Schneider VF, et al. Rapid detection of microorganisms in blood cultures of newborn infants utilizing an automated blood culture system. Pediatrics 2000;105(3):523–7.

25. Schelonka RL, Chai MK, Yoder BA, et al. Volume of blood required to detect common neonatal pathogens. J Pediatr 1996;129(2):275–8.

26. Alexander VN, Northrup V, Bizzarro MJ. Antibiotic exposure in the newborn intensive care unit and the risk of necrotizing enterocolitis. J Pediatr 2011;159(3): 392–7.

27. Centers for Disease Control and Prevention (CDC). Prevention of perinatal group B streptococcal disease: revised guidelines from the CDC. MMWR Recomm Rep 2002;51:1–22.

28. Van Dyke MK, Phares CR, Lynfield R, et al. Evaluation of universal antenatal screening for group B streptococcus. N Engl J Med 2009;360(25):2626–36.

29. Muller AE, Mouton JW, Oostvogel PM, et al. Pharmacokinetics of clindamycin in pregnant women in the peripartum period. Antimicrob Agents Chemother 2010; 54(5):2175–81.

30. Philipson A, Sabath LD, Charles D. Transplacental passage of erythromycin and clindamycin. N Engl J Med 1973;288(23):1219–21.

31. Borchardt S, DeBusscher J, Tallman P, et al. Frequency of antimicrobial resistance among invasive and colonizing group B streptococcal isolates. BMC Infect Dis 2006;6(1):57.

32. Castor ML, Whitney CG, Como-Sabetti K, et al. Antibiotic resistance patterns in invasive group B streptococcal isolates. Infect Dis Obstet Gynecol 2008;2008: 727505.

33. Phares CR, Lynfield R, Farley MM, et al. Epidemiology of invasive group B streptococcal disease in the United States, 1999–2005. JAMA 2008;299(17):2056–65.

The Use of Antiviral Drugs During the Neonatal Period

Richard J. Whitley, MD

KEYWORDS

• Viral infections • Neonates • Acyclovir • Ganciclovir

Parenteral therapy of viral infections of the newborn and infant became a reality with the introduction of vidarabine (adenine arabinoside) for the treatment of neonatal herpes simplex virus (HSV) infections in the early 1980s. Since then, acyclovir has become the treatment of choice for neonatal HSV infections, as well as a variety of other herpesvirus infections. Similarly, ganciclovir has been established as beneficial for the treatment of congenital cytomegalovirus (CMV) infections that involve the central nervous system (CNS). This article reviews the lessons learned from treating neonatal HSV and congenital CMV infections in relation to the use of acyclovir and ganciclovir. Although the natural history of these diseases is reviewed elsewhere in this issue, a brief summary precedes a detailed discussion of available established and alternative therapeutics. The reader is referred to more extensive reviews of antiviral therapy in children and adults.[1,2]

THERAPY FOR HSV INFECTIONS

Neonatal HSV infections occur in approximately 1 in 3200 deliveries in the United States[3] and, of these, approximately two-thirds develop some form of CNS disease.[4] Most cases are caused by HSV-2.[5] The risk of transmission is increased with primary maternal infection during the third trimester, being 30% to 50%, and can be decreased by cesarean delivery if HSV has been isolated from the cervix or external genitalia near the time of delivery.[3] As reviewed by Kimberlin,[6] 85% of neonatal HSV cases occur because of peripartum transmission, whereas 10% occur via postnatal transmission, and only 5% are caused by transmission in utero.

Infants with intrauterine HSV infection are characterized by the triad of cutaneous findings (active lesions, scarring), neurologic findings (microcephaly, hydranencephaly), and eye findings (chorioretinitis, microphthalmia) present at birth. Intrauterine

Department of Pediatrics, The University of Alabama at Birmingham, 1600 7th Avenue South, Birmingham, AL 35233-1711, USA
E-mail address: RWhitley@peds.uab.edu

Clin Perinatol 39 (2012) 69–81
doi:10.1016/j.clp.2011.12.004
0095-5108/12/$ – see front matter © 2012 Elsevier Inc. All rights reserved.

HSV infection has been found to occur with both primary and recurrent maternal HSV infections,[7] although the risk from a recurrent infection is less.

HSV infection acquired in the peripartum or postpartum period can be categorized as skin, eye, and/or mouth (SEM) disease, CNS disease, or disseminated disease. By definition, SEM disease does not involve the CNS. Disseminated disease may involve the CNS (75% of cases) along with multiple other organ systems including the liver; adrenals; gastrointestinal tract; and the skin, eyes, or mouth.[8] CNS disease may also have a component of SEM involvement, but does not involve other organ systems. Of all infants with neonatal HSV infections, approximately 33% have CNS disease, whereas about 25% have disseminated disease.[9] Thus, about 50% of infants with neonatal HSV infection have CNS disease.

The pathogenesis of CNS involvement in neonatal HSV infections differs depending on whether or not the infection is disseminated. Encephalitis associated with dissemination is caused by hematogenous spread, whereas isolated encephalitis or encephalitis associated with only SEM involvement likely occurs because of retrograde intraneuronal transport of HSV.[4] This difference corresponds with the clinical presentations of disseminated versus CNS disease in that the blood-borne spread of disseminated disease presents earlier (9–11 days of life on average) and causes more diffuse brain involvement with multiple areas of hemorrhagic necrosis, whereas CNS disease occurring via slower axonal transport presents later (around 16–17 days of life) and typically causes more focal CNS involvement.[10]

The early era of antiviral therapy for neonatal HSV infection was marked by improved mortality with intravenous vidarabine as well as with standard-dose (SD) intravenous acyclovir (30 mg/kg/d in 3 divided doses). The 1-year mortality for disseminated disease decreased from 85% with no therapy to 50% with vidarabine and 61% with SD acyclovir, whereas the 1-year mortality for CNS disease dropped from 35% with no therapy to 14% for both vidarabine and SD acyclovir.[11] More recently, high-dose (HD) acyclovir has been shown to further improve these mortality figures. Using HD intravenous acyclovir (60 mg/kg/d in 3 divided doses for 21 days), the 1-year mortalities were 29% and 4% for disseminated and CNS diseases, respectively.[12] Although HD acyclovir improved morbidity for infants with disseminated disease (83% of survivors had normal neurodevelopmental outcomes), infants with CNS disease did not have a significant improvement in morbidity (31% of survivors had normal neurodevelopmental outcomes).

Babies with SEM involvement have the best prognosis and, as noted later, only require 14 days of HD intravenous acyclovir therapy.

Recently, acyclovir suppressive therapy for babies with CNS disease after completing intravenous treatment significantly improved neurologic outcome as measured by Bailey Developmental Scores.[13] This regimen led to approximately 60% (as opposed to 31%) of children with CNS disease developing normally or with mild impairment. Treatment was administered at a dosage of 300/mg/m^2 by mouth 3 times a day for 6 months.

Therapy for Neonatal Varicella-Zoster Virus Infections

Women who experience primary varicella-zoster virus (VZV) infections within 48 hours of delivery have children at risk for the development of chickenpox within the first 3 weeks of life. Newborns delivered to these women traditionally receive zoster immune globulin (ZIG) to prevent disease. However, with sporadic shortages of ZIG, some newborns experience neonatal disease. No controlled clinical trials have evaluated acyclovir therapy for this disease; however, experts recommend this drug for the treatment of newborn disease.

AVAILABLE THERAPIES FOR HSV AND VZV INFECTIONS
Acyclovir (Acycloguanosine)

Acyclovir is the most frequently prescribed antiviral agent for the management of HSV infections of the newborn and infant. It has been available for clinical use for nearly 3 decades and has shown remarkable safety and efficacy against mild to severe infections caused by HSV and VZV in both normal and immunocompromised patients, including the newborn.

Chemistry and Mechanism of Action

Acyclovir is a deoxyguanosine analog. After preferential uptake by viral-infected cells, acyclovir is phosphorylated by virus-encoded thymidine kinase (TK). Subsequent diphosphorylation and triphosphorylation are catalyzed by host cell enzymes. Acyclovir triphosphate prevents viral DNA synthesis by both inhibiting viral DNA polymerase and being a chain terminator.

Spectrum and Resistance

Acyclovir is most active against HSV; activity against VZV is also substantial but approximately tenfold less. Acyclovir is considered the treatment of choice for both neonatal HSV and VZV infections. Activity against CMV is poor because CMV does not have TK activity and CMV DNA polymerase is poorly inhibited by acyclovir triphosphate.

Resistance of HSV and VZV to acyclovir has become an important clinical problem among immunocompromised patients exposed to long-term therapy.[14] Viral resistance to acyclovir usually results from mutations in the viral TK gene, although mutations in the viral DNA polymerase gene also occur rarely. Resistant isolates can cause severe, progressive, debilitating mucosal disease in adults and, rarely, visceral dissemination.[15,16] Isolates of HSV resistant to acyclovir have also been reported in normal hosts, most commonly in patients with frequently recurrent genital infection who have been treated with chronic acyclovir.[17]

Indications

Acyclovir is effective for the treatment of infections caused by HSV and VZV in both immunocompetent and immunocompromised hosts, including the newborn. For the treatment of neonatal HSV infections, the recommended dose is 20 mg/kg every 8 hours. The duration of therapy for SEM disease is 14 days, whereas, for those babies with either CNS or disseminated disease, therapy should be extended for 21 days.

Oral acyclovir is an experimental approach to suppressive therapy and is not currently approved by the US Food and Drug Administration (FDA).

Pharmacokinetics

After intravenous doses of 2.5 to 15 mg/kg, steady-state concentrations of acyclovir range from 6.7 to 20.6 μg/mL. Acyclovir is widely distributed; high concentrations are attained in kidneys, lung, liver, heart, and skin vesicles; concentrations in the cerebrospinal fluid (CSF) are about 50% of those in the plasma.[18] Acyclovir crosses the placenta and accumulates in breast milk. Protein binding ranges from 9% to 33%, and less than 20% of the drug is metabolized to biologically inactive metabolites. No pharmacokinetic data are available in the newborn for the use of 20 mg/kg/dose.

In the absence of compromised renal function, the half-life of acyclovir is 2 to 3 hours in older children and adults and 2.5 to 5 hours in neonates with normal creatinine clearance. More than 60% of administered drug is excreted in the urine.[18] Elimination is prolonged in patients with renal dysfunction; the half-life is approximately 20 hours in persons with end-stage renal disease, necessitating dose modifications for those with creatinine clearance less than 50 mL/min/1.73 m^2.[19] Acyclovir is effectively removed by hemodialysis but not by continuous ambulatory peritoneal dialysis.[20,21]

Adverse effects

Acyclovir generally is a safe drug. Renal dysfunction results from obstructive nephropathy caused by the formation of acyclovir crystals precipitating in renal tubules. Occasionally administration of acyclovir by the intravenous route is associated with rash, sweating, nausea, headache, hematuria, and hypotension. High doses of intravenous acyclovir (60 mg/kg/d) in neonates have been associated with neutropenia.[12,22]

Neurotoxicity can occur in subjects with compromised renal function who attain high serum concentrations of drug.[23] Neurotoxicity is manifest as lethargy, confusion, hallucinations, tremors, myoclonus, seizures, extrapyramidal signs, and changes in state of consciousness, developing within the first few days of initiating therapy. These signs and symptoms usually resolve spontaneously within several days of discontinuing acyclovir.

Although acyclovir is mutagenic at high concentrations in some in vitro assays, it is not teratogenic in animals. Limited human data suggest that acyclovir use in pregnant women is not associated with congenital defects or other adverse pregnancy outcomes.

Drug interactions

The likelihood of renal toxicity of acyclovir is increased when administered with nephrotoxic drugs such as cyclosporine or amphotericin B.

Therapy for Congenital CMV Infection

CMV commonly infects humans worldwide, with a seroprevalence of approximately 40% in adolescents and approaching 90% in adults with poor socioeconomic status.[24,25] Congenital CMV infection is the most common congenital infection in the developed world, found in about 1% of live-born infants in the United States.[26] Congenital CMV infections most commonly occur via intrauterine transmission, but because the virus is shed in bodily fluids, transmission can also be acquired perinatally during delivery or postnatally through breast milk.

Of all infants born with congenital CMV infection, approximately 7% to 10% have clinically evident disease at birth.[27] Clinical characteristics of intrauterine infection include intrauterine growth restriction, hepatosplenomegaly, jaundice, thrombocytopenia, microcephaly, periventricular calcifications, and chorioretinitis. As reviewed by Dollard and colleagues,[28] true mortalities are difficult to obtain and have been reported to be as high as 30% for symptomatic infants, but more likely average about 5% to 10%.[29] Death usually is caused by of non-CNS manifestations of the infection, such as hepatic dysfunction or bleeding. An estimated 40% to 58% of infants with symptomatic congenital CMV infection have permanent sequelae, whereas infants who are asymptomatic at birth suffer permanent sequelae nearly 14% of the time.[28] Sensorineural hearing loss (SNHL), mental retardation, seizures, psychomotor and speech delays, learning disabilities, chorioretinitis, optic nerve atrophy, and defects in dentition are the most common long-term consequences.[30] As opposed to intrauterine infections, perinatally acquired CMV infections are not typically associated with long-term sequelae, although acute illness has been reported in premature very low birth weight infants.[31] In full-term infants, perinatal infections are commonly asymptomatic, but may present with pneumonitis within the first few months of life.[32]

Congenital CMV infection is the consequence of maternal-fetal infection, with most symptomatic congenital cases occurring because of asymptomatic maternal infection. With maternal primary infection, there seems to be compromise of the placental blood flow following infection of the placental villae.[33] The pathogenesis of CNS involvement in congenital CMV infection begins with disseminated viremic spread, including the endothelial cells of the brain and epithelial cells of the choroid plexus. From the endothelial cells of the brain, the virus spreads to contiguous astrocytes. From the choroid plexus, the virus then moves to the ependymal surfaces via the CSF. Once these cells are infected, the virus undergoes continuous replication, which leads to characteristic intranuclear inclusion bodies and cell death. As antibodies are produced in the face of continuous viral replication, immune complexes form as well, leading to further immune-mediated damage.[30] Although the specific pathogenesis of CMV-mediated SNHL has not been elucidated, histology has shown evidence of infection in the cells of both the cochlear and vestibular endolabyrinth.[34] CMV has also been isolated from the cochlear perilymph on autopsy of infants with congenital CMV infection.[35]

Recent studies of ganciclovir treatment of congenital CMV infections involving the CNS have been promising. Administering ganciclovir at doses of 12 mg/kg/d divided every 12 hours for a duration of 6 weeks improved hearing outcomes in neonates with symptomatic congenital CMV infections involving the CNS (as shown by microcephaly, intracranial calcifications, abnormal CSF for age, chorioretinitis, and/or hearing deficits).[36] The primary endpoint was improved brainstem-evoked response (BSER) between baseline and 6-month follow-up (or no deterioration at the 6-month follow-up if the baseline BSER was normal). For total evaluable ears, 69% of patients who received ganciclovir met the primary endpoint, as opposed to 39% of the control group. No patients receiving ganciclovir had worsening of their hearing between baseline and 6 months. Ganciclovir recipients also had more rapid resolution of alanine aminotransferase abnormalities than did the control group, although they were significantly more likely to become neutropenic. Additional analyses of this randomized controlled trail suggest that ganciclovir may also reduce neurodevelopment delays.[37] Improvement of mortality has not yet been shown with ganciclovir therapy.

TREATMENT OF CMV INFECTIONS
Ganciclovir

Ganciclovir was the first antiviral available for the therapy and prevention of infections caused by CMV. It has proved to be a valuable drug for immunocompromised patients, particularly hematopoietic stem cell transplant recipients, who suffer substantial morbidity and mortality from CMV infections, and, more recently, in children with congenital CMV infection, although it is not approved by the FDA at this time.

Chemistry and Mechanism of Action

Ganciclovir is structurally similar to acyclovir except for a hydroxymethyl group on its acyclic side chain. The initial phosphorylation step is performed by pUL97, which is a viral protein kinase. Cellular kinases then phosphorylate the agent 2 additional times to convert it to its triphosphate derivative, which is able to inhibit the CMV DNA polymerase encoded by *UL97* as well as incorporate into and terminate viral DNA.

Ganciclovir triphosphate is a competitive inhibitor of herpesviral DNA polymerases, resulting in cessation of DNA chain elongation.[1,20]

Spectrum and Resistance

Ganciclovir has similar activity to acyclovir against HSV-1, HSV-2, and VZV but, in contrast with acyclovir, its greatest activity is against CMV. Resistance of CMV isolates usually results from mutations in the UL97 gene.[38] Mutations in the CMV DNA polymerase gene occur less often.

Indications

Ganciclovir is licensed for several indications outside the newborn. Several reviews summarize these clinical outcomes.[2] For the treatment of neonates congenitally infected with CMV, a controlled trial has been performed.[36] As noted earlier, compared with no treatment, ganciclovir therapy prevented hearing deterioration at 2 years, although about two-thirds of treated infants developed neutropenia, often requiring dose modification.

Pharmacokinetics

Oral bioavailability of ganciclovir is poor, with less than 10% of the drug being absorbed following oral administration.[39,40] The oral formulation of ganciclovir is no longer marketed. Peak serum concentrations of ganciclovir after 6 mg/kg (newborn dose) of intravenously administered drug range from 8 to 11 µg/mL, with concentrations sufficient to inhibit sensitive strains of CMV in aqueous humor, subretinal fluid, CSF, and brain tissue.[1] The elimination half-life of ganciclovir is 2 to 3 hours and most of the drug is eliminated unchanged in the urine. The pharmacokinetics of ganciclovir in the neonatal population are similar to those in adults.[41,42] Dose reduction, proportional to the degree of reduction in creatinine clearance, is necessary for persons with impaired renal function. A supplemental dose is recommended after dialysis because it is efficiently removed by hemodialysis.[43]

Adverse effects

Myelosuppression is the most common adverse effect of ganciclovir; dose-related neutropenia (<1000 white blood cells/µL) is the most consistent hematologic aberration, with an incidence of about 40%.[40] Neutropenia is dose limiting in about 1 of 7 courses and reverses after the drug is stopped. Neutropenia is less frequent following oral administration of ganciclovir. Thrombocytopenia (<50,000 platelets/µL) occurs in approximately 20% and anemia in about 2% of ganciclovir recipients. Between 2% and 5% of ganciclovir recipients experience headache, confusion, altered mental status, hallucinations, nightmares, anxiety, ataxia, tremors, seizures, fever, rash, and abnormal levels of serum hepatic enzymes, either singly or in some combination.

Dosage

The dose of ganciclovir for therapy for symptomatic congenital CMV infection is 12 mg/kg/d, given by intravenous infusion twice a day for 6 weeks.

Investigational Drug

Valganciclovir

Valganciclovir was approved by the FDA in March, 2001, for the treatment of CMV retinitis. Because it is well absorbed after oral administration, it may represent a favorable alternative to intravenously administered ganciclovir for the treatment of congenital CMV infection. Currently, it is licensed for the treatment of CMV infections in selected transplant populations and for CMV retinitis in patients with human immunodeficiency virus (HIV)/acquired immune deficiency syndrome (AIDS).

Chemistry, mechanism of action, spectrum, and resistance

Valganciclovir is the L-valine ester prodrug of ganciclovir and, as such, has the same mechanism of action, antiviral spectrum, and potential for development of resistance as ganciclovir.[1,20]

Indications

Valganciclovir has similar indications to ganciclovir. However, based on limited controlled trials published to date, it currently is approved for the induction and maintenance therapy for CMV retinitis and select transplant populations.[44] It is currently being investigated for the treatment of congenital CMV infection. This randomized controlled trial, being performed by the National Institute of Allergy and Infectious Diseases (NIAID) Collaborative Antiviral Study Group (CASG), uses SNHL as its primary endpoint.

Pharmacokinetics

Valganciclovir is rapidly converted to ganciclovir, with a mean plasma half-life of about 30 minutes.[44] The absolute bioavailability of valganciclovir exceeds 60% and is enhanced by about 30% with concomitant administration of food.[45] The area under the curve of ganciclovir after oral administration of valganciclovir is one-third to one-half of that attained after intravenous administration of ganciclovir. Patients with impaired renal function require dosage reduction that is roughly proportional to their reduction in creatinine clearance.

Adverse effects

The most common side effects associated with valganciclovir therapy in adult populations include diarrhea (41%), nausea (30%), neutropenia (27%), anemia (26%), and headache (22%).[44] Only a limited number of newborns have received valganciclovir therapy. The only significant finding was that of neutropenia in 15% of patients.

Dosage

The dose of valganciclovir is tailored to the patient's age and renal function. At this time, the drug is not approved for administration to newborns with congenital CMV infection.

Unproven and Untested Therapies for Neonatal HSV, VZV, and Congenital CMV Infections

The following 2 medications are used to treat HSV, VZV, and CMV infections in older children and adults. Data on these medications are provided should antiviral resistance occur with either HSV or CMV infections of the newborn. Neither drug has been evaluated in proof-of principle studies in the newborn, and both are associated with significant toxicity. In addition, valacyclovir may become available for pediatric administration, particularly for babies with HSV infection limited to the skin, eye, and mouth.

Cidofovir (hydroxy-2-phosphonomethoxypropylcytosine)

Cidofovir was first approved for use in the United States for the therapy for AIDS-associated retinitis caused by CMV, which remains the main indication for this antiviral.

Chemistry and mechanism of action

Cidofovir is a novel acyclic phosphonate nucleoside analog with a mechanism of action similar to that of other nucleoside analogs. In contrast with acyclovir, viral enzymes are not required for initial phosphorylation because native cidofovir has a single phosphate group already attached. Following diphosphorylation by cellular kinases, cidofovir competitively inhibits DNA polymerase.[46] The active form of cidofovir exhibits a 25-fold to 50-fold greater affinity for viral DNA polymerase compared with the cellular DNA polymerase.

Spectrum and resistance
Cidofovir is active against HSV and CMV, including acyclovir-resistant and foscarnet-resistant HSV isolates and ganciclovir-resistant and foscarnet-resistant CMV mutants.[47] It is also active in vitro against VZV, EBV, human herpesvirus-6, human herpesvirus-8, polyomaviruses, adenovirus, and human HPV.

A small number of cidofovir-resistant CMV isolates have been described that also are resistant to ganciclovir because of mutations within the DNA polymerase gene.[48] A CMV mutant resistant to ganciclovir, foscarnet, and cidofovir has also been reported.[49]

Indications
Cidofovir delays retinal disease progression in patients with AIDS.[50,51] Cidofovir has also been useful in the management of disease caused by acyclovir-resistant HSV isolates.[52] Anecdotal reports of improvement of laryngeal papillomatosis following intralesional injection of cidofovir have been published, but a definitive conclusions regarding efficacy is not possible based on this limited experience.[53,54]

Pharmacokinetics
Only 2% to 26% of cidofovir is absorbed after oral administration, therefore it is given intravenously. The plasma half-life of cidofovir is 2.6 hours, but active intracellular metabolites of cidofovir have half-lives of 17 to 48 hours.[55] Ninety percent of the drug is excreted in the urine, primarily by renal tubular secretion.[56] The drug does not cross the blood-brain barrier and, therefore, should not be used to treat CNS infections.

Adverse effects
Because cidofovir concentrates in renal cells in amounts 100 times greater than in other tissues, nephrotoxicity is the main adverse effect, especially if hydration is not well maintained.[55,56] Manifestations of renal toxicity include proteinuria and glycosuria. Aggressive intravenous prehydration, coadministration of probenecid, and avoidance of other nephrotoxic agents reduce the likelihood of toxicity. Cidofovir is contraindicated in patients with a serum creatinine less than 1.5 mg/dL, a calculated creatinine clearance less than or equal to 55 mL/min, or a urine protein greater than or equal to 100 mg/dL, and the drug should be discontinued if serum creatinine increases to greater than or equal to 0.5 mg/dL more than baseline.

Dosage
Cidofovir is administered intravenously to older children and adults as a dose of 5 mg/kg once per week with probenecid. Patients with compromised renal (calculated creatinine clearance <55 mL/min) are treated every 2 weeks. The dose should be reduced from 5 mg/kg to 3 mg/kg if serum creatinine increases to greater than 0.3 mg/dL more than baseline. There are no data for dosing the newborn with cidofovir.

Foscarnet (Phosphonoformic Acid)
Foscarnet is the only antiherpes drug that is not a nucleoside analog. It is not a first-line drug but is useful for the treatment of infections caused by resistant herpes viruses.

Chemistry and mechanism of action

Foscarnet is an inorganic pyrophosphate analog that directly inhibits DNA polymerase by blocking the pyrophosphate binding site.[20,57]

Spectrum and resistance

Foscarnet inhibits all known human herpesviruses, including most ganciclovir-resistant CMV isolates and acyclovir-resistant HSV and VZV strains. It also is active against HIV. Resistance occurs as a result of DNA polymerase mutations. Strains of CMV, HSV, and VZV with reduced sensitivity to foscarnet have been reported.[57,58]

Indications

Foscarnet is as effective as ganciclovir for therapy for sight-threatening chorioretinitis caused by CMV in adult patients with AIDS.[59] Because of its inherent activity against HIV, it may even offer a survival advantage for treated patients.[60] Refractory cases of chorioretinitis may respond to a combination of foscarnet and ganciclovir. Foscarnet also is effective in the therapy for CMV infections caused by ganciclovir-resistant strains of virus.[60] Limited data also suggest that foscarnet may be of benefit when administered to patients with AIDS who have gastrointestinal and pulmonary infections caused by CMV.

Infections caused by acyclovir-resistant strains of HSV and VZV have been successfully controlled with foscarnet.[61,62]

Pharmacokinetics

Only about 20% of foscarnet is absorbed after oral administration. Maximum serum concentration attained after an intravenous dose of 60 mg/kg is approximately 500 μmol/L.[57] CSF concentrations are about two-thirds of those in serum. The half-life of foscarnet is about 48 hours and 80% of an administered dose is eliminated unchanged in the urine. Dose reduction, proportional to reduction in creatinine clearance, is necessary. Hemodialysis efficiently eliminates foscarnet and therefore a supplemental dose is recommended after dialysis.[63] There are no data on the use of foscarnet in the newborn.

Adverse effects

The most common adverse effects of foscarnet are nephrotoxicity and metabolic derangements. Evidence of nephrotoxicity includes azotemia, proteinuria, acute tubular necrosis, crystalluria, and interstitial nephritis. Serum creatinine concentrations increase in up to 50% of patients. Renal function returns to normal within 2 to 4 weeks of discontinuing therapy. Preexisting renal disease, concurrent use of other nephrotoxic drugs, dehydration, rapid injection, or continuous intravenous infusion of drug are risk factors for developing renal dysfunction.[64]

Metabolic disturbances associated with foscarnet therapy include hypocalcemia and hypercalcemia and hypophosphatemia and hyperphosphatemia.[65] Hypocalcemia can be associated with paresthesias, tetany, seizures, and arrhythmias. Metabolic disturbances are minimized if foscarnet is administered by slow infusion. CNS symptoms associated with foscarnet therapy include headache, tremor, irritability, seizures, and hallucinations. Fever, nausea, vomiting, abnormal serum hepatic enzymes, anemia, granulocytopenia, and genital ulcerations also have been reported.

Drug interactions

Concomitant use of amphotericin B, cyclosporine, gentamicin, and other nephrotoxic drugs increases the likelihood of renal dysfunction. Coadministration of pentamidine increases the risk of hypocalcemia. Anemia and neutropenia are more common when patients also are receiving zidovudine.

Dosage

The usual dose of foscarnet for CMV infection is 180 mg/kg/d in 3 divided doses for 14 to 21 days, followed by a daily maintenance dose of 90 to 120 mg/kg. The dosage of foscarnet used for infections caused by acyclovir-resistant HSV and VZV infections is 120 mg/kg/d in 3 divided doses.

SUMMARY

Although significant progress has been achieved in the management of congenital CMV and neonatal HSV infections, further advances are needed. With the appearance of new antiviral drugs that have a different mechanism of action, the opportunity for combination therapy arises, so long as medications can be proved safe.

ACKNOWLEDGMENTS

This project has been funded in whole or in part with federal funds from the National Institute of Allergy and Infectious Diseases, National Institutes of Health, Department of Health and Human Services, under contract no. N01-AI-30,025.

REFERENCES

1. Kimberlin D. Antiviral agents. In: Long S, Pickering L, Prober C, editors. Principles and practice of pediatric infectious diseases. 3rd edition. New York: Elsevier; 2008. p. 1470–88.
2. Rha B, Kimberlin DW, Whitley R. Antiviral drugs. In: Jerome K, editor. Laboratory diagnosis of viral infections. 3rd edition. New York: Informa Healthcare; 2009. p. 519–29.
3. Brown ZA, Wald A, Morrow RA, et al. Effect of serologic status and cesarean delivery on transmission rates of herpes simplex virus from mother to infant. JAMA 2003;289(2):203–9.
4. Whitley RJ. Herpes simplex virus. In: Scheld MW, Whitley RJ, Marra CM, editors. Infections in the central nervous system. 3rd edition. Philadelphia: Lippincott Williams & Wilkins; 2004. p. 123–44.
5. Kimberlin DW, Lin CY, Jacobs RF, et al. Natural history of neonatal herpes simplex virus infections in the acyclovir era. Pediatrics 2001;108(2):223–9.
6. Kimberlin DW. Management of HSV encephalitis in adults and neonates: diagnosis, prognosis and treatment. Herpes 2007;14(1):11–6.
7. Hutto C, Arvin A, Jacobs R, et al. Intrauterine herpes simplex virus infections. J Pediatr 1987;110(1):97–101.
8. Whitley RJ. Herpes simplex virus infections. In: Remington JS, Klein JO, editors. Infectious diseases of the fetus and newborn infants. 3rd edition. Philadelphia: WB Saunders; 1990. p. 282–305.
9. Whitley RJ, Corey L, Arvin A, et al. Changing presentation of herpes simplex virus infection in neonates. J Infect Dis 1988;158(1):109–16.
10. Whitley RJ, Roizman B. Herpes simplex viruses. In: Richman DD, Whitley RJ, Hayden FG, editors. Clinical virology. 2nd edition. Washington, DC: ASM Press; 2004. p. 375–401.
11. Whitley R, Arvin A, Prober C, et al. A controlled trial comparing vidarabine with acyclovir in neonatal herpes simplex virus infection. N Engl J Med 1991;324(7): 444–9.

12. Kimberlin DW, Lin CY, Jacobs RF, et al. Safety and efficacy of high-dose intravenous acyclovir in the management of neonatal herpes simplex virus infections. Pediatrics 2001;108(2):230–8.
13. Kimberlin D, Whitley R, Wan W, et al. Impact of oral acyclovir suppression on neurodevelopmental outcomes and skin recurrences following neonatal herpes simplex virus disease. N Engl J Med 2011;365(14):1284–92.
14. Englund JA, Zimmerman ME, Swierkosz EU, et al. Herpes simplex virus resistant to acyclovir. A study in a tertiary care center. Ann Intern Med 1990;112:416–22.
15. Field AK, Biron KK. "The end of innocence" revisited: resistance of herpesviruses to antiviral drugs. Clin Microbiol Rev 1994;7(1):1–13.
16. Lyall EG, Ogilvie MM, Smith NM, et al. Acyclovir resistant varicella zoster and HIV infection. Arch Dis Child 1994;70(2):133–5.
17. Morfin F, Thouvenot D. Herpes simplex virus resistance to antiviral drugs. J Clin Virol 2003;26(1):29–37.
18. Wagstaff AJ, Faulds D, Goa KL. Aciclovir. A reappraisal of its antiviral activity, pharmacokinetic properties and therapeutic efficacy. Drugs 1994;47:153–205.
19. Laskin OL, Longstreth JA, Whelton A, et al. Effect of renal failure on the pharmacokinetics of acyclovir. Am J Med 1982;73(1A):197–201.
20. Yin M, Brust J, Tieu H, et al. Anti-hepatitis virus and anti-respiratory virus agents. In: Richman D, Whitley R, Hayden F, editors. Clinical virology. Washington, DC: ASM Press; 2009. p. 217–64.
21. Krasny HC, Liao SH, de Miranda P, et al. Influence of hemodialysis on acyclovir pharmacokinetics in patients with chronic renal failure. Am J Med 1982;73(1A):202–4.
22. Kimberlin D, Powell D, Gruber W, et al. Administration of oral acyclovir suppressive therapy following neonatal herpes simplex virus disease limited to the skin, eyes, and mouth: results of a phase I/II trial. Pediatr Infect Dis J 1996;15:247–54.
23. Revankar SG, Applegate AL, Markovitz DM. Delirium associated with acyclovir treatment in a patient with renal failure. Clin Infect Dis 1995;21(2):435–6.
24. Griffiths PD, Emery VC. Cytomegalovirus. In: Richman DD, Whitley RJ, Hayden FG, editors. Clinical virology. 2nd edition. Washington, DC: ASM Press; 2002. p. 433–61.
25. Staras SA, Dollard SC, Radford KW, et al. Seroprevalence of cytomegalovirus infection in the United States, 1988-1994. Clin Infect Dis 2006;43(9):1143–51.
26. Demmler GJ. Infectious Diseases Society of America and Centers for Disease Control. Summary of a workshop on surveillance for congenital cytomegalovirus disease. Rev Infect Dis 1991;13(2):315–29.
27. Conboy TJ, Pass RF, Stagno S, et al. Early clinical manifestations and intellectual outcome in children with symptomatic congenital cytomegalovirus infection. J Pediatr 1987;111(3):343–8.
28. Dollard SC, Grosse SD, Ross DS. New estimates of the prevalence of neurological and sensory sequelae and mortality associated with congenital cytomegalovirus infection. Rev Med Virol 2007;17(5):355–63.
29. Ross SA, Boppana SB. Congenital cytomegalovirus infection: outcome and diagnosis. Semin Pediatr Infect Dis 2005;16(1):44–9.
30. Griffiths PD, McLaughlin JE. Cytomegalovirus. In: Scheld WM, Whitley RJ, Marra CM, editors. Infections of the central nervous system. Philadelphia: Lippincott Williams & Wilkins; 2004. p. 159–73.
31. Maschmann J, Hamprecht K, Dietz K, et al. Cytomegalovirus infection of extremely low-birth weight infants via breast milk. Clin Infect Dis 2001;33(12):1998–2003.

32. Brasfield DM, Stagno S, Whitley RJ, et al. Infant pneumonitis associated with cytomegalovirus, chlamydia, pneumocystis, and ureaplasma. Pediatrics 1987; 79:76–83.

33. Pereira L, Maidji E. Cytomegalovirus infection in the human placenta: maternal immunity and developmentally regulated receptors on trophoblasts converge. Curr Top Microbiol Immunol 2008;325:383–95.

34. Strauss M. Human cytomegalovirus labyrinthitis. Am J Otolaryngol 1990;11(5): 292–8.

35. Davis LE, Johnsson LG, Kornfeld M. Cytomegalovirus labyrinthitis in an infant: morphological, virological, and immunofluorescent studies. J Neuropathol Exp Neurol 1981;40(1):9–19.

36. Kimberlin DW, Lin CY, Sanchez PJ, et al. Effect of ganciclovir therapy on hearing in symptomatic congenital cytomegalovirus disease involving the central nervous system: a randomized, controlled trial. J Pediatr 2003;143(1):16–25.

37. Oliver S, Cloud G, Sánchez P, et al. Effect of ganciclovir (GCV) therapy on neuro-developmental outcomes in symptomatic congenital cytomegalovirus (CMV) infections involving the central nervous system (CNS): a randomized, controlled study. Society for Pediatric Research (SPR) Annual Meeting. San Francisco, CA, April 29, 2006. p. [abstract: 752908].

38. Markham A, Faulds D. Ganciclovir: an update of its therapeutic use in cytomeg-alovirus infection. Drugs 1994;48:455.

39. Reddy V, Hao Y, Lipton J, et al. Management of allogeneic bone marrow trans-plant recipients at risk for cytomegalovirus disease using a surveillance bron-choscopy and prolonged pre-emptive ganciclovir therapy. J Clin Virol 1999; 13(3):149–59.

40. Jacobson MA, Gambertoglio JG, Aweeka FT, et al. Foscarnet-induced hypocal-cemia and effects of foscarnet on calcium metabolism. J Clin Endocrinol Metab 1991;72(5):1130–5.

41. Frenkel LM, Capparelli EV, Dankner WM, et al. Oral ganciclovir in children: phar-macokinetics, safety, tolerance, and antiviral effects. The Pediatric AIDS Clinical Trials Group. J Infect Dis 2000;182(6):1616–24.

42. Trang JM, Kidd L, Gruber W, et al. Linear Single-dose pharmacokinetics of gan-ciclovir in newborns with congenital cytomegalovirus infections. Clin Pharmacol Ther 1993;53:15–21.

43. Swan SK, Munar MY, Wigger MA, et al. Pharmacokinetics of ganciclovir in a patient undergoing hemodialysis. Am J Kidney Dis 1991;17(1):69–72.

44. Cocohoba JM, McNicholl IR. Valganciclovir: an advance in cytomegalovirus ther-apeutics. Ann Pharmacother 2002;36(6):1075–9.

45. Jung D, Dorr A. Single-dose pharmacokinetics of valganciclovir in HIV- and CMV-seropositive subjects. J Clin Pharmacol 1999;39(8):800–4.

46. Ho HT, Woods KL, Bronson JJ, et al. Intracellular metabolism of the antiherpes agents (S)-1-{3-hydroxy-2-(phosphonylmethoxy)propyl}cytosine. Mol Pharmacol 1992;41:197–202.

47. Safrin S, Cherrington J, Jaffe HS. Clinical uses of cidofovir. Rev Med Virol 1997; 7(3):145–56.

48. Lurain N, Spafford LE, Thompson KD. Mutation in the UL97 open reading frame of human cytomegalovirus strains resistant to ganciclovir. J Virol 1994;68: 4427–31.

49. Cherrington JM, Miner R, Allen SJ, et al. Sensitivities of human cytomegalovirus (HCMV) clinical isolates to cidofovir. Eighth International Conference on Antiviral Research. Santa Fe (New Mexico); 1995.

50. The Studies of Ocular Complications of AIDS Research Group in collaboration with the AIDS Clinical Trials Group. Cidofovir (HPMPC) for the treatment of cytomegalovirus retinitis in patients with AIDS: the HPMPC peripheral cytomegalovirus retinitis trial. Ann Intern Med 1997;126:264–74.

51. Lalezari JP, Staagg RJ, Kuppermann BD, et al. Intravenous cidofovir for peripheral cytomegalovirus retinitis in patients with AIDS: a randomized, controlled trial. Ann Intern Med 1997;126:257–63.

52. Lalezari JP, Drew WL, Glutzer E, et al. Treatment with intravenous (S)-1-[3-hydroxy-2-(phosphonylmethoxy)propyl)-cytosine of acyclovir-resistant mucocutaneous infection with herpes simplex virus in a patient with AIDS. J Infect Dis 1994;170:570–2.

53. Kimberlin DW, Malis DJ. Juvenile onset recurrent respiratory papillomatosis: possibilities for successful antiviral therapy. Antiviral Res 2000;45(2):83–93.

54. Pransky SM, Magit AE, Kearns DB, et al. Intralesional cidofovir for recurrent respiratory papillomatosis in children. Arch Otolaryngol Head Neck Surg 1999; 125(10):1143–8.

55. Cundy KC, Petty BG, Flaherty J, et al. Clinical pharmacokinetics of cidofovir in human immunodeficiency virus-infected patients. Antimicrob Agents Chemother 1995;39:1247–52.

56. Lalezari JP, Drew WL, Glutzer E, et al. (S)-1{3-hydroxy-2-(phosphonylmethoxy)propyl}cytosine (cidofoviir): results of a phase I/II study of a novel antiviral nucleotide analogue. J Infect Dis 1995;171:788–96.

57. Wagstaff AJ, Bryson HM. Foscarnet: a reappraisal of its antiviral activity, pharmacokinetic properties and therapeutic use in immunocompromised patients with viral infectious. Drugs 1994;48:199–226.

58. Safrin S, Kemmerly S, Plotkin B, et al. Foscarnet-resistant herpes simplex virus infection in patients with AIDS. J Infect Dis 1994;169:193–6.

59. Snoeck R, Andrei G, Gerard M, et al. Successful treatment of progressive mucocutaneous infection due to acyclovir- and foscarnet-resistant herpes simplex virus with (S)-1-(3-hydroxy-2-phosphonylmethoxypropyl)cytosine (HPMPC). Clin Infect Dis 1994;18(4):570–8.

60. Jacobson MA, Drew WL, Feinberg J, et al. Foscarnet therapy for ganciclovir-resistant cytomegalovirus retinitis in patients with AIDS. J Infect Dis 1991;163: 1348–51.

61. Safrin S, Berger TG, Gilson I. Foscarnet therapy in five patients with AIDS and acyclovir-resistant varicella zoster virus infection. Ann Intern Med 1991;115: 19–21.

62. Studies of Ocular Complications of AIDS Research Group. Mortality in patients with the acquired immunodeficiency syndrome treated with either foscarnet or ganciclovir for cytomegalovirus retinitis. N Engl J Med 1992;326:213–20.

63. Safrin S, Crumpacker C, Chatis P, et al. A controlled trial comparing foscarnet with vidarabine for acyclovir-resistant mucocutaneous herpes simplex in the acquired immunodeficiency syndrome. N Engl J Med 1991;325:551–5.

64. MacGregor RR, Graziani AL, Weiss R, et al. Successful foscarnet therapy for cytomegalovirus retinitis in an AIDS patient undergoing hemodialysis: rationale for empiric dosing and plasma level monitoring. J Infect Dis 1991;164(4):785–7.

65. Deray G, Martinez F, Katlama C, et al. Foscarnet nephrotoxicity: mechanism, incidence and prevention. Am J Nephrol 1989;9(4):316–21.

The Use of Antifungal Therapy in Neonatal Intensive Care

Daniela Testoni, MD[a], P. Brian Smith, MD, MHS, MPH[a,b],
Daniel K. Benjamin Jr, MD, PhD, MPH[a,b],*

KEYWORDS

- Invasive candidiasis • Amphotericin B deoxycholate
- Flucytosine • Fluconazole • Voriconazole • Posaconazole
- Micafungin • Anidulafungin • Caspofungin

Invasive candidiasis in extremely premature infants is the second most common cause of infectious disease-related death.[1] Birth weight is strongly related to the incidence of invasive candidiasis (1% of infants born weighing 1000–1500 g vs up to 12% of infants born weighing 401–750 g).[2] The morbidity and mortality of premature infants with invasive candidiasis are high.[3,4] In a cohort of 320 extremely-low-birth-weight (ELBW, <1000 g birth weight) infants with invasive candidiasis, 73% died or were neurodevelopmentally impaired at 18 to 22 months' corrected age.[3]

A unique characteristic of invasive candidiasis in infants is the frequent involvement of the central nervous system (CNS). The incidence of *Candida* meningitis among infants with candidemia varies from 5% to 25%.[3,5,6] Meningitis is not the only manifestation of CNS disease; parenchymal abscesses and vasculitis are also frequent in infants with invasive candidiasis.[7] Therefore, CNS involvement in invasive candidiasis among infants can best be termed meningoencephalitis. In meningoencephalitis due to *Candida*, cerebrospinal fluid (CSF) culture results are often negative, CSF parameters (eg, white blood cell count) are often normal,[5] and imaging is unreliable.

Given the high incidence of meningoencephalitis in the setting of candidemia and the lack of reliability of testing, the presence of meningoencephalitis should be assumed in the neonate with candidemia. This assumption influences length of therapy, dosing, and other key components of antifungal drug development and selection.

Disclosure: See last page of article.
a Duke Clinical Research Institute, Duke University Medical Center, 2400 Pratt Street, Durham, NC 27705, USA
b Department of Pediatrics, Duke University Medical Center, Duke University, Box 3352, Durham, NC 27710, USA
* Corresponding author. Duke University Medical Center, Duke Clinical Research Institute, 2400 Pratt Street, Durham, NC 27705.
E-mail address: danny.benjamin@duke.edu

Clin Perinatol 39 (2012) 83–98
doi:10.1016/j.clp.2011.12.008
0095-5108/12/$ – see front matter © 2012 Elsevier Inc. All rights reserved.

Although antifungals have long been used in infants, their efficacy in this population is based on extrapolation from trials performed in adults.[8] Randomized trials to evaluate prophylactic systemic antifungal agents in very-low-birth-weight (VLBW, <1500 g birth weight) and ELBW infants exist, but no well-powered trials exist to guide treatment of invasive fungal infection in preterm infants.[9–13] However, several pharmacokinetic (PK) antifungal studies have been completed (**Table 1**). In this article, we summarize those findings.

POLYENES
Amphotericin B Deoxycholate

Amphotericin B deoxycholate was approved for use in adults in 1958 and is now approved for use in children and adults. It acts by binding to a cytoplasmic membrane ergosterol of the fungus, thereby creating pores in cell membranes.[14] Amphotericin B deoxycholate is poorly absorbed after oral administration and is highly protein bound (95%).[15] It is widely distributed in the body and can be detected in the liver, spleen, and kidneys.[15]

Amphotericin B deoxycholate has a longer half-life in infants (15 hours) than in adults and greater potential for drug accumulation.[16] The half-life, volume of distribution, and clearance are highly variable in infants.[16] CSF penetration in infants is higher than in

Table 1
Pediatric antifungal dosing

Drug	Formulation	Infants (31 d–2 y)	Neonates (0–30 d)	FDA Label
Polyenes				
Amphotericin B deoxycholate	IV	1 mg/kg/d	1 mg/kg/d	Children and adults
Amphotericin B lipid complex	IV	Unknown	Unknown	>16 mo
Amphotericin B colloidal dispersion	IV	Unknown	Unknown	Children and adults
Liposomal amphotericin B	IV	5 mg/kg/d	5 mg/kg/d	≥1 mo
Nucleoside analogues				
5-Flucytosine	PO	50–150 mg/kg/d q 6 h	50–150 mg/kg/d q 6 hr	Adults
Triazoles				
Fluconazole	IV, PO	12 mg/kg/d (25 mg/kg/loading dose)	12 mg/kg/d (25 mg/kg load)	≥6 mo
Voriconazole	IV, PO	Unknown	Unknown	≥12 y
Posaconazole	PO	Unknown	Unknown	≥13 y
Echinocandins				
Caspofungin	IV	50 mg/m²/d	25 mg/m²/d	>3 mo
Micafungin	IV	10 mg/kg/d	10 mg/kg/d	Adults
Anidulafungin	IV	1.5 mg/kg/d (3 mg/kg/loading dose)	1.5 mg/kg/d (3 mg/kg/load)	Adults

Abbreviations: IV, intravenous; PO, oral.
Data from Refs.[16,20,25,37,40,86,89,92,97,101,109,110]

adults, with concentrations at 40% to 90% of the serum concentrations[16]; importantly, the amphotericin products tend to have substantial brain tissue penetration.

Nephrotoxicity is an important side effect observed with use of amphotericin B deoxycholate.[16–18] In a retrospective study evaluating 92 infants with a median gestational age of 26 weeks (range, 23–41 weeks), 16% experienced nephrotoxicity and 17% had hypokalemia.[19] However, in another study designed to compare the effectiveness and tolerability of 3 antifungal preparations, amphotericin B deoxycholate, liposomal amphotericin B (L-amB), and amphotericin B colloidal dispersion (ABCD), no infant (n = 56) experienced renal function deterioration during treatment.[20]

Amphotericin Lipid Formulations

Three lipid formulations of amphotericin are available: L-amB (or AmBisome), amphotericin B lipid complex (ABLC or Abelcet), and ABCD (or Amphotec). The Food and Drug Administration (FDA) has approved L-amB for use in children aged 1 month or more, ABLC for children aged 16 months or more, and ABCD for children and adults.

L-amB at a dose of 1 mg/kg daily demonstrated cumulative dose effect, and the peak plasma concentrations were higher in adults than children and infants.[21] Accumulation of amphotericin B in rabbits' kidneys after 5 mg/kg/d of L-amB was only 0.87 µg/g compared with 12.7 µg/g after 1 mg/kg/d of amphotericin B deoxycholate.[22] The clearance of ABLC in infants was similar to that observed in older patients.[23] The recommended dose for ABLC is 2.5 to 5 mg/kg/d.[23]

Infants in a prospective single-center study were given 1 mg/kg/d of amphotericin B deoxycholate (n = 34) if their serum creatinine level was less than 1.2 mg/dL; otherwise, they were given either 5 mg/kg/d of L-amB (n = 6) or 3 mg/kg/d of ABCD (n = 16). No statistical difference in mortality was noted among the 3 groups.[20] In a study of 46 VLBW infants who received L-amB at a dose of 1 to 3 mg/kg/d (26 infants) or amphotericin B deoxycholate at a dose of 0.5 to 1.0 mg/kg/d (20 infants), the fungal eradication rate was similar between groups: 84% of the L-amB group and 89% of the amphotericin B deoxycholate group.[14] Effectiveness of L-amB was 73% (n = 44) in a prospective cohort of infants with invasive candidiasis and 63% (n = 21) among VLBW infants.[24] L-amB was effective in 95% of infants (n = 41) with invasive candidiasis (28 were ELBW) treated with a high dose (5–7 mg/kg/d). The infection cleared faster if the target dose was reached earlier.[25]

In a prospective cohort of 21 VLBW infants receiving L-amB, hypokalemia was the only side effect observed and was supplementation responsive.[24] The number of studies of ABLC and ABCD in pediatric populations is small, but both agents were well tolerated.[23,26,27] In a prospective study comparing the 3 formulations, no significant renal or hepatic toxicities were noted with any of the preparations.[20] Because renal penetration is limited with lipid formulations, the clinician should document negative urine cultures in infants for whom these preparations are used as monotherapy.[22]

NUCLEOSIDE ANALOGUES
Flucytosine

Flucytosine (5-FC), through its antimetabolite 5-fluoracil, alters RNA and DNA synthesis of the mycotic cell. 5-FC is converted to 5-fluoracil by cytosine deaminase, a fungi enzyme absent from human cells.[28] 5-FC is active against *Candida* sp, *Aspergillus* sp, and *Cryptococcus* sp.[28] The occurrence of resistance with the use of 5-FC as monotherapy precludes its use as a single agent.[29] 5-FC is highly bioavailable and has excellent penetration of body fluids, with CSF concentrations at 74% of plasma levels.[28] 5-FC is FDA approved only for use in adults.[30] The recommended dose is

25 to 100 mg/kg/d.[16] In 13 infants (24–40 weeks' gestational age), the median half-life was twice that of adults, with considerable interindividual variability.[16] 5-FC can be toxic and can result in hepatic injury, bone marrow suppression, and gastrointestinal intolerance.[31] The risk for developing toxic events increases when 5-FC levels exceed 100 mg/L; therefore, therapeutic drug monitoring is necessary.[31,32]

The PK data in infants are limited, and there has been no clinical trial to evaluate 5-FC efficacy in this population. A cohort study of 27 ELBW infants with meningoencephalitis showed that time to clear infection was longer in infants given combination 5-FC and amphotericin B deoxycholate than that in those treated with amphotericin B deoxycholate alone.[3] 5-FC use is limited by its toxicities and the need for oral dosing, and we typically discourage its use except in rare circumstances.

TRIAZOLES
Fluconazole

Fluconazole is a water-soluble triazole whose mode of action is inhibition of the demethylase enzyme that is involved in the synthesis of ergosterol.[33] Fluconazole is available in both oral and intravenous formulations, with oral bioavailability greater than 90%. Fluconazole is labeled by the FDA for use in children aged 6 months or more. The volume of distribution in adults is 0.7 L/kg with a low plasma protein binding (12%). Plasma half-life is approximately 30 hours in adults.[34]

The PK properties of fluconazole are well described in children. The volume of distribution varies with age; it is greatest during the neonatal period and decreases by young adulthood. In children, fluconazole clearance is more rapid than in adults, with a mean half-life of 20 hours. Fluconazole is eliminated renally; therefore, dosing adjustments are necessary in patients with substantial renal impairment.[35,36] In the premature infant, we typically reserve dose adjustment for the infant with substantially impaired urine output and elevated creatinine level.[37]

Fluconazole is commonly used to treat candidiasis in infants and is active against the most frequently isolated species of *Candida*.[38] Infants with invasive candidiasis should receive 12 mg/kg/d of fluconazole to achieve an area under the curve greater than 400 mg × h/L.[39] A loading dose of 25 mg/kg on the first day is likely to provide optimal exposure; otherwise, infants may not reach target exposures for several days.[40] Fluconazole is also well absorbed in infants[41] and is found in the CSF at 80% of the levels observed in plasma.[42]

Fluconazole seems to be safe in infants. Laboratory abnormalities in patients receiving fluconazole are uncommon; a transient increase in liver enzymes was seen in less than 5% of children (n = 564; from premature neonatal age to 17 years).[43] Fluconazole was given to 493 infants in clinical trials to evaluate fluconazole prophylaxis, and no serious adverse events were found.[9–13,44] One trial showed differences in liver enzyme levels for patients administered fluconazole compared with controls (alanine transaminase 18 IU/mL and 15 IU/mL for treated vs controls, respectively), but levels returned to baseline levels after the end of therapy.[11]

Several randomized trials and several prospective cohort studies found that antifungal prophylaxis with fluconazole decreased the incidence of invasive candidiasis (**Table 2**).[9–13,45–51] Although fluconazole prophylaxis decreases invasive candidiasis in high-risk populations, it is unknown if prophylaxis decreases overall mortality and decreases candidiasis in low-incidence settings or what the effects of prophylaxis may be on long-term neurodevelopment. There are also concerns that antifungal prophylaxis may increase the incidence of fluconazole-resistant *Candida*.[52]

Voriconazole

Voriconazole, a second-generation triazole, exhibits broad-spectrum antifungal activity against fungal pathogens such as *Candida* spp, *Aspergillus* spp, and *Cryptococcus neoformans* and less common mold pathogens, including several species of *Fusarium* and *Penicillium marneffei*.[53] Voriconazole has high oral bioavailability (90%) and a mean half-life of 6 hours.[53] It is FDA approved for children aged 12 years or more. CSF penetration is high, and the drug is metabolized by the liver cytochrome P4502C19; genetic polymorphisms of this enzyme play a role in its PK.[53,54]

Walsh and colleagues[55] demonstrated a nonlinear elimination for the dose range of 4 mg/kg every 12 hours and 8 mg/kg every 12 hours. The clearance in children is higher than in adults, and the bioavailability is lower (65%); a dose of 7 mg/kg may provide plasma concentrations comparable to exposures in adults given 4 mg/kg.[55,56] Plasma levels of voriconazole in children are highly variable; this is especially true in young infants. Plasma levels should therefore be monitored in a neonate who receives this product.[57–59] In a study of 10 children with a median age of 17 months (range, 2 weeks–35 months), voriconazole trough concentrations were highly variable and did not correlate with the dose administered.[60]

Voriconazole is safe in adults. Children and adults experience the same adverse effects: transient visual disturbances and photosensitivity.[55,58,61–63] Mild transient elevation of hepatic enzyme levels has also been observed.[55,58] Voriconazole clinical trials have not been performed in infants.[64] This product should be reserved as a second-line (or third-line) agent, primarily in the context of resistance or in the rare case of invasive aspergillosis in the nursery.

Posaconazole

Posaconazole is available in an oral formulation and has extended activity against *Candida* spp, *Aspergillus* spp, *C neoformans*, and zygomycetes.[65,66] Posaconazole is approved for prophylaxis of invasive *Aspergillus* and *Candida* infections and for treatment of oropharyngeal candidiasis in patients aged 13 years or more.

Posaconazole has a half-life of 25 hours[67] and is excreted unchanged in the feces; renal elimination is minor, and the drug is not a substrate for the cytochrome P450 enzymatic system.[68]

Experience with posaconazole in children is limited. In a retrospective study including 15 patients aged 3 to 17 years, posaconazole was used as salvage therapy for invasive fungal infections in immunocompromised children and adolescents.[69] In a PK study that included 12 patients younger than 18 years, posaconazole concentrations in plasma were similar for juvenile and adult patients, following a dose of 400 mg/kg twice daily.[70] There are no published studies in infants, but higher doses are likely needed for younger patients.

ECHINOCANDINS

Echinocandins are noncompetitive inhibitors of $1,3-\beta-D-glucan$ synthase, an enzyme that is necessary for the synthesis of $1,3-\beta-D$ glucan. Without this component, the fungal wall cell is compromised.[71] The echinocandins have a large molecular weight and poor penetration into the CSF[72]; however, micafungin and anidulafungin can be given in dosages in which the products successfully achieve maximum killing concentrations inside the CNS. These studies have been conducted in a series of animal model experiments followed by neonatal PK trials.[73,74]

Table 2
Fluconazole prophylaxis studies

References	Study Design	Population	N	Drug Regimen	Outcomes
Aydemir et al,[9] 2010	RCT	VLBW	93, FP; 94, NP; 91, placebo	Fluconazole, 3 mg/kg, q 3 d; nystatin, 1 mL, q 8 h	IC rate: 3%, FP; 4%, NP; 17%, placebo (P<.001) Similar mortality: 9%, FP; 9%, NP; 12%, placebo
Rueda et al,[50] 2010	Retrospective cohort	<1250 g	252, FP; 272, control	3 mg/kg, q 48 h	IC rate decreased: 8%, control; 1%, FP (P = .007) IC-related mortality decreased: 6%–1% (P = .003)
Aziz et al,[45] 2010	Retrospective cohort	ELBW	163, FP; 99, control	3 mg/kg, q 48–72 h	IC rate decreased: 7%, control; 2%, FP (P = .045)
Weitkamp et al,[51] 2008	Retrospective cohort	<750 g	42, FP; 44, control	3 mg/kg twice weekly	IC rate decreased: 20%, control; 0%, FP (P = .004) Similar mortality: 20%, control; 26%, FP
Healy et al,[47] 2008	Retrospective cohort	ELBW	362, FP; 206, control	3 mg/kg, q 24–72 h	IC rate decreased: 7%, control; 2%, FP (P = .003) IC-related mortality: 2%, control; 0%, FP (P = .1)
Parikh et al,[13] 2007	RCT	VLBW	60, FP; 60, placebo	3 mg/kg, q 24–72 h	IC rate: 25%, placebo; 26%, FP (P = .835) Same mortality: 28% in both groups
Manzoni et al,[12] 2007	RCT	VLBW	112, HD; 104, LD; 106, placebo	6 mg/kg (HD); 3 mg/kg (LD), q 48–72 h	IC rate decreased: 13%, placebo, and 3%, HD (P = .05); 13.2%, placebo, and 3.8%, LD (P = .002) Similar mortality: 8%, HD; 10%, LD; 9%, placebo

Study	Design	Birth weight	N	Dosage	Results
McCrossan et al,[49] 2007	Retrospective cohort	VLBW	31, FP; 33, control	6 mg/kg, q 24–72 h	IC rate decreased: 6%, control; 0%, FP (P = .03); IC-related mortality: 12%, control; 0%, FP (P = .11)
Manzoni et al,[48] 2006	Retrospective cohort	VLBW	225, FP; 240, control	6 mg/kg, q 48–72 h	IC rate decreased: 17%, control; 5%, FP (P<.0001); Similar mortality: 11%, control; 11%, FP
Kaufman et al,[44] 2005	RCT	ELBW	41, FP previous; 40, FP twice/wk	3 mg/kg twice weekly or q 24–72 h	IC rate: 5% previous; –3%, twice a wk (P = .68); Similar mortality: 13%, control; 8%, FP (P = 8.1%)
Bertini et al,[46] 2005	Retrospective cohort	VLBW	136, FP; 119, control	6 mg/kg, q 24–72 h	IC rate decreased: 8%, control; l–0%, FP (P = .003)
Healy et al,[117] 2005	Retrospective cohort	ELBW	240, FP; 206, control	3 mg/kg, q 24–72 h	IC rate decreased: 7%, control; 2%, FP (P = .01); IC-related mortality: 12%, control; 0%, FP (P = .4)
Kicklighter et al,[11] 2001	RCT	VLBW	53, FP; 50, placebo	6 mg/kg, q 24–72 h	Fungal colonization decreased: 46%, placebo; 15%, FP (P = .0005); IC rate or mortality not related
Kaufman et al,[10] 2001	RCT	ELBW	50, FP; 50, placebo	3 mg/kg, q 24–72 h	IC rate decreased: 20%, placebo; 0%, FP (P = .008); Similar mortality: 20%, placebo; 8%, FP (P = .22)

Abbreviations: FP, fluconazole prophylaxis group; HD, high-dosage group; IC, invasive candidiasis; LD, low-dosage group; NP, nystatin prophylaxis group; RCT, randomized controlled trial.

Micafungin

Micafungin exhibits broad-spectrum activity against clinically important pathogens including azole-resistant *Candida albicans*.[75] It is fungicidal against *Candida* spp and fungistatic in vitro against *Aspergillus* spp.[75,76] Micafungin is an intravenous antifungal approved in the United States for adult patients and has been approved for use in children (including infants) in Europe for treatment of invasive candidiasis.[77] Trials in patients older than 16 years (and 1 including children from 0 week to 16 years of age) found that micafungin has the same efficacy against invasive candidiasis as amphotericin B,[78–80] fluconazole,[81] or caspofungin,[82] with fewer adverse events than amphotericin B deoxycholate.[78,79]

Micafungin has a half-life of approximately 12 hours in adults; the highest drug concentrations are detected in the lungs, liver, spleen, and kidneys.[83,84] Micafungin is highly plasma protein bound. Metabolism occurs mainly in the liver, but, because the echinocandins are poor substrates for the cytochrome P450 enzymes, few drug interactions are described. Fecal excretion is the major route of elimination.[72]

Of the echinocandins, the PK of micafungin is the best described across all pediatric age groups. In children with fever and neutropenia, micafungin (0.5–4.0 mg/kg/d) demonstrated linear PK, and clearance was inversely related to age.[85] To achieve micafungin exposures equivalent to adults, children require dosages greater than 3 mg/kg.[86] However, the clearance of micafungin in premature infants is faster than in older children and adults; age-dependent serum protein binding of micafungin might be responsible for its higher clearance.[87]

Elevated dosing in the premature infant is thought to be critical for getting micafungin into the CNS.[73] After administration of more than 2 mg/kg of micafungin to rabbits, micafungin was detected in most brain compartments (meninges, spinal cord, choroid, cerebrum, cerebellum, and aqueous humor).[73] For lower doses (0.5–1.0 mg/kg), micafungin was not detected.[73] PK data obtained in 12 premature infants (mean gestational age of 27 weeks) suggest that a micafungin dose of 15 mg/kg/d achieves similar exposures to those observed in adults receiving 5 mg/kg/d.[88] A dose of 10 mg/kg/d provided target systemic exposure corresponding to levels adequate to provide CNS penetration and is thought to be the optimal dose for premature and term infants.[89,90]

The most common adverse events related to micafungin include gastrointestinal tract manifestations (nausea, diarrhea), hypersensitivity reactions, elevation of liver enzymes, and hypokalemia.[80,85] King and colleagues[91] presented a case of hepatitis related to micafungin in a 44-day-old infant. Micafungin doses from 0.75 to 15.00 mg/kg/d have been studied in children.[88,92,93]

Anidulafungin

Anidulafungin has activity against *Candida* and *Aspergillus* sp in adults. It has been used in the treatment of esophageal and systemic candidiasis[94–96] and is FDA approved for use in adults. Anidulafungin demonstrates linear PK with a long half-life, approximately 26 hours for adults and 20 hours for children.[97,98] Clearance of anidulafungin seems to be primarily due to slow chemical degradation, and it is eliminated in the feces predominantly as a degradation product. Fecal elimination likely occurs via biliary excretion. Once anidulafungin is degraded in the blood, it does not require dosage adjustment in individuals with hepatic or renal impairment.[99] The tissue concentrations after multiple dosing are highest in the lungs, liver, spleen, and kidneys, with measurable concentrations in the brain tissue.[100]

Children aged 2 to 17 years with neutropenia were given anidulafungin (1.5–3 mg/kg loading dose, 0.75–1.5 mg/kg/d maintenance dose) and had exposures similar to adult patients receiving the same weight-adjusted dose; they achieved steady-state plasma concentrations after administration of a loading dose.[97] Anidulafungin was administered to 15 patients younger than 18 months intravenously as a loading dose of 3 mg/kg on day 1, with daily maintenance dosages of 1.5 mg/kg. Among the patients, there were 8 newborns with a median gestational age of 27 weeks (range, 26–39 weeks), median birth weight of 1120 g (770–3730 g), and median postnatal age of 28 days (range, 2–451 days).[101] Infants receiving 1.5 mg/kg/d had similar anidulafungin exposures compared with children receiving similar weight-based dosing and adult patients receiving 100 mg/d.[94,97,101] Two patients supported by extracorporeal membrane oxygenation had lower drug exposure.[101,102] High-dose anidulafungin (10 mg/kg/d) reduced fungal load in murine brains, but a lower dose (5 mg/kg/d) in the same animal model was not effective.[74] The adequate dose for infants to achieve CNS penetration with anidulafungin is unknown.

Anidulafungin is well tolerated in the pediatric population.[97,101] Adverse events occurred in few patients; the most commonly reported adverse event was transient liver function test elevations, and 2 infants showed worsening of baseline bilirubin levels.[97,101]

Caspofungin

Caspofungin has activity against both *Candida* sp and *Aspergillus* sp.[103] Caspofungin is FDA approved for adults and children older than 3 months. The typical adult dose is 50 mg daily after a 70 mg loading dose.[104,105] The metabolism of caspofungin is hepatic, and its half-life is 9 to 10 hours.[106] Patients with renal insufficiency do not need dose adjustments[107]; however, decrease of daily dosage is necessary in patients with hepatic insufficiency.[108]

The PK of caspofungin was first evaluated in children in a study of 39 patients aged 2 to 17 years (29 patients younger than 1 year); a dose of 50 mg/m^2/d provided similar exposures to an adult dose of 50 mg/kg.[109] Caspofungin clearance is increased in children, as demonstrated by lower exposures and shorter half-life (8 hours) compared with adults.[109] At the same time, the maximum concentration is higher after a loading dose.[110] In children, the main use of caspofungin has been in refractory cases of invasive candidiasis as a salvage or combination therapy.[111,112] Most recently, some studies have made use of the medication as the primary treatment of invasive candidiasis[113] or for empiric antifungal therapy.[114]

In infants and toddlers with fever and neutropenia, caspofungin, 50 mg/m^2/d, produced similar steady-state exposures as those observed in older children with the same dose.[115] A dose of 25 mg/m^2/d in 18 infants younger than 3 months resulted in peak concentrations lower than those in older children given 50 mg/m^2/d and similar concentrations to those seen in adults administered 50 mg/d.[110]

The efficacy of caspofungin against CNS candidiasis has not yet been demonstrated.

The most common adverse events are fever, headache, and rash. Increase of hepatic transaminases and hypokalemia was found in few patients.[109,114] In a cohort of 18 infants (gestational age 24–41 weeks), 94% of the patients presented 1 or more clinical adverse events; none were considered to be related to caspofungin.[110] In a retrospective study with infants (≤3 months of age), caspofungin was not associated with any serious adverse events.[66,80,84,85,87,88,91,116]

SUMMARY

Invasive fungal infections remain a significant cause of infection-related mortality and morbidity in preterm infants. CNS involvement is the hallmark of neonatal candidiasis, differentiating the disease's impact on young infants as compared with all other patient populations. As such, CNS involvement substantially influences candidiasis treatment in infants. Over the past decade, the number of antifungal agents in development has grown exponentially, but most are not labeled for use in newborns. More clinical trials and PK studies are required for the new antifungals to be used in infants.

DISCLOSURES

Dr Benjamin receives support from the United States government for his work in pediatric and neonatal clinical pharmacology (1R01HD057956-02, 1R01FD003519-01, 1K24HD058735-01, and Government Contract HHSN-267200700051C and HHSN275201000003I), the nonprofit organization Thrasher Research Foundation for his work in neonatal candidiasis (http://www.thrasherresearch.org), and from industry for neonatal and pediatric drug development (http://www.dcri.duke.edu/research/coi.jsp). Dr Smith receives support from NICHD 1K23HD060040-01 and DHHS-1R18AE000028-01 and from industry for neonatal and pediatric drug development (http://www.dcri.duke.edu/research/coi.jsp). Dr Testoni has no disclosures to report.

REFERENCES

1. Benjamin DK Jr, Stoll BJ, Gantz MG, et al. Neonatal candidiasis: epidemiology, risk factors, and clinical judgment. Pediatrics 2010;126(4):e865–73.
2. Smith PB, Steinbach WJ, Benjamin DK Jr. Neonatal candidiasis. Infect Dis Clin North Am 2005;19(3):603–15.
3. Benjamin DK Jr, Stoll BJ, Fanaroff AA, et al. Neonatal candidiasis among extremely low birth weight infants: risk factors, mortality rates, and neurodevelopmental outcomes at 18 to 22 months. Pediatrics 2006;117(1):84–92.
4. Smith PB, Morgan J, Benjamin JD, et al. Excess costs of hospital care associated with neonatal candidemia. Pediatr Infect Dis J 2007;26(3):197–200.
5. Cohen-Wolkowiez M, Smith PB, Mangum B, et al. Neonatal Candida meningitis: significance of cerebrospinal fluid parameters and blood cultures. J Perinatol 2007;27(2):97–100.
6. Fernandez M, Moylett EH, Noyola DE, et al. Candidal meningitis in neonates: a 10-year review. Clin Infect Dis 2000;31(2):458–63.
7. Benjamin DK Jr, Poole C, Steinbach WJ, et al. Neonatal candidemia and end-organ damage: a critical appraisal of the literature using meta-analytic techniques. Pediatrics 2003;112(3 Pt 1):634–40.
8. Watt K, Benjamin DK Jr, Cohen-Wolkowiez M. Pharmacokinetics of antifungal agents in children. Early Hum Dev 2011;87(Suppl 1):S61–5.
9. Aydemir C, Oguz SS, Dizdar EA, et al. Randomised controlled trial of prophylactic fluconazole versus nystatin for the prevention of fungal colonisation and invasive fungal infection in very low birth weight infants. Arch Dis Child Fetal Neonatal Ed 2011;96(3):F164–8.
10. Kaufman D, Boyle R, Hazen KC, et al. Fluconazole prophylaxis against fungal colonization and infection in preterm infants. N Engl J Med 2001;345(23):1660–6.

11. Kicklighter SD, Springer SC, Cox T, et al. Fluconazole for prophylaxis against candidal rectal colonization in the very low birth weight infant. Pediatrics 2001;107(2):293–8.
12. Manzoni P, Stolfi I, Pugni L, et al. A multicenter, randomized trial of prophylactic fluconazole in preterm neonates. N Engl J Med 2007;356(24):2483–95.
13. Parikh TB, Nanavati RN, Patankar CV, et al. Fluconazole prophylaxis against fungal colonization and invasive fungal infection in very low birth weight infants. Indian Pediatr 2007;44(11):830–7.
14. Jeon GW, Koo SH, Lee JH, et al. A comparison of AmBisome to amphotericin B for treatment of systemic candidiasis in very low birth weight infants. Yonsei Med J 2007;48(4):619–26.
15. Janknegt R, de Marie S, Bakker-Woudenberg IA, et al. Liposomal and lipid formulations of amphotericin B. Clinical pharmacokinetics. Clin Pharmacokinet 1992;23(4):279–91.
16. Baley JE, Meyers C, Kliegman RM, et al. Pharmacokinetics, outcome of treatment, and toxic effects of amphotericin B and 5-fluorocytosine in neonates. J Pediatr 1990;116(5):791–7.
17. Holler B, Omar SA, Farid MD, et al. Effects of fluid and electrolyte management on amphotericin B-induced nephrotoxicity among extremely low birth weight infants. Pediatrics 2004;113(6):e608–16.
18. Makhoul IR, Kassis I, Smolkin T, et al. Review of 49 neonates with acquired fungal sepsis: further characterization. Pediatrics 2001;107(1):61–6.
19. Le J, Adler-Shohet FC, Nguyen C, et al. Nephrotoxicity associated with amphotericin B deoxycholate in neonates. Pediatr Infect Dis J 2009;28(12): 1061–3.
20. Linder N, Klinger G, Shalit I, et al. Treatment of candidaemia in premature infants: comparison of three amphotericin B preparations. J Antimicrob Chemother 2003;52(4):663–7.
21. Kotwani RN, Gokhale PC, Bodhe PV, et al. A comparative study of plasma concentrations of liposomal amphotericin B (L-AMP-LRC-1) in adults, children and neonates. Int J Pharm 2002;238(1–2):11–5.
22. Lee JW, Amantea MA, Francis PA, et al. Pharmacokinetics and safety of a unilamellar liposomal formulation of amphotericin B (AmBisome) in rabbits. Antimicrob Agents Chemother 1994;38(4):713–8.
23. Wurthwein G, Groll AH, Hempel G, et al. Population pharmacokinetics of amphotericin B lipid complex in neonates. Antimicrob Agents Chemother 2005; 49(12):5092–8.
24. Scarcella A, Pasquariello MB, Giugliano B, et al. Liposomal amphotericin B treatment for neonatal fungal infections. Pediatr Infect Dis J 1998;17(2):146–8.
25. Juster-Reicher A, Flidel-Rimon O, Amitay M, et al. High-dose liposomal amphotericin B in the therapy of systemic candidiasis in neonates. Eur J Clin Microbiol Infect Dis 2003;22(10):603–7.
26. Anaissie EJ, Mattiuzzi GN, Miller CB, et al. Treatment of invasive fungal infections in renally impaired patients with amphotericin B colloidal dispersion. Antimicrob Agents Chemother 1998;42(3):606–11.
27. White MH, Bowden RA, Sandler ES, et al. Randomized, double-blind clinical trial of amphotericin B colloidal dispersion vs. amphotericin B in the empirical treatment of fever and neutropenia. Clin Infect Dis 1998;27(2):296–302.
28. Bennet JE. Flucytosine. Ann Intern Med 1977;86(3):319–21.
29. Polak A, Scholer HJ. Mode of action of 5-fluorocytosine and mechanisms of resistance. Chemotherapy 1975;21(3-4):113–30.

30. Smego RA Jr, Perfect JR, Durack DT. Combined therapy with amphotericin B and 5-fluorocytosine for Candida meningitis. Rev Infect Dis 1984;6(6):791–801.

31. Vermes A, van Der Sijs H, Guchelaar HJ. Flucytosine: correlation between toxicity and pharmacokinetic parameters. Chemotherapy 2000;46(2):86–94.

32. Soltani M, Tobin CM, Bowker KE, et al. Evidence of excessive concentrations of 5-flucytosine in children aged below 12 years: a 12-year review of serum concentrations from a UK clinical assay reference laboratory. Int J Antimicrob Agents 2006;28(6):574–7.

33. Galgiani JN. Fluconazole, a new antifungal agent. Ann Intern Med 1990;113(3): 177–9.

34. Brammer KW, Farrow PR, Faulkner JK. Pharmacokinetics and tissue penetration of fluconazole in humans. Rev Infect Dis 1990;12(Suppl 3):S318–26.

35. Berl T, Wilner KD, Gardner M, et al. Pharmacokinetics of fluconazole in renal failure. J Am Soc Nephrol 1995;6(2):242–7.

36. Brammer KW, Coates PE. Pharmacokinetics of fluconazole in pediatric patients. Eur J Clin Microbiol Infect Dis 1994;13(4):325–9.

37. Wade KC, Wu D, Kaufman DA, et al. Population pharmacokinetics of fluconazole in young infants. Antimicrob Agents Chemother 2008;52(11):4043–9.

38. Hajjeh RA, Sofair AN, Harrison LH, et al. Incidence of bloodstream infections due to Candida species and in vitro susceptibilities of isolates collected from 1998 to 2000 in a population-based active surveillance program. J Clin Microbiol 2004;42(4):1519–27.

39. Wade KC, Benjamin DK Jr, Kaufman DA, et al. Fluconazole dosing for the prevention or treatment of invasive candidiasis in young infants. Pediatr Infect Dis J 2009;28(8):717–23.

40. Piper L, Smith PB, Hornik CP, et al. Fluconazole loading dose pharmacokinetics and safety in infants. Pediatr Infect Dis J 2011;30(5):375–8.

41. Nahata MC, Tallian KB, Force RW. Pharmacokinetics of fluconazole in young infants. Eur J Drug Metab Pharmacokinet 1999;24(2):155–7.

42. Wildfeuer A, Laufen H, Schmalreck AF, et al. Fluconazole: comparison of pharmacokinetics, therapy and in vitro susceptibility. Mycoses 1997;40(7–8): 259–65.

43. Novelli V, Holzel H. Safety and tolerability of fluconazole in children. Antimicrob Agents Chemother 1999;43(8):1955–60.

44. Kaufman D, Boyle R, Hazen KC, et al. Twice weekly fluconazole prophylaxis for prevention of invasive Candida infection in high-risk infants of <1000 grams birth weight. J Pediatr 2005;147(2):172–9.

45. Aziz M, Patel AL, Losavio J, et al. Efficacy of fluconazole prophylaxis for prevention of invasive fungal infection in extremely low birth weight infants. Pediatr Infect Dis J 2010;29(4):352–6.

46. Bertini G, Perugi S, Dani C, et al. Fluconazole prophylaxis prevents invasive fungal infection in high-risk, very low birth weight infants. J Pediatr 2005; 147(2):162–5.

47. Healy CM, Campbell JR, Zaccaria E, et al. Fluconazole prophylaxis in extremely low birth weight neonates reduces invasive candidiasis mortality rates without emergence of fluconazole-resistant Candida species. Pediatrics 2008;121(4): 703–10.

48. Manzoni P, Arisio R, Mostert M, et al. Prophylactic fluconazole is effective in preventing fungal colonization and fungal systemic infections in preterm neonates: a single-center, 6-year, retrospective cohort study. Pediatrics 2006;117(1): e22–32.

49. McCrossan BA, McHenry E, O'Neill F, et al. Selective fluconazole prophylaxis in high-risk babies to reduce invasive fungal infection. Arch Dis Child Fetal Neonatal Ed 2007;92(6):F454–8.
50. Rueda K, Moreno MT, Espinosa M, et al. Impact of routine fluconazole prophylaxis for premature infants with birth weights of less than 1250 grams in a developing country. Pediatr Infect Dis J 2010;29(11):1050–2.
51. Weitkamp JH, Ozdas A, LaFleur B, et al. Fluconazole prophylaxis for prevention of invasive fungal infections in targeted highest risk preterm infants limits drug exposure. J Perinatol 2008;28(6):405–11.
52. Manzoni P, Leonessa M, Galletto P, et al. Routine use of fluconazole prophylaxis in a neonatal intensive care unit does not select natively fluconazole-resistant Candida subspecies. Pediatr Infect Dis J 2008;27(8):731–7.
53. Sheehan DJ, Hitchcock CA, Sibley CM. Current and emerging azole antifungal agents. Clin Microbiol Rev 1999;12(1):40–79.
54. Walsh TJ, Karlsson MO, Driscoll T, et al. Pharmacokinetics and safety of intravenous voriconazole in children after single- or multiple-dose administration. Antimicrob Agents Chemother 2004;48(6):2166–72.
55. Walsh TJ, Driscoll T, Milligan PA, et al. Pharmacokinetics, safety, and tolerability of voriconazole in immunocompromised children. Antimicrob Agents Chemother 2010;54(10):4116–23.
56. Michael C, Bierbach U, Frenzel K, et al. Voriconazole pharmacokinetics and safety in immunocompromised children compared to adult patients. Antimicrob Agents Chemother 2010;54(8):3225–32.
57. Spriet I, Cosaert K, Renard M, et al. Voriconazole plasma levels in children are highly variable. Eur J Clin Microbiol Infect Dis 2011;30(2):283–7.
58. Shima H, Miharu M, Osumi T, et al. Differences in voriconazole trough plasma concentrations per oral dosages between children younger and older than 3 years of age. Pediatr Blood Cancer 2010;54(7):1050–2.
59. Bruggemann RJ, van der Linden JW, Verweij PE, et al. Impact of therapeutic drug monitoring of voriconazole in a pediatric population. Pediatr Infect Dis J 2011;30(6):533–4.
60. Doby EH, Benjamin DK Jr, Blaschke AJ, et al. Therapeutic drug monitoring of voriconazole in children less than 3 years of age: a case report and summary of pharmacokinetic data for 10 children. Pediatr Infect Dis J, in press.
61. Cowen EW, Nguyen JC, Miller DD, et al. Chronic phototoxicity and aggressive squamous cell carcinoma of the skin in children and adults during treatment with voriconazole. J Am Acad Dermatol 2010;62(1):31–7.
62. Rubenstein M, Levy ML, Metry D. Voriconazole-induced retinoid-like photosensitivity in children. Pediatr Dermatol 2004;21(6):675–8.
63. Purkins L, Wood N, Greenhalgh K, et al. The pharmacokinetics and safety of intravenous voriconazole—a novel wide-spectrum antifungal agent. Br J Clin Pharmacol 2003;56(Suppl 1):2–9.
64. Kohli V, Taneja V, Sachdev P, et al. Voriconazole in newborns. Indian Pediatr 2008;45(3):236–8.
65. Uchida K, Yokota N, Yamaguchi H. In vitro antifungal activity of posaconazole against various pathogenic fungi. Int J Antimicrob Agents 2001;18(2):167–72.
66. Sun QN, Fothergill AW, McCarthy DI, et al. In vitro activities of posaconazole, itraconazole, voriconazole, amphotericin B, and fluconazole against 37 clinical isolates of zygomycetes. Antimicrob Agents Chemother 2002;46(5):1581–2.

67. Courtney R, Pai S, Laughlin M, et al. Pharmacokinetics, safety, and tolerability of oral posaconazole administered in single and multiple doses in healthy adults. Antimicrob Agents Chemother 2003;47(9):2788–95.
68. Krieter P, Flannery B, Musick T, et al. Disposition of posaconazole following single-dose oral administration in healthy subjects. Antimicrob Agents Chemother 2004;48(9):3543–51.
69. Lehrnbecher T, Attarbaschi A, Duerken M, et al. Posaconazole salvage treatment in paediatric patients: a multicentre survey. Eur J Clin Microbiol Infect Dis 2010;29(8):1043–5.
70. Krishna G, AbuTarif M, Xuan F, et al. Pharmacokinetics of oral posaconazole in neutropenic patients receiving chemotherapy for acute myelogenous leukemia or myelodysplastic syndrome. Pharmacotherapy 2008;28(10):1223–32.
71. Sucher AJ, Chahine EB, Balcer HE. Echinocandins: the newest class of antifungals. Ann Pharmacother 2009;43(10):1647–57.
72. Denning DW. Echinocandin antifungal drugs. Lancet 2003;362(9390):1142–51.
73. Hope WW, Mickiene D, Petraitis V, et al. The pharmacokinetics and pharmacodynamics of micafungin in experimental hematogenous Candida meningoencephalitis: implications for echinocandin therapy in neonates. J Infect Dis 2008;197(1):163–71.
74. Kang CI, Rouse MS, Mandrekar JN, et al. Anidulafungin treatment of candidal central nervous system infection in a murine model. Antimicrob Agents Chemother 2009;53(8):3576–8.
75. Tawara S, Ikeda F, Maki K, et al. In vitro activities of a new lipopeptide antifungal agent, FK463, against a variety of clinically important fungi. Antimicrob Agents Chemother 2000;44(1):57–62.
76. Hatano K, Morishita Y, Nakai T, et al. Antifungal mechanism of FK463 against Candida albicans and Aspergillus fumigatus. J Antibiot (Tokyo) 2002;55(2):219–22.
77. Infante-Lopez ME, Rojo-Conejo P. Micafungin for the treatment of neonatal invasive candidiasis. Rev Iberoam Micol 2009;26(1):56–61 [in Spanish].
78. Dupont BF, Lortholary O, Ostrosky-Zeichner L, et al. Treatment of candidemia and invasive candidiasis in the intensive care unit: post hoc analysis of a randomized, controlled trial comparing micafungin and liposomal amphotericin B. Crit Care 2009;13(5):R159.
79. Kuse ER, Chetchotisakd P, da Cunha CA, et al. Micafungin versus liposomal amphotericin B for candidaemia and invasive candidosis: a phase III randomised double-blind trial. Lancet 2007;369(9572):1519–27.
80. Queiroz-Telles F, Berezin E, Leverger G, et al. Micafungin versus liposomal amphotericin B for pediatric patients with invasive candidiasis: substudy of a randomized double-blind trial. Pediatr Infect Dis J 2008;27(9):820–6.
81. van Burik JA, Ratanatharathorn V, Stepan DE, et al. Micafungin versus fluconazole for prophylaxis against invasive fungal infections during neutropenia in patients undergoing hematopoietic stem cell transplantation. Clin Infect Dis 2004;39(10):1407–16.
82. Pappas PG, Rotstein CM, Betts RF, et al. Micafungin versus caspofungin for treatment of candidemia and other forms of invasive candidiasis. Clin Infect Dis 2007;45(7):883–93.
83. Groll AH, Mickiene D, Petraitis V, et al. Compartmental pharmacokinetics and tissue distribution of the antifungal echinocandin lipopeptide micafungin (FK463) in rabbits. Antimicrob Agents Chemother 2001;45(12):3322–7.

84. Yamada N, Kumada K, Kishino S, et al. Distribution of micafungin in the tissue fluids of patients with invasive fungal infections. J Infect Chemother 2011; 17(5):731–4.

85. Seibel NL, Schwartz C, Arrieta A, et al. Safety, tolerability, and pharmacokinetics of micafungin (FK463) in febrile neutropenic pediatric patients. Antimicrob Agents Chemother 2005;49(8):3317–24.

86. Hope WW, Seibel NL, Schwartz CL, et al. Population pharmacokinetics of micafungin in pediatric patients and implications for antifungal dosing. Antimicrob Agents Chemother 2007;51(10):3714–9.

87. Yanni SB, Smith PB, Benjamin DK Jr, et al. Higher clearance of micafungin in neonates compared with adults: role of age-dependent micafungin serum binding. Biopharm Drug Dispos 2011;32(4):222–32.

88. Smith PB, Walsh TJ, Hope W, et al. Pharmacokinetics of an elevated dosage of micafungin in premature neonates. Pediatr Infect Dis J 2009;28(5):412–5.

89. Benjamin DK Jr, Smith PB, Arrieta A, et al. Safety and pharmacokinetics of repeat-dose micafungin in young infants. Clin Pharmacol Ther 2010;87(1):93–9.

90. Hope WW, Smith PB, Arrieta A, et al. Population pharmacokinetics of micafungin in neonates and young infants. Antimicrob Agents Chemother 2010;54(6): 2633–7.

91. King KY, Edwards MS, Word BM. Hepatitis associated with micafungin use in a preterm infant. J Perinatol 2009;29(4):320–2.

92. Heresi GP, Gerstmann DR, Reed MD, et al. The pharmacokinetics and safety of micafungin, a novel echinocandin, in premature infants. Pediatr Infect Dis J 2006;25(12):1110–5.

93. Natarajan G, Lulic-Botica M, Aranda JV. Refractory neonatal candidemia and high-dose micafungin pharmacotherapy. J Perinatol 2009;29(11):738–43.

94. Pfaller MA, Diekema DJ, Boyken L, et al. Effectiveness of anidulafungin in eradicating Candida species in invasive candidiasis. Antimicrob Agents Chemother 2005;49(11):4795–7.

95. Vazquez JA, Schranz JA, Clark K, et al. A phase 2, open-label study of the safety and efficacy of intravenous anidulafungin as a treatment for azole-refractory mucosal candidiasis. J Acquir Immune Defic Syndr 2008;48(3):304–9.

96. Reboli AC, Rotstein C, Pappas PG, et al. Anidulafungin versus fluconazole for invasive candidiasis. N Engl J Med 2007;356(24):2472–82.

97. Benjamin DK Jr, Driscoll T, Seibel NL, et al. Safety and pharmacokinetics of intravenous anidulafungin in children with neutropenia at high risk for invasive fungal infections. Antimicrob Agents Chemother 2006;50(2):632–8.

98. Dowell JA, Knebel W, Ludden T, et al. Population pharmacokinetic analysis of anidulafungin, an echinocandin antifungal. J Clin Pharmacol 2004;44(6): 590–8.

99. Dowell JA, Stogniew M, Krause D, et al. Anidulafungin does not require dosage adjustment in subjects with varying degrees of hepatic or renal impairment. J Clin Pharmacol 2007;47(4):461–70.

100. Damle B, Stogniew M, Dowell J. Pharmacokinetics and tissue distribution of anidulafungin in rats. Antimicrob Agents Chemother 2008;52(7):2673–6.

101. Cohen-Wolkowiez M, Benjamin DK Jr, Piper L, et al. Safety and pharmacokinetics of multiple-dose anidulafungin in infants and neonates. Clin Pharmacol Ther 2011;89(5):702–7.

102. Leitner JM, Meyer B, Fuhrmann V, et al. Multiple-dose pharmacokinetics of anidulafungin during continuous venovenous haemofiltration. J Antimicrob Chemother 2011;66(4):880–4.

103. Vazquez JA, Lynch M, Boikov D, et al. In vitro activity of a new pneumocandin antifungal, L-743,872, against azole-susceptible and -resistant Candida species. Antimicrob Agents Chemother 1997;41(7):1612–4.

104. Arathoon EG, Gotuzzo E, Noriega LM, et al. Randomized, double-blind, multicenter study of caspofungin versus amphotericin B for treatment of oropharyngeal and esophageal candidiases. Antimicrob Agents Chemother 2002;46(2):451–7.

105. Villanueva A, Arathoon EG, Gotuzzo E, et al. A randomized double-blind study of caspofungin versus amphotericin for the treatment of candidal esophagitis. Clin Infect Dis 2001;33(9):1529–35.

106. Stone JA, Holland SD, Wickersham PJ, et al. Single- and multiple-dose pharmacokinetics of caspofungin in healthy men. Antimicrob Agents Chemother 2002;46(3):739–45.

107. Sable CA, Nguyen BY, Chodakewitz JA, et al. Safety and tolerability of caspofungin acetate in the treatment of fungal infections. Transpl Infect Dis 2002;4(1):25–30.

108. Mistry GC, Migoya E, Deutsch PJ, et al. Single- and multiple-dose administration of caspofungin in patients with hepatic insufficiency: implications for safety and dosing recommendations. J Clin Pharmacol 2007;47(8):951–61.

109. Walsh TJ, Adamson PC, Seibel NL, et al. Pharmacokinetics, safety, and tolerability of caspofungin in children and adolescents. Antimicrob Agents Chemother 2005;49(11):4536–45.

110. Saez-Llorens X, Macias M, Maiya P, et al. Pharmacokinetics and safety of caspofungin in neonates and infants less than 3 months of age. Antimicrob Agents Chemother 2009;53(3):869–75.

111. Cesaro S, Giacchino M, Locatelli F, et al. Safety and efficacy of a caspofungin-based combination therapy for treatment of proven or probable aspergillosis in pediatric hematological patients. BMC Infect Dis 2007;7:28.

112. Merlin E, Galambrun C, Ribaud P, et al. Efficacy and safety of caspofungin therapy in children with invasive fungal infections. Pediatr Infect Dis J 2006;25(12):1186–8.

113. Zaoutis TE, Jafri HS, Huang LM, et al. A prospective, multicenter study of caspofungin for the treatment of documented Candida or Aspergillus infections in pediatric patients. Pediatrics 2009;123(3):877–84.

114. Maertens JA, Madero L, Reilly AF, et al. A randomized, double-blind, multicenter study of caspofungin versus liposomal amphotericin B for empiric antifungal therapy in pediatric patients with persistent fever and neutropenia. Pediatr Infect Dis J 2010;29(5):415–20.

115. Neely M, Jafri HS, Seibel N, et al. Pharmacokinetics and safety of caspofungin in older infants and toddlers. Antimicrob Agents Chemother 2009;53(4):1450–6.

116. Natarajan G, Lulic-Botica M, Rongkavilit C, et al. Experience with caspofungin in the treatment of persistent fungemia in neonates. J Perinatol 2005;25(12):770–7.

117. Healy CM, Baker CJ, Zaccaria E, et al. Impact of fluconazole prophylaxis on incidence and outcome of invasive candidiasis in a neonatal intensive care unit. J Pediatr 2005;147(2):166–71.

Metoclopramide, H$_2$ Blockers, and Proton Pump Inhibitors: Pharmacotherapy for Gastroesophageal Reflux in Neonates

William F. Malcolm, MD, C. Michael Cotten, MD, MHS*

KEYWORDS

• Gastroesophageal reflux • Neonate • Proton pump inhibitor
• H$_2$ blocker • Metoclopramide

Gastroesophageal reflux (GER) is defined as the retrograde movement of stomach contents into the esophagus. Pharmacotherapy aimed at interfering with this physiologic process and potentially reducing the negative sequelae that providers often attribute to GER consists primarily of drugs that increase the viscosity of feeds, reduce stomach acidity, or improve gut motility. Medications used to treat clinical signs thought to be from GER, such as apnea, bradycardia, or feeding intolerance, are among the most commonly prescribed medications in neonatal intensive care units (NICUs) in the United States.[1]

GER is a normal, developmentally appropriate process that occurs during infancy. Reflux occurs with at least one feed daily among 50% of infants younger than 3 months.[2] Most infants tolerate and outgrow this process without the need for medications.[3] However, when GER is thought to be associated with complications (eg, pain, respiratory disease, poor growth), it is described as *gastroesophageal reflux disease* (GERD) and often compels medical providers to prescribe treatment. In the NICU, where most infants at some point encounter physical discomfort, respiratory difficulties, and problems with growth, many clinicians attribute these signs to GERD. In fact, 25% of extremely low-birth-weight infants are discharged home on medications used to treat GERD; this number increases to nearly 50% if the infant has a prolonged NICU hospitalization.[4] The natural history of GER in infants is that it improves with time. Thus, clinical trials must take into account the developmental maturation of infants,

Division of Neonatal-Perinatal Medicine, Department of Pediatrics, Duke University, Durham, NC, USA
* Corresponding author.
E-mail address: Charles.Cotten@duke.edu

Clin Perinatol 39 (2012) 99–109
doi:10.1016/j.clp.2011.12.015
0095-5108/12/$ – see front matter © 2012 Elsevier Inc. All rights reserved.
perinatology.theclinics.com

especially for preterm infants in the NICU, whose pulmonary status, gastrointestinal tract, and nervous systems all undergo significant maturation, impacting their feeding pattern and potential tolerance to reflux events.

When discussing pharmacotherapy for GERD in neonates, the difficulties in accurately diagnosing the condition in this population must be addressed. Several investigators have explored a cause-and-effect clinical relationship between GERD and apnea, bradycardia, chronic lung disease, or behavior in preterm infants without finding a definitive correlation.[5–10] Di Fiore and colleagues[9] showed that fewer than 3% of all cardiorespiratory events in preterm infants are preceded by a reflux episode, and that reflux did not prolong or increase the severity of the event. Furthermore, the use of diagnostic tools considered to be the standard approach in older children with symptoms of GERD is controversial in this population. Radiographic testing, such as an upper gastrointestinal series or nuclear medicine scintigraphy, may appropriately describe anatomic risks, detect aspiration, or quantify gastric emptying; however, the results may not accurately reflect the clinical picture because testing is not performed under physiologic conditions. Continuous esophageal monitoring using pH probe with or without impedance measurements may also be difficult to interpret in the smallest babies with the buffering of frequent or continuous feeds, lack of standard reference values, and unavailable technology in many NICUs. Thus, without a definitive diagnostic test and evaluation tool, efficacy studies of therapeutic interventions for GERD in neonates are challenging.

Not only is GERD poorly diagnosed in preterm infants but also no standard treatment approach exists in this population. As written, the North American Society for Pediatric Gastroenterology and Nutrition (NASPGHAN) clinical practice guidelines for the evaluation and treatment of infants and children with suspected GER are "not intended to be used for premature infants."[11] This lack of a standardized approach for diagnosing and treating GERD in preterm infants is well demonstrated by the extreme variability among centers regarding the use of medications for treating GERD in extremely low-birth-weight infants. Among infants discharged home from NICUs participating in the NICHD Neonatal Research Network at a postmenstrual age of less than 42 weeks, the center range for treatment with antireflux medications (acid reducers or prokinetics) was 2% to 46%, compared with 22% to 90% among infants discharged from the hospital at an age greater than 42 weeks.[4]

THICKENING AGENTS

Feed thickeners are commonly used in both hospital and community settings to reduce reflux episodes with or without aspiration. Although most common thickeners such as baby cereal are considered food products, some commercial thickeners are sold in pharmacies either over the counter or by prescription. Systematic reviews and meta-analyses of thickening agents used to treat GERD in infants show reduction in regurgitation and emesis but no significant reduction in reflux indices.[12,13] A variety of thickening agents were included in the reviews, with no particular thickener proving to be more effective. More recent studies using combined pH-impedance monitoring showed a reduction in non–acid reflux episodes in term infants receiving thickened formula; however, further studies showed no difference in reflux episodes in preterm infants fed thickened human milk.[14,15]

Alginates

Gaviscon® Infant contains sodium and magnesium alginate and is used primarily as a thickener, as opposed to the Gaviscon® more commonly used in adults, which also contains sodium and potassium bicarbonate and also acts as an antacid. Used primarily outside of the United States, alginates have been shown to be effective in reducing the number, duration, and height of acid reflux episodes in term and preterm infants.[16,17] Caution must be taken, however, in preterm infants, because this treatment has been shown to be associated with intestinal obstruction, and the extra sodium may be a concern.

SimplyThick®

Because thickening of breast milk with starch additives is ineffective in reducing GERD in infants, a xanthan gum product (SimplyThick®) has been used as a nondigestible complex carbohydrate additive to evenly thicken human milk. In May 2011, however, the U.S. Food and Drug Administration (FDA) advised health care professionals that the product not be used in preterm infants because of an association with necrotizing enterocolitis, and a voluntary recall followed shortly thereafter. The National Institute of Child Health and Human Development (NICHD) Neonatal Research Network and FDA continue to collect data regarding this association.

MOTILITY AGENTS

Prokinetics are medications used to increase gastrointestinal motility, leaving less liquid in the stomach to reflux proximally into the esophagus. Prokinetic agents act primarily to increase acetylcholine concentrations via the 5-HT$_4$ receptor mechanism, thereby promoting intestinal peristalsis and increasing lower esophageal sphincter tone. This mechanism is also the reason for their adverse side effect profile.

Cisapride

Cisapride is an effective 5-HT$_4$ agonist that has nonspecific affinity to enteric serotonin receptors and, therefore, increases the risk for cardiac and neurologic side effects. Because of these complications, the drug was taken off the market in the United States when it was found to increase the risk of long QT syndrome, predisposing infants to cardiac arrhythmias.[18,19]

Metoclopramide

Metoclopramide binds dopamine D2 receptors, acting as a receptor antagonist, in addition to being a mixed 5-HT$_3$ antagonist and 5-HT$_4$ agonist, with a combined anti-emetic and prokinetic effect. Its use in the NICU dramatically increased in 2000, when cisapride was taken off the market.[1,20] Unlike many medications used in neonates, pharmacokinetic studies performed in preterm infants show a developmental dose dependency and a need for higher dosing in infants younger than 31 weeks.[21]

A paucity of large, well-conducted trials have evaluated the safety and efficacy of metoclopramide in preterm or term infants. Several studies have suggested that metoclopramide is effective in reducing gastric residuals in preterm infants, although its effect on GER is less clear.[22–25] Again, this result may be from poor ability to diagnose and monitor GER as much as it relates to a drug effect. A systematic review of metoclopramide for the treatment of GER in neonates concluded that the literature provides insufficient evidence to support its use in infants.[26] A Cochrane review including older children showed metoclopramide to be effective in reducing daily symptoms of GER and reflux index by physiologic measurements, although its use was associated with increased side effects.[27]

The potential neurologic side effects of metoclopramide are well documented and warrant serious consideration when prescribing long-term treatment for infants with

GER. The drug acts on D2 receptors in the central nervous system, leading to adverse neurologic effects. Irritability, restlessness, drowsiness, apnea, emesis, and dystonia have all been reported in infants receiving metoclopramide.[28–30] The risk of extrapyramidal effects with high dose or prolonged use, including the potentially irreversible movement disorder known as *tardive dyskinesia*, prompted the FDA to issue a black box warning in 2009.[31,32]

A common use for metoclopramide in the NICU may also occur on the maternal side, improving lactation by increasing prolactin concentrations through central dopamine receptor antagonist response. Likewise, neonates have been reported to have a similar response with galactorrhea and gynecomastia.[33]

Erythromycin

Erythromycin is a macrolide antibiotic that also has a gastrointestinal motility effect through acting as a motilin receptor agonist. Motilin is a peptide that stimulates gut propulsion through phase III migratory motor complexes and nonpropagating contractions. Some studies suggest the absence of motilin receptor activity before 32 weeks' gestation, yet improved feeding tolerance has been shown in these younger infants.[34] Lower doses are usually prescribed when given as a prokinetic agent; however, safety and efficacy have not been established for prolonged use in neonates with GERD. Most studies of erythromycin use in preterm infants aim to evaluate gastric emptying and feeding intolerance. A systematic review of erythromycin evaluating effectiveness in promoting motility and feeding tolerance in preterm infants, in addition to assessing its safety, concluded that the drug may help establish full enteral feeds, and no significant short-term adverse events were associated with its use, although insufficient evidence prevented definitive recommendation.[35] A randomized controlled study of low-dose erythromycin use in preterm infants showed improved reflux over the treatment period, as determined with pH probe; however, improvement was shown in both erythromycin and placebo groups, and no statistically significant differences were found between groups in terms of GER or time to full feeds.[36]

Erythromycin use has been associated with the development of hypertrophic pyloric stenosis in term and preterm infants. Although more commonly seen in infants receiving antibiotic doses of erythromycin, case reports have documented pyloric stenosis in extremely low-birth-weight infants receiving low-dose therapy for feeding intolerance.[37] Clinical trials and meta-analyses have not reported pyloric stenosis as a potential side effect when erythromycin is used for this indication in preterm infants. Hypertrophic pyloric stenosis has also been described in breastfeeding infants of mothers undergoing erythromycin therapy.[38]

Erythromycin is metabolized by enzymes of the cytochrome P450 system, as an inhibitor of CYP3A. Therefore, the potential for interactions and altering drug concentrations for the many medications associated with this system for metabolism must be considered. Erythromycin use has also been associated with a prolonged QT interval and cardiac arrhythmias, especially when used in combination with other CYP3A inhibitors.[39] Furthermore, prolonged use of any antibiotic warrants concern for antimicrobial resistance and interference with the establishment of healthy gut flora.

Domperidone

Domperidone is an antidopaminergic medication used for nausea, vomiting, and poor gastrointestinal motility. Several small studies have shown improved reflux episodes and clinical symptoms in children with GER taking domperidone compared with placebo or metoclopramide.[40–42] A systematic review of domperidone use in children concluded that evidence of its efficacy is insufficient to recommend its use considering the benign nature of GER and the potential risk of side effects.[43] The North American Society for Pediatric Gastroenterology , Hepatology and Nutrition (NASPGHAN) Working Group also concluded that its effectiveness in infants and children is unproven.[11]

Unlike metoclopramide, domperidone is not believed to cross the blood–brain barrier, and therefore is less likely to cause the same neurologic side effects. However, a few case reports have linked its use to extrapyramidal adverse effects.[44] Domperidone is currently not approved for prescription in the United States because of additional concerns of QT prolongation and hypernatremia.

GASTRIC ACID REDUCERS

Gastric acid suppression in infants is primarily accomplished by the use of histamine2 (H_2) receptor antagonists and proton pump inhibitors (PPIs). Through decreasing stomach acidity, these medications are believed to decrease pain and some of the suspected complications of GERD in infants, including apnea, respiratory disease, upper airway edema, esophagitis, and feeding difficulties. In adults, acid suppression has been shown to be beneficial in Barrett's esophagus or erosive disease, often requiring long-term treatment because GERD is considered to be ongoing in this population. In infants, especially preterm, many have suggested that the acid-producing parietal cells are immature, and that acid reflux contributes less to the suspected comorbidities than nonacidic liquid reflux. Also, the frequent and continuous feedings seen in the NICU constantly buffer the acidity of stomach contents, making esophageal reflux less likely to be acidic. Several studies have shown that most reflux episodes in infants are nonacidic, and one study using combined pH-impedance monitoring supported this theory in showing that postprandial reflux is less acidic in preterm infants.[45] Nonetheless, some infants experience reflux events with an esophageal pH measuring less than four; however, whether a true link exists between reflux acidity and the complications described earlier remains a matter of debate.

Gastric acidity plays an important role in the immune system and selective intestinal colonization; therefore, use of acid suppression therapy may increase risk for infection. Both H_2 receptor antagonists and PPIs have been shown to alter gastrointestinal flora directly through allowing for upper gastrointestinal tract colonization and indirectly through interfering with naturally occurring bacterial and fungal H^+-ATPase enzymes.[46] One study of infants being treated with ranitidine documented an increase in gastric colonization of bacteria and yeast, without showing a significant increase in infection.[47] A large, multicenter, retrospective study of H_2 receptor blocker use in very low-birth-weight infants showed an association with necrotizing enterocolitis.[48] Similarly, a large observational study of ranitidine use in the NICU was associated with an increased risk for late-onset sepsis, although a causal relationship could not be determined.[49] Several studies have examined acid suppression in the intensive care environment and shown an increased risk in ventilator-associated pneumonia, sepsis, and nasogastric tube colonization.[50–52]

Gastric acid suppression may also affect nutrition. Stomach acid is necessary for pepsin activation, thereby participating in protein metabolism. Other nutritional roles of gastric acidity include vitamin B_{12} and calcium absorption. Several studies in adults have raised the concern of poor bone density in the setting of long-term use of gastric acid reducers.[53–55] In preterm infants already at risk for osteopenia, this type of therapy warrants serious consideration. Lastly, decreasing stomach acidity may decrease the bioavailability and effect of other oral medications that require the normal low-pH environment for their effective absorption.

H₂ Receptor Antagonists

H_2 receptor antagonists block the H_2 receptor in gastric parietal cells, thereby decreasing hydrochloric acid secretion and reducing the effect of other acid-stimulating substances (eg, gastrin). H_2 blockers have traditionally been considered first-line treatment for suspected acid reflux in infants, and their use in the NICU primarily includes ranitidine, famotidine, and cimetidine.

Several studies in older children have documented improved esophageal acid exposure and esophagitis associated with H_2 blockers. In a blinded, randomized, controlled trial of cimetidine in 33 symptomatic children as young as 2 months, Cucchiara and colleagues[56] showed improved symptoms, as well as reduced acid exposure on pH probe and esophagitis on endoscopy. In a double-blinded randomized controlled trial, Orenstein and colleagues[57] studied famotidine in low and high doses in infants aged 1.3 to 10.5 months. Infants receiving either dose regimen had improved regurgitation compared with placebo, whereas those taking higher doses also had decreased crying time. However, several babies receiving the study drug showed signs of agitation and headache. NASPGHAN concluded that "H_2 receptor antagonists produce relief of symptoms and mucosal healing" in children with GERD.[11]

Wheatley and Kennedy[58] conducted a crossover trial of ranitidine and metoclopramide therapy in preterm infants with bradycardia events suspected to be caused by GERD. In this study, infants receiving medications actually had a significant increase in the number of bradycardiac events compared with those receiving placebo. Although the crossover design was able to account for normal developmental maturation of the infant, with both groups showing a decrease in bradycardia episodes over time, the correlation with reflux is debatable.

H_2 receptor antagonists have been reported to cause several other possible side effects. H_2 blockers have been found to have cardiovascular effects, including bradyarrhythmia, because of histamine receptors found in the heart.[59,60] Ranitidine has also been noted to cause reversible bone marrow suppression and central nervous system side effects, including headache.[61] Histamine blockers, especially cimetidine, are inhibitors of several isoenzymes of the cytochrome P450 system, and interactions with other medications metabolized similarly must be considered.

PPIs

PPIs are effective gastric acid reducers through inactivation of the hydrogen/potassium adenosine triphosphatase pump, responsible for transporting hydrogen ions across the parietal cell membrane into the stomach. Therefore, PPIs are considered more potent than H_2 blockers in increasing gastric pH through actually decreasing the volume of gastric acid secretions. FDA-approved drugs in this class of acid suppressors include omeprazole, pantoprazole, lansoprazole, rabeprazole, and esomeprazole. Although no PPIs are currently labeled for use in infants younger than 1 year, their use in this population is increasing given their proven effect in older children and adults with reflux esophagitis.[62] Omeprazole and lansoprazole are the most commonly used and best-studied PPIs in infants.

Several studies have shown improvements with omeprazole therapy on pH probe or endoscopy in children with GERD with or without esophagitis, especially when refractory to histamine receptor antagonists. In a double-blinded, randomized, controlled trial, Cucchiara and colleagues[63] showed omeprazole to be effective in reducing symptoms, esophageal acid exposure on pH probe, and endoscopic signs of esophagitis in children aged 6 months to 13 years with GERD refractory to ranitidine. However, two randomized controlled trials of omeprazole use in preterm and term infants showed no improvement in GERD symptoms compared with placebo, although both showed improved esophageal acidity on pH probe.[64,65] Lansoprazole was more effective than hydrolyzed formula in reducing GERD symptoms in another study.[66] A recent systematic review concluded that PPIs are not effective in reducing GERD symptoms in infants, although they are effective in reducing gastric acidity in all age groups.[67] Two placebo-controlled trials were designed to account for a developmental maturation effect, showing no difference between lansoprazole or omeprazole and placebo in reflux symptoms, although both groups showed symptomatic improvement with time.

Evidence is lacking to ensure safety, with most studies involving infants showing an increase in adverse events associated with PPI therapy compared with placebo. Like other acid suppressors, PPIs may put infants at risk for infection. One study cited an increase in serious adverse events, including lower respiratory tract infections, in infants receiving lansoprazole treatment.[68] PPIs have also been associated with infectious diarrhea, including *Clostridium difficile*, with a greater risk compared with H_2 receptor antagonists.[69]

Both PPIs and histamine blockers may interfere with calcium absorption and bone health. Recently, the FDA issued a safety alert and class labeling change for PPIs, citing data suggesting an increased fracture risk in adults receiving long-term therapy. Long-term safety studies of PPI use in infants and children are not available, although its use in infants at risk for vitamin D deficiency and preterm infants at risk for osteopenia of prematurity warrants consideration.

SUMMARY

The use of medications for suspected GERD in the NICU continues to be common, without definitive evidence for accurate diagnostic tests or effective and safe treatment strategies in these at-risk infants. No drugs currently used for GERD in infants, especially those born prematurely, are proven to be safe and effective. When studying infants with symptoms of GERD in this population, most clinical trials use subjective entry criteria and evaluation tools, or use primary clinical end points that have been shown to be poorly associated with GERD, such as apnea, bradycardia, or irritability. Furthermore, few studies take into account the normal developmental maturation that occurs in neonates, because both physiologic GER and the many signs and symptoms suggestive of GERD that occur in the NICU will improve over time.

What is clear is that infants receiving medications for the treatment of GERD experience a significant increase in adverse events, with some being serious or irreversible. What remains unknown is the long-term impact that some of these medications have on overall gut health, the immune system, and a developing nervous system.

Supportive measures, such as positioning or removal of nasogastric tubes, have been documented as effective measures for reducing GER in infants. For infants apparently refractory to nonpharmacologic measures, other diagnoses must be seriously considered and evaluated before medical therapy is prescribed. If the clinician initiates pharmacotherapy for GERD in the NICU, ongoing evaluation and documentation of clinical effect should occur. If the infant shows little improvement after a trial period, the medication should be discontinued, whereas if an improvement is documented, then a short-term course of therapy should be planned and a trial off the medication considered after a set period, because the condition will naturally improve and long-term safety data are lacking.

REFERENCES

1. Clark RH, Bloom BT, Spitzer AR, et al. Reported medication use in the neonatal intensive care unit: data from a large national data set. Pediatrics 2006;117(6): 1979–87.
2. Nelson SP, Chen EH, Syniar GM, et al. Prevalence of symptoms of gastroesophageal reflux during infancy: a pediatric practice-based survey. Arch Pediatr Adolesc Med 1997;151:569–72.
3. Martin AJ, Pratt N, Kennedy JD, et al. Natural history and familial relationships of infant spilling to 9 years of age. Pediatrics 2002;109:1061–7.
4. Malcolm WF, Gantz M, Martin RJ, et al. National Institute of Child Health and Human Development Neonatal Research Network. Use of medications for gastroesophageal reflux at discharge among extremely low birth weight infants. Pediatrics 2008;121(1):22–7.
5. Peter CS, Sprodowski N, Bohnhorst B, et al. Gastroesophageal reflux and apnea of prematurity: no temporal relationship. Pediatrics 2002;109:8–11.
6. Barrington KJ, Tan K, Rich W. Apnea at discharge and gastro-esophageal reflux in the preterm infant. J Perinatol 2002;22:8–11.
7. Molloy EJ, Di Fiore JM, Martin RJ. Does gastroesophageal reflux cause apnea in preterm infants? Biol Neonate 2005;87:254–61.
8. Kimball AL, Carlton DP. Gastroesophageal reflux medications in the treatment of apnea in premature infants. J Pediatr 2001;138:355–60.
9. Di Fiore J, Arko M, Herynk B, et al. Characterization of cardiorespiratory events following gastroesophageal reflux in preterm infants. J Perinatol 2010;10:683–7.
10. Snel A, Barnett CP, Cresp TL, et al. Behavior and gastroesophageal reflux in the premature neonate. J Pediatr Gastroenterol Nutr 2000;30:18–21.
11. Rudolph CD, Mazur LJ, Liptak GS, et al. Guidelines for evaluation and treatment of gastroesophageal reflux in infants and children: recommendations of the North American Society for Pediatric Gastroenterology and Nutrition. J Pediatr Gastroenterol Nutr 2001;32(Suppl 2):S1–31.
12. Horvath A, Dziechciarz P, Szajewska H. The effect of thickened-feed interventions on gastroesophageal reflux in infants: systematic review and meta-analysis of randomized, controlled trials. Pediatrics 2008;122(6):e1268–77.
13. Craig WR, Hanlon-Dearman A, Sinclair C, et al. Metoclopramide, thickened feedings, and positioning for gastro-oesophageal reflux in children under two years. Cochrane Database Syst Rev 2004;4:CD003502.
14. Wenzl TG, Schneider S, Scheele F, et al. Effects of thickened feeding on gastroesophageal reflux in infants: a placebo-controlled crossover study using intraluminal impedance. Pediatrics 2003;111(4 Pt 1):e355–9.
15. Corvaglia L, Ferlini M, Rotatori R, et al. Starch thickening of human milk is ineffective in reducing the gastroesophageal reflux in preterm infants: a crossover study using intraluminal impedance. J Pediatr 2006;148(2):265–8.
16. Miller S. Comparison of the efficacy and safety of a new aluminum-free paediatric alginate preparation and placebo in infants with recurrent gastro-oesophageal reflux. Curr Med Res Opin 1999;15(3):160–8.
17. Corvaglia L, Aceti A, Mariani E, et al. The efficacy of sodium alginate (Gaviscon) for the treatment of gastro-oesophageal reflux in preterm infants. Aliment Pharmacol Ther 2011;33(4):466–70.

18. Henney JE. Withdrawal of troglitazone and cisapride. JAMA 2000;283:2228.
19. Dubin A, Kikkert M, Mirmiran M, et al. Cisapride associated with QTc prolongation in very low birth weight preterm infants. Pediatrics 2001;107(6):1313–6.
20. Du W, Warrier I, Tutag Lehr V, et al. Changing patterns of drug utilization in a neonatal intensive care population. Am J Perinatol 2006;23(5):279–85.
21. Kearns GL, van den Anker JN, Reed MD, et al. Pharmacokinetics of metoclopramide in neonates. J Clin Pharmacol 1998;38(2):122–8.
22. Hyman PE, Abrams C, Dubois A. Effect of metoclopramide and bethanechol on gastric emptying in infants. Pediatr Res 1985;19:1029–32.
23. Hyman PE, Abrams CE, Dubois A. Gastric emptying in infants: response to metoclopramide depends on the underlying condition. J Pediatr Gastroenterol Nutr 1988;7:181–4.
24. Kearns GL, Butler HL, Lane JK, et al. Metoclopramide pharmacokinetics and pharmacodynamics in infants with gastroesophageal reflux. J Pediatr Gastroenterol Nutr 1988;7:823–9.
25. Harlev D, Mimouni F, Dollberg S. A clinical pilot trial of metoclopramide therapy for gastric residuals in preterm infants. Acta Paediatr 2007;96(8): 1239–41.
26. Hibbs AM, Lorch SA. Metoclopramide for the treatment of gastroesophageal reflux disease in infants: a systematic review. Pediatrics 2006;118(2):746–52.
27. Craig WR, Hanlon-Dearman A, Sinclair C, et al. Metoclopramide, thickened feedings, and positioning for gastro-oesophageal reflux in children under two years. Cochrane Database Syst Rev 2010;5:CD003502.
28. Hyams JS, Leichtner AM, Zamett LO, et al. Effect of metoclopramide on prolonged intraesophageal pH testing in infants with gastroesophageal reflux. J Pediatr Gastroenterol Nutr 1986;5:716–20.
29. Leung AK, Lai PC. Use of metoclopramide for the treatment of gastroesophageal reflux in infants and children. Curr Ther Res Clin Exp 1984;36:911–5.
30. Machida HM, Forbes DA, Gall DG, et al. Metoclopramide in gastroesophageal reflux of infancy. J Pediatr 1988;112:483–7.
31. Shaffer D, Butterfield M, Pamer C, et al. Tardive dyskinesia risks and metoclopramide use before and after U.S. market withdrawal of cisapride. J Am Pharm Assoc (Wash DC) 2004;44:661–5.
32. Mejia NI, Jankovic J. Metoclopramide-induced tardive dyskinesia in an infant. Mov Disord 2005;20:86–9.
33. Madani S, Tolia V. Gynecomastia with metoclopramide use in pediatric patients. J Clin Gastroenterol 1997;24:79–81.
34. Ng PC, So KW, Fung KS, et al. Randomised controlled study of oral erythromycin for treatment of gastrointestinal dysmotility in preterm infants. Arch Dis Child Fetal Neonatal Ed 2001;84(3):F177–82.
35. Ng E, Shah VS. Erythromycin for the prevention and treatment of feeding intolerance in preterm infants. Cochrane Database Syst Rev 2008;3:CD001815.
36. Ng SC, Gomez JM, Rajadurai VS, et al. Establishing enteral feeding in preterm infants with feeding intolerance: a randomized controlled study of low-dose erythromycin. J Pediatr Gastroenterol Nutr 2003;37(5):554–8.
37. Shoji H, Suganuma H, Daigo M, et al. Hypertrophic pyloric stenosis in monoovular extremely preterm twins after use of erythromycin. Pediatr Int 2008; 50(5):701–2.
38. Mahon BE, Rosenman MB, Kleiman MB. Maternal and infant use of erythromycin and other macrolide antibiotics as risk factors for infantile hypertrophic pyloric stenosis. J Pediatr 2001;139(3):380–4.

39. Ray WA, Murray KT, Meredith S, et al. Oral erythromycin and the risk of sudden death from cardiac causes. N Engl J Med 2004;351:1089–96.
40. Bines J, Quinlan JE, Treves S, et al. Efficacy of domperidone in infants and children with gastro-oesophageal reflux. J Pediatr Gastroenterol Nutr 1992;14: 400–5.
41. De Loore I, Van Ravenstein, Ameryckx L. Domperidone drops in the symptomatic treatment of chronic paediatric vomiting and regurgitation: a comparison with metoclopramide. Postgrad Med J 1979;55:40–2.
42. Grill BB, Hillemeier C, Semeraro LA, et al. Effects of domperidone therapy on symptoms and upper gastrointestinal motility in infants with gastroesophageal reflux. J Pediatr 1985;106(2):311–6.
43. Pritchard DS, Baber N, Stephenson T. Should domperidone be used for the treatment of gastro-oesophageal reflux in children? Systematic review of randomized controlled trials in children aged 1 month to 11 years old. Br J Clin Pharmacol 2005;59(6):725–9.
44. Franckx J, Noel P. Acute extrapyramidal dysfunction after domperidone administration. Helv Paediatr Acta 1984;39:285–8.
45. Slocum C, Arko M, Di Fiore J, et al. Apnea, bradycardia and desaturation in preterm infants before and after feeding. J Perinatol 2009;29(3):209–12.
46. Williams C. Occurrence and significance of gastric colonization during acid-inhibitory therapy. Best Pract Res Clin Gastroenterol 2001;15(3):511–21.
47. Cothran DS, Borowitz SM, Sutphen JL, et al. Alteration of normal gastric flora in neonates receiving ranitidine. J Perinatol 1997;17(5):383–8.
48. Guillet R, Stoll BJ, Cotten CM, et al. National Institute of Child Health and Human Development Neonatal Research Network. Association of H2-blocker therapy and higher incidence of necrotizing enterocolitis in very low birth weight infants. Pediatrics 2006;117(2):e137–42.
49. Bianconi S, Gudavalli M, Sutija VG, et al. Ranitidine and late-onset sepsis in the neonatal intensive care unit. J Perinat Med 2007;35(2):147–50.
50. Messori A, Trippoli S, Vaiani M, et al. Bleeding and pneumonia in intensive care patients given ranitidine and sucralfate for prevention of stress ulcer: meta-analysis of randomized controlled trials. BMJ 2000;321:1103.
51. Mehall JR. Prospective study of the incidence and complications of bacterial contamination of enteral feeding in neonates. J Pediatr Surg 2002;37(8):1177–82.
52. Levy J. Enteral nutrition: an increasingly recognized cause of nosocomial bloodstream infection. Infect Control Hosp Epidemiol 1989;10:395–7.
53. Yang YX, Lewis JD, Epstein S, et al. Long-term proton pump inhibitor therapy and risk of hip fracture. JAMA 2006;296:2947–53.
54. Gray SL, LaCroix AZ, Larson J, et al. Proton pump inhibitor use, hip fracture, and change in bone mineral density in postmenopausal women: results from the Women's Health Initiative. Arch Intern Med 2010;170:765–71.
55. Kaye JA, Jick H. Proton pump inhibitor use and risk of hip fractures in patients without major risk factors. Pharmacotherapy 2008;28:951–9.
56. Cucchiara S, Staiano A, Romaniello G, et al. Antacids and cimetidine treatment for gastro-oesophageal reflux and peptic oesophagitis. Arch Dis Child 1984; 59(9):842–7.
57. Orenstein SR, Shalaby TM, Devandry SN, et al. Famotidine for infant gastro-oesophageal reflux: a multi-centre, randomized, placebo-controlled, withdrawal trial. Aliment Pharmacol Ther 2003;17(9):1097–107.
58. Wheatley E, Kennedy KA. Cross-over trial of treatment for bradycardia attributed to gastroesophageal reflux in preterm infants. J Pediatr 2009;155(4):516–21.

59. Nault MA, Milne B, Parlow JL. Effects of the selective H1 and H2 histamine receptor antagonists loratadine and ranitidine on autonomic control of the heart. Anesthesiology 2002;96:336–41.
60. Ooie T, Saikawa T, Hara M, et al. H_2-blocker modulates heart rate variability. Heart Vessels 1999;14:137–42.
61. Amos RJ, Kirk B, Amess JA, et al. Bone marrow hypoplasia during intensive care: bone marrow culture studies implicating ranitidine in the suppression of haemopoiesis. Hum Toxicol 1987;6(6):503–6.
62. Barron JJ, Tan H, Spalding J, et al. Proton pump inhibitor utilization patterns in infants. J Pediatr Gastroenterol Nutr 2007;45(4):421–7.
63. Cucchiara S, Minella R, Iervolino C, et al. Omeprazole and high dose ranitidine in the treatment of refractory reflux oesophagitis. Arch Dis Child 1993;69(6):655–9.
64. Omari TI, Haslam RR, Lundborg P, et al. Effect of omeprazole on acid gastroesophageal reflux and gastric acidity in preterm infants with pathological acid reflux. J Pediatr Gastroenterol Nutr 2007;44(1):41–4.
65. Moore DJ, Tao BS, Lines DR, et al. Double-blind placebo-controlled trial of omeprazole in irritable infants with gastroesophageal reflux. J Pediatr 2003;143(2):219–23.
66. Khoshoo V, Dhume P. Clinical response to 2 dosing regimens of lansoprazole in infants with gastroesophageal reflux. J Pediatr Gastroenterol Nutr 2008;46(3):352–4.
67. van der Pol RJ, Smits MJ, van Wijk MP, et al. Efficacy of proton-pump inhibitors in children with gastroesophageal reflux disease: a systematic review. Pediatrics 2011;127(5):925–35.
68. Orenstein SR, Hassall E, Furmaga-Jablonska W, et al. Multicenter, double-blind, randomized, placebo-controlled trial assessing the efficacy and safety of proton pump inhibitor lansoprazole in infants with symptoms of gastroesophageal reflux disease. J Pediatr 2009;154(4):514–20.
69. Turco R, Martinelli M, Miele E, et al. Proton pump inhibitors as a risk factor for paediatric Clostridium difficile infection. Aliment Pharmacol Ther 2010;31(7):754–9.

Evidence-Based Use of Indomethacin and Ibuprofen in the Neonatal Intensive Care Unit

Palmer G. Johnston, MD[a], Maria Gillam-Krakauer, MD[a],
M. Paige Fuller, PharmD, BCPS[b], Jeff Reese, MD[a,c],*

KEYWORDS

- Patent ductus arteriosus (PDA)
- Hemodynamically significant PDA (hsPDA) • Indomethacin
- Ibuprofen • Prematurity • Intraventricular hemorrhage (IVH)
- Necrotizing enterocolitis (NEC)
- Spontaneous intestinal perforation (SIP)

Pioneers in the care of premature infants recognized that a patent ductus arteriosus (PDA) could result in symptomatic hemodynamic changes with left-to-right circulatory shunt, and increased incidence of pulmonary hemorrhage,[1] parenchymal lung disease, necrotizing enterocolitis (NEC), intraventricular hemorrhage (IVH), and death.[2] The prevalence of hemodynamically significant PDA (hsPDA) is inversely related to maturity. Although it affects 42% to 60% of infants born weighing less than 1000 g, the incidence decreases to 5% in infants weighing 1500 to 1750 g at birth.[3,4] From 1939 to 1976, the primary treatment of a symptomatic PDA was surgical ligation. In 1969, Arcilla and colleagues[5] reported a case of an infant born with heart failure from suspected in utero ductus closure following maternal treatment with salicylates late in pregnancy. Subsequent animal studies examining the relationship

Financial support: Supported by NIH grants HL77395, HL96967, and HL109199 (Reese).
The authors have nothing to disclose.

[a] Neonatal-Perinatal Medicine, Division of Neonatology, Department of Pediatrics, Vanderbilt University Medical Center, 2200 Children's Way, Doctor's Office Tower 11111, Nashville, TN 37232-9544, USA
[b] Department of Pharmacy, Monroe Carell Jr. Children's Hospital at Vanderbilt, 2200 Children's Way, Room 4508, Nashville, TN 37232, USA
[c] Department of Cell and Developmental Biology, Vanderbilt University Medical Center, U-3218 MRB III Building, Nashville, TN 37232-8240, USA
* Corresponding author. Department of Cell and Developmental Biology, Vanderbilt University Medical Center, U-3218 MRB III Building, Nashville, TN 37232-8240.
E-mail address: jeff.reese@vanderbilt.edu

Clin Perinatol 39 (2012) 111–136
doi:10.1016/j.clp.2011.12.002   perinatology.theclinics.com

between the ductus arteriosus and prostaglandins led to clinical studies in neonates showing the effectiveness of prostaglandin synthesis inhibitors as a treatment for PDA.[6,7]

In the same 1976 issue of the *New England Journal of Medicine*, both Friedman and colleagues[6] and Heymann and colleagues[7] presented the cases of 6 and 18 premature infants, respectively, each with a large PDA, most of which were successfully closed with a single dose of rectal or enteral indomethacin. These reports were the first clinical trials of indomethacin use in human premature infants. Although Coceani and colleagues[8,9] studied the effects of ibuprofen on ductus patency in a lamb model in the late 1970s, it would take another 2 decades for clinical studies evaluating the effectiveness of ibuprofen for ductus closure to be published.[10–12]

PHARMACOLOGY OF INDOMETHACIN AND IBUPROFEN

Within the body, synthesis of prostaglandins occurs when arachidonic acid is freed from lipid storage by phospholipase A_2. Subsequently, cyclooxygenase (COX) converts arachidonic acid to PGG_2 and PGH_2. PGH_2 is the precursor to multiple types of prostaglandins, including PGE_2, PGD_2, $PGF_{2\alpha}$, and PGI_2 and thromboxane.[13] Prostaglandins are known to play a critical role in the pathophysiology of PDA, thus, inhibiting the production of these vasoactive substances has been the goal of pharmacologic approaches for many years.[14] Two particular prostaglandin inhibitors, indomethacin and ibuprofen, have been the most studied for the prophylaxis and treatment of PDA because of their ability to enter the COX hydrophobic channel, competing with arachidonic acid for binding at the catalytic site and blocking the production of prostaglandins.[15,16]

Indomethacin

Although both are classified as nonsteroidal antiinflammatory drugs (NSAIDs), indomethacin and ibuprofen have different kinetics and pharmacologic properties. Indomethacin first became available in 1963[17] and belongs to a group of drugs called indoleacetic acids. Synthetically derived from arylacetic acid,[18] indomethacin inhibits COX in a competitive, time-dependent, slowly reversible manner.[15,16,18] Indomethacin nonselectively inhibits COX enzymes, resulting in decreased synthesis of all prostaglandin types. The nonselective mechanism of COX inhibition is responsible for the various unwanted side effects that can occur with administration.[14] From 1976 until 2004, indomethacin was the standard medication for the pharmacologic closure of PDA until the arrival of intravenous (IV) formulations of ibuprofen on the market (**Fig. 1**).

Ibuprofen

Ibuprofen was the first drug in the propionic class to become used routinely by the general public in its oral form.[17] It is a chiral compound derived from arylpropionic acid.[18] Ibuprofen exerts its effect in a simple, competitive, rapidly reversible manner.[15,16,18] Like indomethacin, ibuprofen inhibits COX in a nonselective manner.[14,17] In 2006, ibuprofen lysine, an IV formulation, became available in the United States for the treatment of PDA (see **Fig. 1**).

Two Cyclooxygenases

In 1991, a second COX enzyme (COX-2) was discovered, which led researchers to study why 2 isoforms, COX-1 and COX-2, exist.[19] Studies in mice suggest that COX-2 has a more important role in the closure of the DA, whereas COX-1 plays

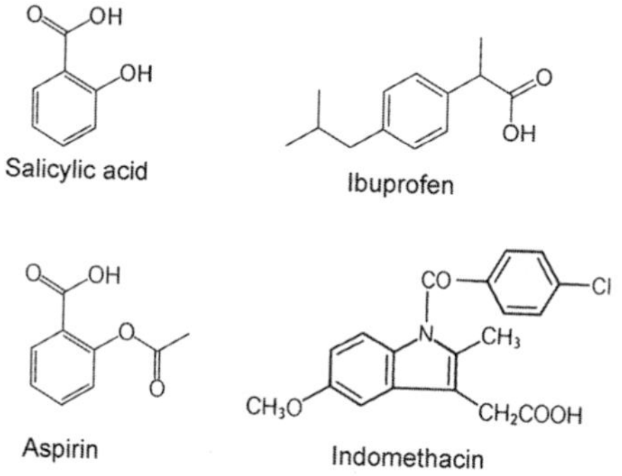

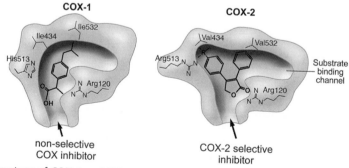

Fig. 1. Structure of common NSAIDs. The NSAID parent compound, salicylic acid, was purified in 1829 and commercially synthesized in the mid-1800s. By 1897, salicylic acid had been successfully acetylated and was marketed as aspirin in 1899. Subsequent NSAID development led to the production of phenacetin (1887), acetaminophen (1888), phenylbutazone (1949), the fenamates (1950s), ibuprofen (1961), and indomethacin (1963).

a more compensatory function.[19–22] Results in the human ductus are less clear; COX-1 expression is greater than COX-2,[23] but selective COX-2 inhibitors can constrict the fetal ductus.[24] The catalytic channel of COX-2 is larger and more accommodating based on the size, charge, and chemical environment versus COX-1 (**Fig. 2**).[15,25,26] All classical NSAIDS (those before 1995) inhibit both COX-1 and COX-2 but in general bind more tightly to COX-1.[15] Indomethacin is more specific for COX-1, thus, resulting in overall greater systemic, nonselective vasoconstriction,[27] although ibuprofen is also somewhat more selective for COX-1 than COX-2 (**Fig. 3**).[18,28] Indomethacin and other NSAIDs may also have effects on noncyclooxygenase pathways that augment ductus constriction or add to their deleterious side effects.[17,29–32]

TREATMENT OF hsPDA
Efficacy when Treatment is Indicated

NSAIDs are an effective measure to induce PDA closure. Following the initial reports of Friedman and Heymann in the mid-1970s, many studies were published in the early

Fig. 2. Structure of COX-1 and COX-2 substrate binding channels. Amino acid residues, Val 434, Arg 513, and Val 523, create a side pocket in COX-2, whereas the larger residues, Ile 434, His 513, and Ile 532, in the COX-1 channel block the bulky side chains of selective COX-2 inhibitors. (*Adapted from* Grosser T, Fries S, FitzGerald GA. Biological basis for the cardiovascular consequences of COX-2 inhibition: therapeutic challenges and opportunities. J Clin Invest 2006;116(1):4–15; with permission.)

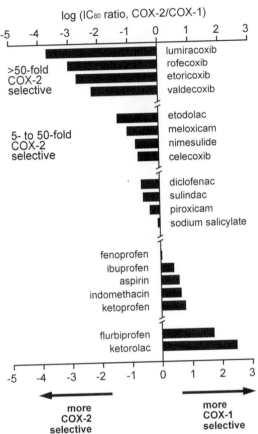

Fig. 3. Relative selectivity of different NSAIDs for COX-1 or COX-2. Values were extrapolated from inhibition curves for each compound against COX-1 and COX-2 that were generated in a human modified whole blood assay. Bars represent the ratio of IC_{80} concentrations, plotted logarithmically. (*Adapted from* Warner TD, Mitchell JA. Cyclooxygenases: new forms, new inhibitors, and lessons from the clinic. FASEB J 2004;18(7):790–804; with permission.)

1980s showing a significant decrease in the presence of PDA after infants were treated with indomethacin compared with control. Rates of initial ductus closure in infants born weighing less than 1750 g range from 60% to 86% after a treatment course of indomethacin.[7,33–39] By comparison, spontaneous closure occurs in just 35% of infants weighing less than 1750 g[33] and is more likely to occur in infants greater than 29 weeks' gestation and 1000 g at birth.[4,40]

Ibuprofen and indomethacin have similar efficacy for primary closure of a PDA. Rates of closure after an initial 3-dose course of ibuprofen range from 66% to 73%.[34,35,39,41] In a randomized controlled trial comparing treatment of PDA with ibuprofen or indomethacin in the first 48 to 72 hours of age, Lago and colleagues[34] reported successful closure after 3 doses of medication in 69% of infants given indomethacin compared with 73% who were given ibuprofen. Between 44% and 48% of infants required 3 additional doses of the same medication, resulting in an overall closure rate of 82% for indomethacin and 86% for ibuprofen (*P* values not significant).

The overall rate of ductus reopening after successful treatment with either indomethacin or ibuprofen is around 21% to 26%.[33,34,42] Infants born at less than or equal to 26 weeks' gestation have a significantly increased risk of ductus reopening compared with infants born at older gestational ages (37% vs 11%, $P<.03$).[42] Treatment failure has been found to be more common in infants with (1) residual flow through the ductus lumen, (2) absence of antenatal steroids, (3) increased severity of respiratory distress syndrome (RDS), (4) exposure to antenatal indomethacin, and (5) chorioamnionitis.[42–49]

Decreased Need for Surgical Ligation

In most studies, treatment of a PDA with indomethacin has been shown to decrease the need for surgical ligation.[7,33,36,50] Mahony and colleagues[50] found a significant decrease ($P<.005$) in the need for surgical ligation of the PDA in infants with less than a 1000-g birth weight who received indomethacin compared with control. One of the first published studies comparing indomethacin versus aspirin for the treatment of PDA by Heymann and colleagues[7] enrolled 18 infants and found that no patients who received indomethacin treatment required surgical ligation of the PDA. Another early study of 59 infants by Merritt and colleagues[36] in 1978 compared indomethacin treatment with primary surgical ligation. Only 4 of 35 (11%) infants in the indomethacin group needed surgical ligation of their ductus secondary to symptoms of heart failure after treatment with indomethacin. Delaying treatment with indomethacin during a brief course of supportive care does not seem to significantly increase the need for later surgical ligation.[33]

In one of only a few studies that examined ibuprofen compared with placebo for the treatment of PDA, Aranda and colleagues[51] (2009) reported a multicenter, double-blinded, randomized, controlled trial in 136 infants who had a hsPDA diagnosed before 72 hours of age. Infants were randomized to receive ibuprofen or placebo initially with indomethacin for rescue therapy and then surgical ligation if needed. Infants who received ibuprofen had a significant decrease in the need for rescue indomethacin as compared with controls ($P = .0003$). Interestingly, there was no difference between the ibuprofen group and control in the need for surgical ligation in the infants who received rescue indomethacin. Rescue indomethacin was given to all infants who failed to have duct closure before proceeding with surgical ligation.

Several randomized, placebo-controlled trials found that ibuprofen was as effective as indomethacin at decreasing the need for surgical ligation.[11,34,41,52] A Cochrane meta-analysis evaluating the efficacy of ibuprofen for PDA closure identified 13 trials (n = 848 infants) that reported ligation as an endpoint. By meta-analysis, there was no significant difference between ibuprofen- and indomethacin-treated groups in the need for ligation.[53]

Indomethacin

Treatment dosing

Determining the optimal dosing regimen, length of treatment, and timing of indomethacin for the management of PDA has been challenging. The response of the PDA to indomethacin depends on the size of the dose and the number of doses.[54] Furthermore, it is known that the success of indomethacin in producing PDA closure wanes with advancing postnatal age.[27,54,55] However, the risks of PDA treatment in the youngest preterm infants should be weighed against the potential benefits. Although one standard regimen may not be optimal for each individual, evidence shows that there are advantages and disadvantages to different approaches.

Prolonged versus short course

Circulating PGE_2 concentrations return to pretreatment levels several days following the completion of an indomethacin course, which may not allow enough time for ductus remodeling in the immature infant.[54] Seyberth and colleagues[56] reported a significant reappearance of PGE_2 after 5.5 days of completed therapy with indomethacin. Thus, prolongation of the more typical 2- to 3-day course of indomethacin has been described.

A 2007 Cochrane meta-analysis sought to determine whether longer courses of indomethacin would increase the success rate of PDA closure. Five trials describing the outcomes of a total of 431 preterm infants were included in the review. On comparison of short ($\leq$3 doses) versus prolonged ($\geq$4 doses) treatment courses, there were no significant effects on closure, re-treatment, reopening, or ligation rates of PDA. Additionally, there was no significant effect on outcomes, such as chronic lung disease, IVH, and mortality. When examining side-effect differences, the prolonged course of indomethacin was linked to an increased possibility of developing NEC, but a decreased risk of renal dysfunction. The investigators concluded that although there is less renal impairment with a prolonged dosing approach, the risk of NEC precludes routine recommendation of prolonged courses of indomethacin.[57]

Continuous infusion versus intermittent bolus

Prolonging the indomethacin infusion time from a short bolus to 20 to 30 minutes reduces the detrimental effects of indomethacin on cerebral blood flow velocity.[14,54] Investigators subsequently hypothesized that a continuous infusion of indomethacin might also alleviate the side effects seen with bolus dosing. In 1995, Hammerman and colleagues[58] published findings of 18 preterm patients: 9 that received continuous indomethacin (0.011 mg/kg/h for 36 hours) and 9 that received bolus dosing (0.2 mg/kg over 60 seconds followed by 0.1 mg/kg doses every 12 hours for 2 additional doses). Fluctuation found in the middle cerebral artery systolic and diastolic flow velocities in the continuous indomethacin group were significantly less than in the bolus group.

A similar trial by Christmann[59] evaluated 32 preterm infants comparing differences in blood flow in the cerebral vasculature. Infants in the continuous indomethacin group received the same total dose of 0.4 mg/kg over 36 hours (0.011 mg/kg/h) as in the Hammerman trial. In the bolus group (given over 30 seconds), doses were divided into 3 injections: 0.2 mg/kg at the first dose, then 0.1 mg/kg at 12 and 36 hours after the first injection. Statistically significant differences between the 2 regimens occurred at various time points during the study regarding cerebral, renal, and mesenteric blood flow velocities.[59] The benefits of continuous indomethacin infusion are tempered by potential drawbacks with this approach: necessity for stable IV access, an infusion time of 36 hours, adequate preservatives for a prolonged infusion time, concerns regarding drug precipitation or incompatibility with other infusions, or excess fluid administration. A standard administration time of at least 20 to 30 minutes is currently favored, until continuous infusion is more thoroughly studied.

Routes of Administration

Over the years, indomethacin has been administered intravenously, intramuscularly, enterally, and rectally for the treatment of PDA.[60,61] Enteral administration is the most studied alternative to the IV formulation. In 1979, Cooke[62] reported an inadequate response to oral indomethacin provided at 0.2 mg/kg/dose every 12 hours for 3 doses; 5 of the 7 treated infants had no clinical response. More concerning than the potential lack of clinical response are the reports of intestinal perforations associated with enteral indomethacin. Alpan and colleagues[63] published a case series in 1985 in which 4 premature infants experienced localized small-bowel perforation after the administration of indomethacin via a nasogastric tube. The investigators speculated that perhaps their findings were related to a locally induced prostaglandin deficiency resulting in less cytoprotection in the gastrointestinal tract. Kuhl and Seyberth[60] hypothesized that the gastrointestinal side effects are not a local effect caused by oral administration, but rather decreased gut perfusion caused by the PDA, coupled with the blockage of mucosal vasodilation and integrity normally provided by prostaglandins. Similar findings were reported in a single case report in a letter to the editor in 1985 and by Nagaraj[61] in 1981 in which 8 of 82 infants given enteral indomethacin developed a focal perforation in various locations in the gastrointestinal tract.[60,61,64] Inadequate and inconsistent drug absorption by the enteral route has also been a concern with this method of administration.[65,66] Determining the optimal formulation of enteral indomethacin has also proved challenging and may affect absorption.[67] Because of the potential side-effect profile and variation in absorption of enteral indomethacin in the literature, the IV formulation is preferred over the enteral formulation at this time.

Ibuprofen

A recent Cochrane review on the use of ibuprofen for the treatment of PDA included a total of 20 trials (n = 1092) that compared ibuprofen with indomethacin, and 1 trial (n = 136) comparing ibuprofen with placebo. Among the 21 trials, 14 used the IV formulation. Of these, 12 used a dosing regimen of 10 mg/kg for the initial dose followed by 5 mg/kg doses every 24 hours for 2 days,[53] which is the dosing regimen outlined by the manufacturers. This regimen was determined by the dose-finding study by Aranda and colleagues[68] in 1997 and confirmed by Desfrere's group in 2005 who found this regimen provides an 80% closure rate balanced with minimal side effects.[69]

Seven trials included in the Cochrane review provided ibuprofen via the enteral route. Five of these studies followed the same dosing regimen that most researchers have used in IV trials: 10 mg/kg for the initial dose followed by 5 mg/kg daily for 2 days. One study used 10 mg/kg/dose for all 3 doses given every 24 hours, whereas one study did not specify an exact dosing regimen. When comparing oral ibuprofen with IV indomethacin, the meta-analysis found no statistically significant difference in the failure to close a PDA after 3 doses, although the investigators commented that enteral ibuprofen seemed less effective than IV indomethacin. It was concluded that both the enteral and IV routes of ibuprofen seem equally effective in the closure of PDA.[53] There have been 2 studies that compared safety and efficacy between IV and oral ibuprofen.[70,71] Both studies found that the oral formulation had a higher success in the PDA closure rate compared with IV, although the Gokmen study[71] comments on the trend of more immature infants in the IV group, which may have affected outcomes.

Several concerns have been raised surrounding the use of enteral ibuprofen, specifically gastrointestinal side effects with the potential for a localized COX-inhibition effect in the gut similar to oral indomethacin. There were no bowel perforations reported in either the Cherif[70] or Gokmen studies in the oral groups.[70,71] In the Gokmen trial, 6.0% of the patients in the IV group and 3.6% of the patients in the oral group experienced NEC, whereas 3.1% of the patients in the IV group and 6.3% of the patients in the oral group were observed to have the same outcome in the Cherif study. One patient in the oral ibuprofen group was found to have a gastrointestinal hemorrhage versus none in the IV group in both trials. Gokmen and colleagues mention 19 other cases of gastrointestinal bleeding out of 191 total patients in other pooled studies and theorizes that that gastrointestinal irritation is caused by the method of administration. Neither study had the power to detect a difference in complications, thus, prompting the need for trials with larger numbers.[70,71]

Other concerns regarding the use of enteral ibuprofen include interpatient pharmacokinetic variability, which can be caused by differences in cytochrome P450 enzyme expression and interactions with other medications that affect protein binding, elimination, or hepatic metabolism of ibuprofen. Additionally, peak plasma concentrations are reportedly not as high as those with IV, suggesting that a higher milligram-per-kilogram dosing regimen might be necessary. However, the longer half-life in infants, larger AUC24, and adequate absorption, all factors that contribute to more contact time with the ductus, may explain the better response rates seen in recent studies investigating enteral ibuprofen.[70–74]

In summary, larger studies with improved design are needed that are powered to detect both closure and complication rates between oral and IV ibuprofen, as well as additional pharmacokinetic data to determine the optimal dosing scheme. More information is also needed on the osmolality of the enteral formulations being used and studied. Until more data are available, the authors cannot recommend using enteral ibuprofen in an off-label fashion for the closure of the PDA unless IV alternatives are not available.

ADVERSE EFFECTS
Gastrointestinal Effects

Untoward gastrointestinal events occur with increased frequency in infants treated with NSAIDs. These adverse effects may be greater with indomethacin than ibuprofen and depend on the mode of administration, with rectal and enteral forms having greater toxicity.[2,75]

Spontaneous intestinal perforation

Early indomethacin exposure has been associated with spontaneous intestinal perforation (SIP), especially when given in close proximity to postnatal corticosteroids. Both Stark and colleagues[76] and Watterberg and colleagues[77] found a significant effect with indomethacin and dexamethasone both given within the first 24 hours of age and indomethacin and hydrocortisone at 48 hours of age. A randomized, placebo-controlled trial of hydrocortisone to prevent bronchopulmonary dysplasia (BPD) was prematurely terminated because of gastrointestinal perforations in the hydrocortisone group that received indomethacin or ibuprofen.[78] A retrospective study by Attridge and colleagues[79] found that one of the independent risk factors for developing SIP was the administration of IV indomethacin within the first 3 days of life (odds ratio 1.86; $P<.0001$). Patients who developed SIP were also more likely to have a significant PDA.

There are case reports of increased incidence of SIP in infants who received either enteral or IV indomethacin as prophylaxis.[61,63,80,81] In a large prospective study, Sharma and colleagues[82] observed that any indomethacin exposure increased the risk for SIP, with increased risk among infants treated at less than 12 hours of age. Although conflicting evidence exists,[82] there is also concern that *antenatal* exposure to indomethacin may also pose a risk for postnatal intestinal perforation.[47,83–85] However, no randomized control trial comparing prophylactic indomethacin to placebo (including a Cochrane meta-analysis) found a significant increase in the incidence of SIP or NEC in infants who received indomethacin for prophylaxis.[86]

Necrotizing enterocolitis

Although the pathogenesis of NEC is multifactorial, there is evidence to suggest that disturbances in gut perfusion leading to ischemia may play an important role in this disease. Several studies identified a correlation between the mere presence of an hsPDA and the development of NEC or increased mortality from NEC, especially among infants with a birth weight less than 1500 g and gestational age less than 28 weeks.[2,87–90] This correlation is thought to be secondary to the mesenteric blood flow disturbances resulting from a left-to-right circulatory shunt.

Using Doppler ultrasonography, multiple studies have shown that indomethacin decreases blood flow velocity in the superior mesenteric artery.[59,91–95] This effect is especially pronounced when indomethacin is given by rapid bolus (duration 20 seconds), but even slow infusion (duration 30–35 minutes) is associated with significantly decreased blood flow velocity compared with continuous infusion.[59] Although compelling, these small studies provide insufficient data to support continuous dosing rather than slow infusion.[59,91,92,94]

There are numerous studies that report NEC as an adverse outcome after treatment with indomethacin.[61,96–100] In a retrospective analysis, Grosfeld and colleagues[97] found a significant increase in the incidence of NEC in infants with a PDA who were treated with indomethacin as compared with infants who did not have a PDA and did not receive indomethacin treatment (35% vs 13%, $P<.5$). In a larger retrospective study involving more than 18,000 infants admitted to 17 level III nurseries in Canada, Sankaran and colleagues[100] observed a similar association between NEC and indomethacin in infants with a birth weight less than 1500 g. In contrast, an observational population study by Dollberg and colleagues[88] did not find an increased risk of NEC with indomethacin treatment of PDA in more than 6000 very-low-birth-weight (VLBW) infants. Moreover, the Trial of Indomethacin Prophylaxis in Preterm Infants (TIPP) involving more than 1000 VLBW infants did not find a significant increase in the risk of NEC associated with the administration of indomethacin as prophylaxis for PDA.[101] Despite the known association between indomethacin and NEC, there is no clear evidence that the incidence or severity of NEC is related to treatment with indomethacin or that a cause-effect relationship exists.[86,102–104]

When ibuprofen was compared with indomethacin for the treatment of hsPDA in a meta-analysis of 15 studies that had NEC as an outcome, there was a decrease in the relative risk (RR) of NEC with the use of ibuprofen (RR 0.68, confidence interval [CI] 0.47–0.99).[53] Pezzati and colleagues[92] compared mesenteric blood flow velocities in 17 infants using Doppler ultrasonography following bolus administration of either indomethacin or ibuprofen and found that, unlike indomethacin, ibuprofen did not significantly reduce mesenteric blood flow. No cases of NEC developed in either group.

Enteral prophylactic ibuprofen may confer a slightly increased risk of gastrointestinal bleeding when compared with control. Two different randomized, placebo-controlled trials by the same investigators enrolled a combination of 104 infants to evaluate the effectiveness of oral ibuprofen for prophylaxis. Neither study found a significant increase in gastrointestinal bleeding in the treatment group. Bleeding only became significant when the studies were analyzed together by meta-analysis (RR = 1.99 [95% CI 1.13–3.50]).[105–107]

Renal Effects

Adverse effects on the kidney, including increased blood urea nitrogen and creatinine, oliguria, and renal failure, have been noted following treatment with indomethacin.

Indomethacin causes water retention and hyponatremia by enhancing vasopressin action and increasing renal vascular resistance and reducing renal blood flow.[108] Ibuprofen does not decrease renal blood flow and, in fact, is associated with increased blood flow velocity at 120 minutes.[92]

Increased creatinine

VLBW infants with hsPDA have a statistically significant increase in serum creatinine concentration following treatment with indomethacin, but no increase occurs following treatment with the first course of ibuprofen.[33,34,92] This effect is transient and usually disappears within 24 hours, although resolution may take up to 7 days.[34,92] However, when infants who receive a second course of either medication are compared, there is no difference between the decrease in urine output and the increase in creatinine.[34,109] In contrast, Katakam and colleagues[110] did not find a significant difference in creatinine between infants treated with indomethacin or ibuprofen. Continuous infusion of indomethacin prevents the increase in creatinine induced by bolus dosing.[58]

Prophylactic ibuprofen may be associated with a brief increase in creatinine levels. Van Overmeire and colleagues[111] randomized 415 infants to receive either placebo or prophylactic ibuprofen and found a transient but significant increase in serum creatinine 24 hours after the third dose of ibuprofen when compared with placebo ($P<.0001$). Gournay and colleagues[112] also noted a significant increase in serum creatinine 4 to 7 days after treatment in the infants who received prophylactic ibuprofen ($P<.002$). A meta-analysis of 5 trials that reported creatinine level as an outcome indicated that prophylactic use of ibuprofen compared with placebo is associated with a statistically significant increase in creatinine levels on the third day of life.[105]

Decreased urine output

Oliguria, defined as urine output less than 1 mL/kg/h, is observed more often in infants receiving indomethacin compared with ibuprofen.[34,39,41,52,92] When compared with placebo, infants weighing greater than 1000 g receiving indomethacin have a significant decrease in mean urine output at 24 to 48 hours after treatment.[50] Bandstra and colleagues[113] reported that oliguria also occurs after prophylactic indomethacin. The infants most affected tended to have a higher birth weight (900–1300 g), but all infants had resolution of oliguria within 72 hours. Bolus indomethacin is more likely to cause oliguria at 12 and 24 hours than continuous infusion.[59]

Although treatment with ibuprofen results in a lower incidence of oliguria than indomethacin, it is not completely free of negative effects on the kidney. In a 2008 study involving 119 infants randomized to ibuprofen or indomethacin for the treatment of a PDA, Su and colleagues[41] found an incidence of oliguria in the ibuprofen group of 6.7%. It was still significantly lower than the rate of oliguria in the indomethacin group (15.3%, $P<.05$). A more recent study by Vieux and colleagues[114] suggests that renal impairment after ibuprofen may not be transient. In this study, ibuprofen-treated infants did not experience the normal postnatal increase in glomerular filtration rate (GFR) on days 2 to 7, and alterations in GFR and tubular function (fractional excretion of sodium) were noted until 28 days of age. In addition, instances of acute renal failure indicate that ibuprofen treatment still poses nephrotoxic risks for preterm infants.[115–119] Thus, although the rate of renal complications is lower with ibuprofen than with indomethacin, they nevertheless deserve consideration.

There is no evidence to support the use of either furosemide or dopamine during treatment with indomethacin to prevent adverse effects on the kidney. Although dopamine does not impair ductus closure[120,121] and may increase urine output,[120] it neither prevents elevation of creatinine nor decreases incidence of oliguria.[120–122]

Hyperbilirubinemia

In vitro studies suggest that high doses of ibuprofen can displace bilirubin from albumin, thus, increasing free bilirubin levels and theoretically increasing the risk of kernicterus.[123] Rheinlaender and colleagues[124] reported that total bilirubin levels were significantly elevated in patients who received ibuprofen compared with indomethacin for treatment of hsPDA (P<.01). However, even with the increase in bilirubin, neither the number of days of phototherapy treatment nor neurodevelopmental outcome at 2 years of age differed between the ibuprofen and indomethacin groups. Zecca and colleagues[125] also detected an association between ibuprofen and increased peak serum bilirubin levels and a longer need for phototherapy. However, both of these reports are retrospective and several clinical studies show that the risks for hyperbilirubinemia are limited.[35,126–128]

Cerebrovascular and Other Effects

Ibuprofen has limited effects on cerebrovascular perfusion.[129–131] In contrast, indomethacin is known to induce significant reductions in cerebral blood flow.[129,130,132–139] Cerebral oxygenation is also affected by indomethacin treatment.[130,133,140,141] Alterations in cerebral perfusion are, therefore, an important concern for indomethacin use in neonates. However, studies indicate that prophylactic indomethacin is protective against high-grade IVH[86,101] and may reduce the incidence of white matter injury.[86] Moreover, neurodevelopmental outcomes of indomethacin-treated infants are no different than controls at 18 months[101] and 36 months[142,143] and may be improved at 4.5 and 8 years of age.[144–146] The accumulated results of numerous studies have not shown an overall increase in the incidence of other potential morbidities, including retinopathy of prematurity and chronic lung disease.[147]

Summary

Indomethacin effectively induces closure of the ductus arteriosus and decreases the need for surgical ligation; but compared with ibuprofen, the use of indomethacin is associated with increased concerns for gastrointestinal complications and decreased renal function. The difference between these drugs may be caused by indomethacin effects on noncyclooxygenase pathways. A transient decrease in urine output and an increase in creatinine can usually be medically supported. However, the complications arising from an episode of SIP or NEC in a very premature infant are often serious and, in the worst scenario, can lead to loss of life. Although indomethacin may have a useful role in *prophylaxis* for PDA (see later discussion),[148] current evidence does not support the routine use of indomethacin over ibuprofen for the treatment of the hsPDA when side effects are considered.

Ibuprofen is as effective as indomethacin in closing a PDA. Although ibuprofen does have some side effects, particularly on renal function, these effects are less when compared with indomethacin. If closure of an hsPDA is warranted, IV ibuprofen is an acceptable treatment option with the realization that there are associated side effects.

PROPHYLACTIC TREATMENT TO PREVENT IVH OR hsPDA

Preventive strategies for IVH co-evolved with efforts to effectively treat PDA. Because the smallest preterm infants are at the greatest risk of developing an hsPDA, both indomethacin and ibuprofen have been used in attempts to prevent progression to an hsPDA, reduce left-to-right shunting of blood away from vital organ systems, and avoid surgery.[149]

Efficacy to Prevent Intraventricular Hemorrhage

The early trials of indomethacin for treatment of PDA occurred as efforts to identify compounds for prevention of IVH in premature infants were taking place. In 1983, the two intersected when Laura Ment and colleagues[150] published the first report of indomethacin successfully preventing IVH in the newborn beagle puppy. The mechanism of action of indomethacin on the cerebral vasculature is not completely known but is likely unrelated to the closure of the ductus arteriosus.[151,152]

This discovery was followed by a series of short-term clinical trials in neonates.[113,151,153,154] Although there was initially conflicting evidence on the effectiveness of IVH prevention, especially in infants weighing less than 1000 g,[154,155] it was subsequently shown that prophylactic indomethacin (administered at <12 hours of age) was effective in reducing higher-grade IVH. In 1988, Bandstra and colleagues[113] randomized almost 200 infants born at less than 1300 g to either receive 3 doses of indomethacin starting within 12 hours of birth or placebo. They found that prophylactic indomethacin significantly reduced the incidence of grade 2 to 4 IVH compared with control (23% vs 46%, $P<.002$). Ment and colleagues[156] reported a multicenter study involving more than 400 infants weighing between 600 and 1250 g given either 3 doses of indomethacin starting within 12 hours of birth or placebo. A significant decrease in all forms of IVH was noted ($P = .03$), but especially in grade 4 IVH. In the placebo group, 10 out of 222 infants experienced grade 4 IVH compared with only 1 out of 209 in the intervention group ($P = .01$). There were no differences in adverse events between the 2 groups and no extension of IVH in infants who already had a grade 1 or 2 hemorrhage by 11 hours of age.

More recently, in a group of 1200 infants born weighing less than 1000 g randomized to either receive indomethacin or placebo, the TIPP trial also reported that prophylactic indomethacin decreases severe (grade 3–4) IVH compared with placebo (9% vs 13%, $P = .02$).[101]

Although prophylactic indomethacin has been shown to decrease severe forms of IVH, the long-term effect on neurodevelopmental outcomes is equivocal or only somewhat improved. Couser and colleagues[142] found comparable head growth and neurodevelopmental outcomes in prophylactic indomethacin- and placebo-treated infants at the 36-month follow-up. In the multicenter trial by Ment and colleagues,[143] there was a decrease in the presence of ventriculomegaly at term in infants who had received prophylactic indomethacin (0% vs 5%, $P = .027$) and no statistically significant difference in survival at 36 months ($P = .09$). At 54 months, there was no difference in the incidence of cerebral palsy between the 2 groups. There was a significantly lower number of children who received indomethacin with an IQ less than 70 on the full-scale Wechsler Preschool and Primary Scale of Intelligence-Revised (9% vs 17%, $P = .035$). Children who received indomethacin also performed better on the Peabody Picture Vocabulary Test-Revised (PPVT-R) ($P = .02$).[144] At 8 years of age, there was no difference between the 2 groups regarding neurologic assessment, school performance, or cognitive functioning. There was no evidence at any age of adverse effects attributable to indomethacin.[145,146] Boys who received prophylactic indomethacin had significantly higher verbal scores on the PPVT-R when compared with control boys ($P = .017$).[145]

Although the TIPP trial also found a significant decrease in severe periventricular and intraventricular hemorrhage in infants given prophylactic indomethacin, there was no difference at 18 months in mortality or severe neurosensory impairment (cerebral palsy, cognitive delay [mental developmental index <70], deafness, and blindness).[101] Controversy exists regarding the study design and the interpretation of these results.[147,148,157]

Ibuprofen does not appear to confer protection against IVH.[112,158] In a trial of 415 infants given either prophylactic ibuprofen or placebo, Van Overmeire and colleagues[111] found no difference in any form of IVH between the 2 groups. This finding was supported by a trial by Dani and colleagues[159] that also found that prophylactic ibuprofen was ineffective in preventing grade 2 to 4 IVH.

Efficacy to Prevent hsPDA

Multiple prospective, randomized, placebo-controlled trials show a statistically significant reduction in PDA when prophylactic indomethacin was given within the first 24 hours of life versus placebo.[101,113,155,156,160] For example, in 199 infants with a birth weight less than 1300 g, Bandstra and colleagues[113] saw a significant reduction in PDA at several days of life in infants who received prophylactic indomethacin (0.2 mg/kg IV × 1 within the first 12 hours of life followed by 2 doses of 0.1 mg/kg IV every 12 hours). PDA was present in 11% of the treatment group compared with 42% of infants who received the placebo (P<.001).

Although only a secondary outcome, the multicenter TIPP trial found a significant reduction (P<.001) in PDA from 50% in infants who received placebo to 24% in infants who received indomethacin prophylaxis.[101] Even a single dose of indomethacin (0.2 mg/kg IV) given within the first 24 hours of life significantly reduced the presence of PDA from 56% in the placebo group to 7% in the treatment group (P<.007).[155] A systematic review of 19 randomized controlled trials showed that prophylactic indomethacin significantly reduced the risks for any reported type of PDA and the need for surgical ligation.[86] Further randomized trials of prophylactic indomethacin were deemed unnecessary. However, prophylactic treatment of PDA was only recommended by the Cochrane investigators in neonatal units without ready access to cardiac services or if cost-benefit analyses were favorable.[86]

In multiple randomized controlled trials in comparison to placebo, patients who received IV ibuprofen prophylaxis had a significant decrease in PDA by 72 hours after treatment.[12,105,111,112,159,161,162] The largest of these studies included 415 infants in a multicenter trial by Van Overmeire.[111] In that study, 84% of the infants who received 3 doses of prophylactic ibuprofen (10 mg/kg IV <6 hours of life, then 5 mg/kg IV at 24 and 48 hours) had closure of their PDA on the third day of life compared with 60% of infants who received placebo (P<.0001). Ibuprofen prophylaxis had the most effect on PDA closure in infants whose birth weight was 500 to 750 g.[111] However, a study by Varvarigou[12] in 1996 involving 34 infants aged less than 31 weeks specified that infants receiving only 1 dose of IV ibuprofen, like placebo, did not have a significant decrease in PDA compared with infants receiving 3 doses.

The use of oral ibuprofen for prophylaxis has been studied. In 2006, one randomized controlled study by Sangtawesin[107] with 42 patients found a significant decrease in the presence of PDA in infants who received 3 doses of ibuprofen suspension 10 mg/kg dose (first dose within first 24 hours of life and then again at 24 and 48 hours after the first dose) administered via gastric tube compared with placebo. However, Gournay and colleagues[112] discontinued a 2004 study because of severe pulmonary hypertension in 3 infants that received prophylactic ibuprofen. These episodes may be related to the acidic formulation of tromethamine ibuprofen; however, a case report in 2006 reported an acute episode of pulmonary hypertension in a patient who received L-lysine ibuprofen for PDA prophylaxis.[163]

Efficacy to Prevent Surgical Ligation

Prophylactic indomethacin is also associated with a significant decrease in the need for surgical ligation of PDA.[50,86,101,160] The TIPP trial investigators found a decreased need for surgical ligation of hsPDA in the patients who received prophylactic indomethacin compared with placebo (12% vs 7%, P<.001) with a number needed to treat of 20.[101]

Although the study was stopped early because of the development of pulmonary hypertension in 3 infants, Gournay and colleagues[112] found a significant decrease in the need for surgical ligation in infants who received prophylactic IV ibuprofen (10 mg/kg within the first 6 hours of life, then a 5 mg/kg dose at 24 and 48 hours) compared with those who received placebo. In a recent retrospective cohort study, Tefft[164] reported that prophylactic ibuprofen administration significantly reduced the need for surgical ligation and observed that numerous other studies found similar results, although they did not reach statistical significance.

In reviewing 19 different trials evaluating the effectiveness of prophylactic indomethacin, no other side effects, such as BPD (oxygen requirement at 28 days of life), days requiring mechanical ventilation, pulmonary hemorrhage, excessive bleeding, thrombocytopenia, visual impairment, hearing impairment, or cerebral palsy, were found more often in patients who received prophylactic indomethacin versus control.[86]

Dosing Regimens for Indomethacin Prophylaxis

There are different opinions regarding dosing regimens for indomethacin when used as prophylaxis. Plasma clearance depends on postnatal age, resulting in a rapid decline in half-life over the first week of life.[165–167] An initial dose of 0.1 to 0.2 mg/kg IV has been used in the first 2 to 24 hours of life, and follow-up doses of 0.1 to 0.2 mg/kg IV have been given every 12 to 24 hours after the initial dose for 1 to 6 total doses. Many studies gave an initial dose of 0.2 mg/kg IV, with follow-up doses of 0.1 mg/kg IV. In the studies that gave more than 3 total doses, a lower dose of 0.1 mg/kg IV was used. Out of 19 trials included in a meta-analysis, 15 used a 3-dose regimen.[86] Three trials used 4, 5, or 6 total doses, whereas Krueger and colleagues[155] provided a single dose based on the pharmacokinetics of indomethacin and the minimization of side effects. The optimal dosing of IV indomethacin for prophylaxis is not currently known.[86]

Summary

Both indomethacin and ibuprofen administered prophylactically reduce the need for later medical or surgical closure of the PDA. There is little evidence to date, however, that prophylactic closure of the PDA improves long-term outcomes or decreases other morbidities. Indomethacin prophylaxis has been shown in multiple studies to decrease the incidence of severe IVH, but there is insufficient long-term data to determine whether this has an impact on neurodevelopmental outcomes.

Although prophylactic ibuprofen does significantly improve the PDA closure rate and decreases the need for surgical ligation, there are well-documented side effects observed in patients who received prophylactic ibuprofen. Prophylactic ibuprofen has not been shown to decrease the incidence of severe IVH, and along with the increased potential risks of pulmonary hypertension and decreased urine output, ibuprofen cannot be recommended for use as prophylactic management of PDA in the preterm infant.

OBSERVATIONAL TREATMENT OF PDA

Justification for PDA treatment was traditionally based on evidence that prolonged exposure to a significant left-to-right shunt was deleterious. Morbidities attributed to the presence of an hsPDA have included BPD, pulmonary hemorrhage, increased RDS severity, NEC, renal impairment, IVH, periventricular leukomalacia, and death.[102] However, numerous investigators have challenged the cause-and-effect relationship between PDA and these outcomes and questioned whether exposure to the risks of medical or surgical interventions is warranted.[101–104,168–170]

Arguments for Treatment

Historical, prospective trials reported increased mortality in preterm infants with a symptomatic PDA compared with those without PDA.[171–174] Thereafter, 2 small, randomized clinical trials that examined the consequences of an untreated, persistent symptomatic PDA demonstrated increased mortality, increased need for respiratory support, and worse outcomes.[175,176]

In one report, Alexander and colleagues[177] compared outcomes among 298 extremely low-birth-weight infants with echocardiographically proven PDA. Infants treated with indomethacin or surgical ligation had significantly better survival rates compared with infants with untreated PDA. Nonsurvival was associated with immaturity, sepsis, and congestive heart failure, but study design did not permit the evaluation of relationships between PDA and other outcomes. In Western Australia, Brooks and colleagues[178] performed a retrospective analysis of 252 infants born at 28 weeks or less in a nursery lacking access to a pediatric surgeon to determine if closure of PDA was necessary. This study revealed that infants who had a persistent PDA despite treatment with indomethacin, even after adjustment for gestational age, had a 4-fold increased risk of death compared with infants who either did not have a PDA or who had PDA closure after indomethacin treatment ($P = .033$). No other morbidities were increased in the group without PDA closure. Noori and colleagues[75] reported another single-center, retrospective analysis evaluating the risk of persistent PDA. The study included 301 infants born at 29 weeks or less with a birth weight less than 1500 g and found a significant 8-fold increase in mortality in infants who had a persistent PDA after 14 days of age compared with infants with a closed PDA. The increase in mortality was still present after adjusting for gestational age ($P<.001$). A third, more recent retrospective study found an increased risk of a combined outcome of mortality and chronic lung disease (CLD) from 40% to 54% in infants who had more conservative management of PDA with decreased use of indomethacin, ibuprofen, or surgical ligation as compared with infants who received traditional treatment of PDA using indomethacin and surgical ligation ($P = .04$).[179] Thus, the presence of a persistent, untreated, symptomatic PDA may be associated with worse outcomes and increased mortality.

Arguments Against Treatment

Herrman and colleagues[180] performed a retrospective, observational cohort study on VLBW infants discharged from their unit with a PDA. Among 310 infants who survived, 21 had a documented PDA at the time of discharge. Two of the 21 infants were discharged on oxygen, with 2 on diuretic therapy and 2 on both. All of the infants survived to 18 months of age, and 18 out of 21 infants had spontaneous closure of their ductus. Two infants required transcatheter coil embolization and one still had a persistent PDA at 18 months chronologic age. Almost all of the infants with PDA at discharge had a small PDA, with 2 infants having a small to moderate PDA.

A recent meta-analysis of 10 trials comparing the use of indomethacin and ibuprofen versus placebo (with rescue therapy if needed) for the treatment of PDA performed by Jones and colleagues[181] found that there was no associated reduction in the risk of major morbidities or mortality with PDA closure. Their risk-to-benefit ratios revealed that treating 100 infants with ibuprofen compared with placebo to achieve PDA closure could cause 14 cases of CLD, 3 cases of IVH, and 1 death, whereas indomethacin could cause 2 cases of CLD and 2 cases of IVH. In contrast to the strict criteria for Cochrane reviews, Benitz[102] recently performed a systematic review of the literature by pooling the results from all available randomized clinical trials of PDA treatment. The intention was to avoid exclusion of any evidence that might be informative. It was concluded that later treatment, if any, might be beneficial; but the absence of improved long-term outcomes should limit all pharmacologic therapies for PDA to patients who are enrolled in on-going clinical trials.[102]

SUMMARY

Symptomatic PDA is a well-documented complication of premature birth and is associated with multiple other morbidities. Studies over the past decade have challenged the seemingly foregone conclusion that a symptomatic PDA should be treated on the grounds that short-term morbidities and long-term outcomes may not be improved by PDA closure and infants are unnecessarily exposed to potentially harmful therapies. Yet, no randomized, double-blinded clinical trials comparing the treatment of symptomatic PDA versus placebo without rescue treatment have been done. The determination of whether or not a PDA should be treated is outside the scope of this review. For clinicians who decide that pharmacologic closure of the ductus is warranted, NSAIDs are currently the only available choice.

The use of indomethacin and ibuprofen for prophylaxis and treatment of PDA has been carefully studied and reported in the literature; however, thoroughly documented adverse effects associated with either medication limit recommendations for treatment. Indomethacin, but not ibuprofen, is an effective agent for the prevention of IVH and should be considered in patient populations in which elevated rates of IVH are a concern. Indomethacin, when used as a *prophylactic* measure for PDA, reduces the risks for development of an hsPDA and prevents pulmonary hemorrhage and the need for surgical ligation. In the smallest premature infants, these seem to be laudable goals, although risk-benefit ratios should be weighed. Indomethacin and ibuprofen, when used in *treatment* mode, are both effective measures to induce closure of an hsPDA. However, optimal treatment regimens require additional study. Recently, Hammerman and colleagues[182] reported the off-label use of enteral paracetamol to successfully close a refractory hsPDA in 5 VLBW infants. With no observed side effects, this report is an exciting new development for the medical treatment of hsPDA, which has not seen a new therapy in more than a decade. The justification for PDA treatment is a topic of current debate but would benefit from additional treatment options that pose fewer risks.

REFERENCES

1. Kluckow M, Evans N. Ductal shunting, high pulmonary blood flow, and pulmonary hemorrhage. J Pediatr 2000;137(1):68–72.
2. Cotton RB, Stahlman MT, Kovar I, et al. Medical management of small preterm infants with symptomatic patent ductus arteriosus. J Pediatr 1978;92(3): 467–73.

3. Ellison RC, Peckham GJ, Lang P, et al. Evaluation of the preterm infant for patent ductus arteriosus. Pediatrics 1983;71(3):364–72.
4. Koch J, Hensley G, Roy L, et al. Prevalence of spontaneous closure of the ductus arteriosus in neonates at a birth weight of 1000 grams or less. Pediatrics 2006;117(4):1113–21.
5. Arcilla RA, Thilenius OG, Ranniger K. Congestive heart failure from suspected ductal closure in utero. J Pediatr 1969;75(1):74–8.
6. Friedman WF, Hirschklau MJ, Printz MP, et al. Pharmacologic closure of patent ductus arteriosus in the premature infant. N Engl J Med 1976;295(10):526–9.
7. Heymann MA, Rudolph AM, Silverman NH. Closure of the ductus arteriosus in premature infants by inhibition of prostaglandin synthesis. N Engl J Med 1976;295(10):530–3.
8. Coceani F, Olley PM, Bishai I, et al. Prostaglandins and the control of muscle tone in the ductus arteriosus. Adv Exp Med Biol 1977;78:135–42.
9. Coceani F, White E, Bodach E, et al. Age-dependent changes in the response of the lamb ductus arteriosus to oxygen and ibuprofen. Can J Physiol Pharmacol 1979;57(8):825–31.
10. Patel J, Marks KA, Roberts I, et al. Ibuprofen treatment of patent ductus arteriosus. Lancet 1995;346(8969):255.
11. Van Overmeire B, Follens I, Hartmann S, et al. Treatment of patent ductus arteriosus with ibuprofen. Arch Dis Child 1997;76(3):F179–84.
12. Varvarigou A, Bardin CL, Beharry K, et al. Early ibuprofen administration to prevent patent ductus arteriosus in premature newborn infants. JAMA 1996; 275(7):539–44.
13. Dubois RN, Abramson SB, Crofford L, et al. Cyclooxygenase in biology and disease. FASEB J 1998;12(12):1063–73.
14. Hammerman C. Patent ductus arteriosus. Clinical relevance of prostaglandins and prostaglandin inhibitors in PDA pathophysiology and treatment. Clin Perinatol 1995;22(2):457–79.
15. Smith WL, DeWitt DL, Garavito RM. Cyclooxygenases: structural, cellular, and molecular biology. Annu Rev Biochem 2000;69:145–82.
16. Reese J, Dey SK. Cyclooxygenases. In: KazazianJr HH, Klein G, Moser HW, et al, editors. Encyclopedia of molecular medicine. 5th edition. New York: John Wiley & Sons, Inc; 2002. p. 961–5.
17. Grosser T, Smyth E, FitzGerald GA. Anti-inflammatory, antipyretic, and analgesic agents; pharmacotherapy of gout. In: Brunton LL, Lazo JS, Parker KL, editors. Goodman & Gilmans's The pharmacological basis of therapeutics. 12th edition. New York (NY): McGraw-Hill; 2011. p. 959–1004. Chapter 34.
18. Romagnoli C, Bersani I, Rubortone SA, et al. Current evidence on the safety profile of NSAIDs for the treatment of PDA. J Matern Fetal Neonatal Med 2011;24(Suppl 3):10–3.
19. Smith WL, Langenbach R. Why there are two cyclooxygenase isozymes. J Clin Invest 2001;107(12):1491–5.
20. Loftin CD, Trivedi DB, Tiano HF, et al. Failure of ductus arteriosus closure and remodeling in neonatal mice deficient in cyclooxygenase-1 and cyclooxygenase-2. Proc Natl Acad Sci U S A 2001;98(3):1059–64.
21. Trivedi DB, Sugimoto Y, Loftin CD. Attenuated cyclooxygenase-2 expression contributes to patent ductus arteriosus in preterm mice. Pediatr Res 2006; 60(6):669–74.
22. Reese J, Anderson JD, Brown N, et al. Inhibition of cyclooxygenase isoforms in late- but not midgestation decreases contractility of the ductus arteriosus and

prevents postnatal closure in mice. Am J Physiol Regul Integr Comp Physiol 2006;291(6):R1717–23.

23. Rheinlaender C, Weber SC, Sarioglu N, et al. Changing expression of cyclooxygenases and prostaglandin receptor EP4 during development of the human ductus arteriosus. Pediatr Res 2006;60(3):270–5.

24. Groom KM, Shennan AH, Jones BA, et al. TOCOX–a randomised, double-blind, placebo-controlled trial of rofecoxib (a COX-2-specific prostaglandin inhibitor) for the prevention of preterm delivery in women at high risk. BJOG 2005; 112(6):725–30.

25. Grosser T, Fries S, FitzGerald GA. Biological basis for the cardiovascular consequences of COX-2 inhibition: therapeutic challenges and opportunities. J Clin Invest 2006;116(1):4–15.

26. Grosser T. The pharmacology of selective inhibition of COX-2. Thromb Haemost 2006;96(4):393–400.

27. Forsey JT, Elmasry OA, Martin RP. Patent arterial duct. Orphanet J Rare Dis 2009;4:17.

28. Warner TD, Mitchell JA. Cyclooxygenases: new forms, new inhibitors, and lessons from the clinic. FASEB J 2004;18(7):790–804.

29. Lehmann T, Day RO, Brooks PM. Toxicity of antirheumatic drugs. Med J Aust 1997;166(7):378–83.

30. Malcolm DD, Segar JL, Robillard JE, et al. Indomethacin compromises hemodynamics during positive-pressure ventilation, independently of prostanoids. J Appl Physiol 1993;74(4):1672–8.

31. Sagi SA, Weggen S, Eriksen J, et al. The non-cyclooxygenase targets of nonsteroidal anti-inflammatory drugs, lipoxygenases, peroxisome proliferator-activated receptor, inhibitor of kappa B kinase, and NF kappa B, do not reduce amyloid beta 42 production. J Biol Chem 2003;278(34):31825–30.

32. Tegeder I, Pfeilschifter J, Geisslinger G. Cyclooxygenase-independent actions of cyclooxygenase inhibitors. FASEB J 2001;15(12):2057–72.

33. Gersony WM, Peckham GJ, Ellison RC, et al. Effects of indomethacin in premature infants with patent ductus arteriosus: results of a national collaborative study. J Pediatr 1983;102(6):895–906.

34. Lago P, Bettiol T, Salvadori S, et al. Safety and efficacy of ibuprofen versus indomethacin in preterm infants treated for patent ductus arteriosus: a randomised controlled trial. Eur J Pediatr 2002;161(4):202–7.

35. Linder N, Bello R, Hernandez A, et al. Treatment of patent ductus arteriosus: indomethacin or ibuprofen? Am J Perinatol 2010;27(5):399–404.

36. Merritt TA, DiSessa TG, Feldman BH, et al. Closure of the patent ductus arteriosus with ligation and indomethacin: a consecutive experience. J Pediatr 1978; 93(4):639–46.

37. Merritt TA, Harris JP, Roghmann K, et al. Early closure of the patent ductus arteriosus in very low-birth-weight infants: a controlled trial. J Pediatr 1981;99(2): 281–6.

38. Rudd P, Montanez P, Hallidie-Smith K, et al. Indomethacin treatment for patent ductus arteriosus in very low birthweight infants: double blind trial. Arch Dis Child 1983;58(4):267–70.

39. Van Overmeire B, Smets K, Lecoutere D, et al. A comparison of ibuprofen and indomethacin for closure of patent ductus arteriosus. N Engl J Med 2000; 343(10):674–81.

40. Nemerofsky SL, Parravicini E, Bateman D, et al. The ductus arteriosus rarely requires treatment in infants > 1000 grams. Am J Perinatol 2008;25(10):661–6.

41. Su BH, Lin HC, Chiu HY, et al. Comparison of ibuprofen and indomethacin for early-targeted treatment of patent ductus arteriosus in extremely premature infants: a randomised controlled trial. Arch Dis Child 2008;93(2):F94–9.
42. Weiss H, Cooper B, Brook M, et al. Factors determining reopening of the ductus arteriosus after successful clinical closure with indomethacin. J Pediatr 1995; 127(3):466–71.
43. Chorne N, Jegatheesan P, Lin E, et al. Risk factors for persistent ductus arteriosus patency during indomethacin treatment. J Pediatr 2007;151(6):629–34.
44. Hermes-DeSantis ER, Clyman RI. Patent ductus arteriosus: pathophysiology and management. J Perinatol 2006;26(Suppl 1):S14–8 [discussion: S22–3].
45. Kim ES, Kim EK, Choi CW, et al. Intrauterine inflammation as a risk factor for persistent ductus arteriosus patency after cyclooxygenase inhibition in extremely low birth weight infants. J Pediatr 2010;157(5):745–50, e741.
46. Narayanan M, Cooper B, Weiss H, et al. Prophylactic indomethacin: factors determining permanent ductus arteriosus closure. J Pediatr 2000;136(3):330–7.
47. Norton ME, Merrill J, Cooper BA, et al. Neonatal complications after the administration of indomethacin for preterm labor. N Engl J Med 1993;329(22): 1602–7.
48. Quinn D, Cooper B, Clyman RI. Factors associated with permanent closure of the ductus arteriosus: a role for prolonged indomethacin therapy. Pediatrics 2002;110(1 Pt 1):e10.
49. Uchiyama A, Nagasawa H, Yamamoto Y, et al. Clinical aspects of very-low-birthweight infants showing reopening of ductus arteriosus. Pediatr Int 2011; 53(3):322–7.
50. Mahony L, Carnero V, Brett C, et al. Prophylactic indomethacin therapy for patent ductus arteriosus in very-low-birth-weight infants. N Engl J Med 1982; 306(9):506–10.
51. Aranda JV, Clyman R, Cox B, et al. A randomized, double-blind, placebo-controlled trial on intravenous ibuprofen L-lysine for the early closure of non-symptomatic patent ductus arteriosus within 72 hours of birth in extremely low-birth-weight infants. Am J Perinatol 2009;26(3):235–45.
52. Su PH, Chen JY, Su CM, et al. Comparison of ibuprofen and indomethacin therapy for patent ductus arteriosus in preterm infants. Pediatr Int 2003;45(6): 665–70.
53. Ohlsson A, Walia R, Shah SS. Ibuprofen for the treatment of patent ductus arteriosus in preterm and/or low birth weight infants. Cochrane Database Syst Rev 2010;4:CD003481.
54. Narayanan-Sankar M, Clyman RI. Pharmacology review: pharmacological closure of patent ductus arteriosus in the neonate. NeoReviews 2003;4:e215–21.
55. Achanti B, Yeh TF, Pildes RS. Indomethacin therapy in infants with advanced postnatal age and patent ductus arteriosus. Clin Invest Med 1986;9(4):250–3.
56. Seyberth HW, Muller H, Wille L, et al. Recovery of prostaglandin production associated with reopening of the ductus arteriosus after indomethacin treatment in preterm infants with respiratory distress syndrome. Pediatr Pharmacol (New York) 1982;2(2):127–41.
57. Herrera C, Holberton J, Davis P. Prolonged versus short course of indomethacin for the treatment of patent ductus arteriosus in preterm infants. Cochrane Database Syst Rev 2007;2:CD003480.
58. Hammerman C, Glaser J, Schimmel MS, et al. Continuous versus multiple rapid infusions of indomethacin: effects on cerebral blood flow velocity. Pediatrics 1995;95(2):244–8.

59. Christmann V, Liem KD, Semmekrot BA, et al. Changes in cerebral, renal and mesenteric blood flow velocity during continuous and bolus infusion of indomethacin. Acta Paediatr 2002;91(4):440–6.

60. Kuhl G, Seyberth HW. Intestinal perforations after enteral administration of indomethacin in premature infants. J Pediatr 1986;108(2):327–8.

61. Nagaraj HS, Sandhu AS, Cook LN, et al. Gastrointestinal perforation following indomethacin therapy in very low birth weight infants. J Pediatr Surg 1981; 16(6):1003–7.

62. Cooke RW, Pickering D. Poor response to oral indomethacin therapy for persistent ductus arteriosus in very low birthweight infants. Br Heart J 1979;41(3): 301–3.

63. Alpan G, Eyal F, Vinograd I, et al. Localized intestinal perforations after enteral administration of indomethacin in premature infants. J Pediatr 1985;106(2): 277–81.

64. Marshall TA, Pai S, Reddy PP. Intestinal perforation following enteral administration of indomethacin. J Pediatr 1985;107(3):484–5.

65. Bhat R, Vidyasagar D, Fisher E, et al. Pharmacokinetics of oral and intravenous indomethacin in preterm infants. Dev Pharmacol Ther 1980;1(2-3):101–10.

66. Evans M, Bhat R, Vidyasagar D, et al. A comparison of oral and intravenous indomethacin dispositions in the premature infant with patent ductus arteriosus. Pediatr Pharmacol (New York) 1981;1(3):251–8.

67. Al Za'abi M, Donovan T, Tudehope D, et al. Orogastric and intravenous indomethacin administration to very premature neonates with patent ductus arteriosus: population pharmacokinetics, absolute bioavailability, and treatment outcome. Ther Drug Monit 2007;29(6):807–14.

68. Aranda JV, Varvarigou A, Beharry K, et al. Pharmacokinetics and protein binding of intravenous ibuprofen in the premature newborn infant. Acta Paediatr 1997; 86(3):289–93.

69. Desfrere L, Zohar S, Morville P, et al. Dose-finding study of ibuprofen in patent ductus arteriosus using the continual reassessment method. J Clin Pharm Ther 2005;30(2):121–32.

70. Cherif A, Khrouf N, Jabnoun S, et al. Randomized pilot study comparing oral ibuprofen with intravenous ibuprofen in very low birth weight infants with patent ductus arteriosus. Pediatrics 2008;122(6):e1256–61.

71. Gokmen T, Erdeve O, Altug N, et al. Efficacy and safety of oral versus intravenous ibuprofen in very low birth weight preterm infants with patent ductus arteriosus. J Pediatr 2011;158(4):549–54, e541.

72. Sharma PK, Garg SK, Narang A. Pharmacokinetics of oral ibuprofen in premature infants. J Clin Pharmacol 2003;43(9):968–73.

73. Barzilay B, Youngster I, Batash D, et al. Pharmacokinetics of oral ibuprofen for patent ductus arteriosus closure in preterm infants. Arch Dis Child 2011. [Epub ahead of print].

74. Gouyon JB, Kibleur Y. Efficacy and tolerability of enteral formulations of ibuprofen in the treatment of patent ductus arteriosus in preterm infants. Clin Ther 2010;32(10):1740–8.

75. Noori S, McCoy M, Friedlich P, et al. Failure of ductus arteriosus closure is associated with increased mortality in preterm infants. Pediatrics 2009;123(1): e138–44.

76. Stark AR, Carlo WA, Tyson JE, et al. Adverse effects of early dexamethasone in extremely-low-birth-weight infants. National Institute of Child Health and Human Development Neonatal Research Network. N Engl J Med 2001;344(2):95–101.

77. Watterberg KL, Gerdes JS, Cole CH, et al. Prophylaxis of early adrenal insufficiency to prevent bronchopulmonary dysplasia: a multicenter trial. Pediatrics 2004;114(6):1649–57.
78. Peltoniemi O, Kari MA, Heinonen K, et al. Pretreatment cortisol values may predict responses to hydrocortisone administration for the prevention of bronchopulmonary dysplasia in high-risk infants. J Pediatr 2005;146(5):632–7.
79. Attridge JT, Clark R, Walker MW, et al. New insights into spontaneous intestinal perforation using a national data set: (1) SIP is associated with early indomethacin exposure. J Perinatol 2006;26(2):93–9.
80. Kuhl G, Wille L, Bolkenius M, et al. Intestinal perforation associated with indomethacin treatment in premature infants. Eur J Pediatr 1985;143(3):213–6.
81. Scholz TD, McGuinness GA. Localized intestinal perforation following intravenous indomethacin for patent ductus arteriosus. J Pediatr Gastroenterol Nutr 1988;7(5):773–5.
82. Sharma R, Hudak ML, Tepas JJ 3rd, et al. Prenatal or postnatal indomethacin exposure and neonatal gut injury associated with isolated intestinal perforation and necrotizing enterocolitis. J Perinatol 2010;30(12):786–93.
83. Major CA, Lewis DF, Harding JA, et al. Tocolysis with indomethacin increases the incidence of necrotizing enterocolitis in the low-birth-weight neonate. Am J Obstet Gynecol 1994;170(1 Pt 1):102–6.
84. Vanhaesebrouck P, Thiery M, Leroy JG, et al. Oligohydramnios, renal insufficiency, and ileal perforation in preterm infants after intrauterine exposure to indomethacin. J Pediatr 1988;113(4):738–43.
85. Gordon PV, Swanson JR, Clark R. Antenatal indomethacin is more likely associated with spontaneous intestinal perforation rather than NEC. Am J Obstet Gynecol 2008;198(6):725 [author reply: 725–6].
86. Fowlie PW, Davis PG, McGuire W. Prophylactic intravenous indomethacin for preventing mortality and morbidity in preterm infants. Cochrane Database Syst Rev 2010;7:CD000174.
87. Cassady G, Crouse DT, Kirklin JW, et al. A randomized, controlled trial of very early prophylactic ligation of the ductus arteriosus in babies who weighed 1000 g or less at birth. N Engl J Med 1989;320(23):1511–6.
88. Dollberg S, Lusky A, Reichman B. Patent ductus arteriosus, indomethacin and necrotizing enterocolitis in very low birth weight infants: a population-based study. J Pediatr Gastroenterol Nutr 2005;40(2):184–8.
89. Milner ME, de la Monte SM, Moore GW, et al. Risk factors for developing and dying from necrotizing enterocolitis. J Pediatr Gastroenterol Nutr 1986;5(3):359–64.
90. Palder SB, Schwartz MZ, Tyson KR, et al. Association of closure of patent ductus arteriosus and development of necrotizing enterocolitis. J Pediatr Surg 1988;23(5):422–3.
91. Coombs RC, Morgan ME, Durbin GM, et al. Gut blood flow velocities in the newborn: effects of patent ductus arteriosus and parenteral indomethacin. Arch Dis Child 1990;65(10 Spec No):1067–71.
92. Pezzati M, Vangi V, Biagiotti R, et al. Effects of indomethacin and ibuprofen on mesenteric and renal blood flow in preterm infants with patent ductus arteriosus. J Pediatr 1999;135(6):733–8.
93. Shimada S, Kasai T, Konishi M, et al. Effects of patent ductus arteriosus on left ventricular output and organ blood flows in preterm infants with respiratory distress syndrome treated with surfactant. J Pediatr 1994;125(2):270–7.

94. Van Bel F, Van Zoeren D, Schipper J, et al. Effect of indomethacin on superior mesenteric artery blood flow velocity in preterm infants. J Pediatr 1990;116(6): 965–70.

95. Yanowitz TD, Yao AC, Werner JC, et al. Effects of prophylactic low-dose indomethacin on hemodynamics in very low birth weight infants. J Pediatr 1998; 132(1):28–34.

96. Fujii AM, Brown E, Mirochnick M, et al. Neonatal necrotizing enterocolitis with intestinal perforation in extremely premature infants receiving early indomethacin treatment for patent ductus arteriosus. J Perinatol 2002;22(7): 535–40.

97. Grosfeld JL, Chaet M, Molinari F, et al. Increased risk of necrotizing enterocolitis in premature infants with patent ductus arteriosus treated with indomethacin. Ann Surg 1996;224(3):350–5 [discussion: 355–7].

98. Rajadurai VS, Yu VY. Intravenous indomethacin therapy in preterm neonates with patent ductus arteriosus. J Paediatr Child Health 1991;27(6):370–5.

99. Ryder RW, Shelton JD, Guinan ME. Necrotizing enterocolitis: a prospective multicenter investigation. Am J Epidemiol 1980;112(1):113–23.

100. Sankaran K, Puckett B, Lee DS, et al. Variations in incidence of necrotizing enterocolitis in Canadian neonatal intensive care units. J Pediatr Gastroenterol Nutr 2004;39(4):366–72.

101. Schmidt B, Davis P, Moddemann D, et al. Long-term effects of indomethacin prophylaxis in extremely-low-birth-weight infants. N Engl J Med 2001;344(26): 1966–72.

102. Benitz WE. Treatment of persistent patent ductus arteriosus in preterm infants: time to accept the null hypothesis? J Perinatol 2010;30(4):241–52.

103. Bose CL, Laughon MM. Patent ductus arteriosus: lack of evidence for common treatments. Arch Dis Child 2007;92(6):F498–502.

104. Clyman RI, Chorne N. Patent ductus arteriosus: evidence for and against treatment. J Pediatr 2007;150(3):216–9.

105. Ohlsson A, Shah SS. Ibuprofen for the prevention of patent ductus arteriosus in preterm and/or low birth weight infants. Cochrane Database Syst Rev 2011; 7:CD004213.

106. Sangtawesin C, Sangtawesin V, Lertsutthiwong W, et al. Prophylaxis of symptomatic patent ductus arteriosus with oral ibuprofen in very low birth weight infants. J Med Assoc Thai 2008;91(Suppl 3):S28–34.

107. Sangtawesin V, Sangtawesin C, Raksasinborisut C, et al. Oral ibuprofen prophylaxis for symptomatic patent ductus arteriosus of prematurity. J Med Assoc Thai 2006;89(3):314–21.

108. Romagnoli C, Zecca E, Papacci P, et al. Furosemide does not prevent indomethacin-induced renal side effects in preterm infants. Clin Pharmacol Ther 1997;62(2):181–6.

109. Kushnir A, Pinheiro JM. Comparison of renal effects of ibuprofen versus indomethacin during treatment of patent ductus arteriosus in contiguous historical cohorts. BMC Clin Pharmacol 2011;11:8.

110. Katakam LI, Cotten CM, Goldberg RN, et al. Safety and effectiveness of indomethacin versus ibuprofen for treatment of patent ductus arteriosus. Am J Perinatol 2010;27(5):425–9.

111. Van Overmeire B, Allegaert K, Casaer A, et al. Prophylactic ibuprofen in premature infants: a multicentre, randomised, double-blind, placebo-controlled trial. Lancet 2004;364(9449):1945–9.

112. Gournay V, Roze JC, Kuster A, et al. Prophylactic ibuprofen versus placebo in very premature infants: a randomised, double-blind, placebo-controlled trial. Lancet 2004;364(9449):1939–44.
113. Bandstra ES, Montalvo BM, Goldberg RN, et al. Prophylactic indomethacin for prevention of intraventricular hemorrhage in premature infants. Pediatrics 1988;82(4):533–42.
114. Vieux R, Desandes R, Boubred F, et al. Ibuprofen in very preterm infants impairs renal function for the first month of life. Pediatr Nephrol 2010;25(2): 267–74.
115. Cataldi L, Leone R, Moretti U, et al. Potential risk factors for the development of acute renal failure in preterm newborn infants: a case-control study. Arch Dis Child 2005;90(6):F514–9.
116. Cuzzolin L, Fanos V, Pinna B, et al. Postnatal renal function in preterm newborns: a role of diseases, drugs and therapeutic interventions. Pediatr Nephrol 2006; 21(7):931–8.
117. Erdeve O, Sarici SU, Sari E, et al. Oral-ibuprofen-induced acute renal failure in a preterm infant. Pediatr Nephrol 2008;23(9):1565–7.
118. Fanos V, Antonucci R, Zaffanello M. Ibuprofen and acute kidney injury in the newborn. Turk J Pediatr 2010;52(3):231–8.
119. Tiker F, Yildirim SV. Acute renal impairment after oral ibuprofen for medical closure of patent ductus arteriosus. Indian Pediatr 2007;44(1):54–5.
120. Baenziger O, Waldvogel K, Ghelfi D, et al. Can dopamine prevent the renal side effects of indomethacin? A prospective randomized clinical study. Klin Padiatr 1999;211(6):438–41.
121. Fajardo CA, Whyte RK, Steele BT. Effect of dopamine on failure of indomethacin to close the patent ductus arteriosus. J Pediatr 1992;121(5 Pt 1):771–5.
122. Barrington K, Brion LP. Dopamine versus no treatment to prevent renal dysfunction in indomethacin-treated preterm newborn infants. Cochrane Database Syst Rev 2002;3:CD003213.
123. Ahlfors CE. Effect of ibuprofen on bilirubin-albumin binding. J Pediatr 2004; 144(3):386–8.
124. Rheinlaender C, Helfenstein D, Walch E, et al. Total serum bilirubin levels during cyclooxygenase inhibitor treatment for patent ductus arteriosus in preterm infants. Acta Paediatr 2009;98(1):36–42.
125. Zecca E, Romagnoli C, De Carolis MP, et al. Does ibuprofen increase neonatal hyperbilirubinemia? Pediatrics 2009;124(2):480–4.
126. Amin SB, Miravalle N. Effect of ibuprofen on bilirubin-albumin binding affinity in premature infants. J Perinat Med 2011;39(1):55–8.
127. Aranda JV, Thomas R. Systematic review: intravenous ibuprofen in preterm newborns. Semin Perinatol 2006;30(3):114–20.
128. Desfrere L, Thibaut C, Kibleur Y, et al. Unbound bilirubin does not increase during ibuprofen treatment of patent ductus arteriosus in preterm infants. J Pediatr 2011. [Epub ahead of print].
129. Mosca F, Bray M, Lattanzio M, et al. Comparative evaluation of the effects of indomethacin and ibuprofen on cerebral perfusion and oxygenation in preterm infants with patent ductus arteriosus. J Pediatr 1997;131(4):549–54.
130. Patel J, Roberts I, Azzopardi D, et al. Randomized double-blind controlled trial comparing the effects of ibuprofen with indomethacin on cerebral hemodynamics in preterm infants with patent ductus arteriosus. Pediatr Res 2000;47(1): 36–42.

131. Romagnoli C, De Carolis MP, Papacci P, et al. Effects of prophylactic ibuprofen on cerebral and renal hemodynamics in very preterm neonates. Clin Pharmacol Ther 2000;67(6):676–83.

132. Austin NC, Pairaudeau PW, Hames TK, et al. Regional cerebral blood flow velocity changes after indomethacin infusion in preterm infants. Arch Dis Child 1992;67(7 Spec No):851–4.

133. Benders MJ, Dorrepaal CA, van de Bor M, et al. Acute effects of indomethacin on cerebral hemodynamics and oxygenation. Biol Neonate 1995;68(2):91–9.

134. Edwards AD, Wyatt JS, Richardson C, et al. Effects of indomethacin on cerebral haemodynamics in very preterm infants. Lancet 1990;335(8704):1491–5.

135. Laudignon N, Chemtob S, Bard H, et al. Effect of indomethacin on cerebral blood flow velocity of premature newborns. Biol Neonate 1988;54(5):254–62.

136. Ohlsson A, Bottu J, Govan J, et al. Effect of indomethacin on cerebral blood flow velocities in very low birth weight neonates with a patent ductus arteriosus. Dev Pharmacol Ther 1993;20(1-2):100–6.

137. Pryds O, Greisen G, Johansen KH. Indomethacin and cerebral blood flow in premature infants treated for patent ductus arteriosus. Eur J Pediatr 1988; 147(3):315–6.

138. Simko A, Mardoum R, Merritt TA, et al. Effects on cerebral blood flow velocities of slow and rapid infusion of indomethacin. J Perinatol 1994;14(1):29–35.

139. Van Bel F, Van de Bor M, Stijnen T, et al. Cerebral blood flow velocity changes in preterm infants after a single dose of indomethacin: duration of its effect. Pediatrics 1989;84(5):802–7.

140. Lemmers PM, Toet MC, van Bel F. Impact of patent ductus arteriosus and subsequent therapy with indomethacin on cerebral oxygenation in preterm infants. Pediatrics 2008;121(1):142–7.

141. McCormick DC, Edwards AD, Brown GC, et al. Effect of indomethacin on cerebral oxidized cytochrome oxidase in preterm infants. Pediatr Res 1993;33(6):603–8.

142. Couser RJ, Hoekstra RE, Ferrara TB, et al. Neurodevelopmental follow-up at 36 months' corrected age of preterm infants treated with prophylactic indomethacin. Arch Pediatr Adolesc Med 2000;154(6):598–602.

143. Ment LR, Vohr B, Oh W, et al. Neurodevelopmental outcome at 36 months' corrected age of preterm infants in the Multicenter Indomethacin Intraventricular Hemorrhage Prevention Trial. Pediatrics 1996;98(4 Pt 1):714–8.

144. Ment LR, Vohr B, Allan W, et al. Outcome of children in the Indomethacin Intraventricular Hemorrhage Prevention Trial. Pediatrics 2000;105(3 Pt 1):485–91.

145. Ment LR, Vohr BR, Makuch RW, et al. Prevention of intraventricular hemorrhage by indomethacin in male preterm infants. J Pediatr 2004;145(6):832–4.

146. Vohr BR, Allan WC, Westerveld M, et al. School-age outcomes of very low birth weight infants in the indomethacin intraventricular hemorrhage prevention trial. Pediatrics 2003;111(4 Pt 1):e340–6.

147. Clyman RI, Saha S, Jobe A, et al. Indomethacin prophylaxis for preterm infants: the impact of 2 multicentered randomized controlled trials on clinical practice. J Pediatr 2007;150(1):46–50, e42.

148. AlFaleh K. Indomethacin prophylaxis revisited: changing practice and supportive evidence. Acta Paediatr 2011;100(5):641–6.

149. Lipman B, Serwer GA, Brazy JE. Abnormal cerebral hemodynamics in preterm infants with patent ductus arteriosus. Pediatrics 1982;69(6):778–81.

150. Ment LR, Stewart WB, Scott DT, et al. Beagle puppy model of intraventricular hemorrhage: randomized indomethacin prevention trial. Neurology 1983;33(2): 179–84.

151. Ment LR, Duncan CC, Ehrenkranz RA, et al. Randomized indomethacin trial for prevention of intraventricular hemorrhage in very low birth weight infants. J Pediatr 1985;107(6):937–43.
152. Ment LR, Duncan CC, Ehrenkranz RA, et al. Randomized low-dose indomethacin trial for prevention of intraventricular hemorrhage in very low birth weight neonates. J Pediatr 1988;112(6):948–55.
153. Bada HS, Green RS, Pourcyrous M, et al. Indomethacin reduces the risks of severe intraventricular hemorrhage. J Pediatr 1989;115(4):631–7.
154. Hanigan WC, Kennedy G, Roemisch F, et al. Administration of indomethacin for the prevention of periventricular-intraventricular hemorrhage in high-risk neonates. J Pediatr 1988;112(6):941–7.
155. Krueger E, Mellander M, Bratton D, et al. Prevention of symptomatic patent ductus arteriosus with a single dose of indomethacin. J Pediatr 1987;111(5):749–54.
156. Ment LR, Oh W, Ehrenkranz RA, et al. Low-dose indomethacin and prevention of intraventricular hemorrhage: a multicenter randomized trial. Pediatrics 1994;93(4):543–50.
157. DeMauro SB, Schmidt B, Roberts RS. Why would a sane clinician not prescribe prophylactic indomethacin? Acta Paediatr 2011;100(5):636.
158. Shah SS, Ohlsson A. Ibuprofen for the prevention of patent ductus arteriosus in preterm and/or low birth weight infants. Cochrane Database Syst Rev 2003;2:CD004213.
159. Dani C, Bertini G, Pezzati M, et al. Prophylactic ibuprofen for the prevention of intraventricular hemorrhage among preterm infants: a multicenter, randomized study. Pediatrics 2005;115(6):1529–35.
160. Couser RJ, Ferrara TB, Wright GB, et al. Prophylactic indomethacin therapy in the first twenty-four hours of life for the prevention of patent ductus arteriosus in preterm infants treated prophylactically with surfactant in the delivery room. J Pediatr 1996;128(5 Pt 1):631–7.
161. Dani C, Bertini G, Reali MF, et al. Prophylaxis of patent ductus arteriosus with ibuprofen in preterm infants. Acta Paediatr 2000;89(11):1369–74.
162. De Carolis MP, Romagnoli C, Polimeni V, et al. Prophylactic ibuprofen therapy of patent ductus arteriosus in preterm infants. Eur J Pediatr 2000;159(5):364–8.
163. Bellini C, Campone F, Serra G. Pulmonary hypertension following L-lysine ibuprofen therapy in a preterm infant with patent ductus arteriosus. CMAJ 2006;174(13):1843–4.
164. Tefft RG. The impact of an early ibuprofen treatment protocol on the incidence of surgical ligation of the ductus arteriosus. Am J Perinatol 2010;27(1):83–90.
165. Brash AR, Hickey DE, Graham TP, et al. Pharmacokinetics of indomethacin in the neonate. Relation of plasma indomethacin levels to response of the ductus arteriosus. N Engl J Med 1981;305(2):67–72.
166. Smyth JM, Collier PS, Darwish M, et al. Intravenous indomethacin in preterm infants with symptomatic patent ductus arteriosus. A population pharmacokinetic study. Br J Clin Pharmacol 2004;58(3):249–58.
167. Yeh TF, Achanti B, Patel H, et al. Indomethacin therapy in premature infants with patent ductus arteriosus–determination of therapeutic plasma levels. Dev Pharmacol Ther 1989;12(4):169–78.
168. Knight DB. Patent ductus arteriosus: how important to which babies? Early Hum Dev 1992;29(1–3):287–92.
169. Knight DB. The treatment of patent ductus arteriosus in preterm infants. A review and overview of randomized trials. Semin Neonatol 2001;6(1):63–73.

170. Laughon MM, Simmons MA, Bose CL. Patency of the ductus arteriosus in the premature infant: is it pathologic? Should it be treated? Curr Opin Pediatr 2004;16(2):146–51.
171. Campbell M. Natural history of persistent ductus arteriosus. Br Heart J 1968; 30(1):4–13.
172. Dudell GG, Gersony WM. Patent ductus arteriosus in neonates with severe respiratory disease. J Pediatr 1984;104(6):915–20.
173. Jacob J, Gluck L, DiSessa T, et al. The contribution of PDA in the neonate with severe RDS. J Pediatr 1980;96(1):79–87.
174. Thibeault DW, Emmanouilides GC, Nelson RJ, et al. Patent ductus arteriosus complicating the respiratory distress syndrome in preterm infants. J Pediatr 1975;86(1):120–6.
175. Cotton RB, Stahlman MT, Bender HW, et al. Randomized trial of early closure of symptomatic patent ductus arteriosus in small preterm infants. J Pediatr 1978; 93(4):647–51.
176. Kaapa P, Lanning P, Koivisto M. Early closure of patent ductus arteriosus with indomethacin in preterm infants with idiopathic respiratory distress syndrome. Acta Paediatr Scand 1983;72(2):179–84.
177. Alexander F, Chiu L, Kroh M, et al. Analysis of outcome in 298 extremely low-birth-weight infants with patent ductus arteriosus. J Pediatr Surg 2009;44(1): 112–7 [disscusion: 117].
178. Brooks JM, Travadi JN, Patole SK, et al. Is surgical ligation of patent ductus arteriosus necessary? The Western Australian experience of conservative management. Arch Dis Child 2005;90(3):F235–9.
179. Kaempf JW, Wu YX, Kaempf AJ, et al. What happens when the patent ductus arteriosus is treated less aggressively in very low birth weight infants? J Perinatol 2011;1–5. DOI: 10.1038/jp.2011.102. Accessed November 11, 2011.
180. Herrman K, Bose C, Lewis K, et al. Spontaneous closure of the patent ductus arteriosus in very low birth weight infants following discharge from the neonatal unit. Arch Dis Child 2009;94(1):F48–50.
181. Jones LJ, Craven PD, Attia J, et al. Network meta-analysis of indomethacin versus ibuprofen versus placebo for PDA in preterm infants. Arch Dis Child 2011;96(1):F45–52.
182. Hammerman C, Bin-Nun A, Markovitch E, et al. Ductal closure with paracetamol: a surprising new approach to patent ductus arteriosus treatment. Pediatrics 2011;e1–4. DOI: 10.1542/peds.2011-0359. Accessed November 11, 2011.

Evidence-Based Methylxanthine Use in the NICU

Alan R. Spitzer, MD

KEYWORDS

• Methylxanthines • Caffeine • Apnea • NICU

Since the introduction of neonatal intensive care units (NICUs) in the United States during the early 1960s, apnea of prematurity (AOP) and apnea of infancy have been problems with which neonatologists and pediatricians have had to frequently contend. For the purposes of this article, references to pathologic apnea are considered as a pause in breathing lasting longer than 20 seconds duration, or a shorter pause that is accompanied by physiologic change (a drop in oxygen saturation <85% or a 30% decline from baseline resting heart rate). These definitions are somewhat arbitrary and other authors have used variations of these numbers, which are noted where appropriate. To a great extent, the frequency of AOP depends on the gestational age and maturity of the infant. In general, however, approximately 70% of infants born before 34 weeks' gestation demonstrate AOP at some point before hospital discharge.[1] In term infants greater than 39 weeks' gestation, approximately 3% to 5% of these infants have prolonged apnea if studied during the first week of life.

Because prolonged apnea is a relatively common event in neonates, two philosophically different points of view have developed regarding its significance: it is a normal developmental process that one need not be concerned with; or, although it is a common process, the physiologic implications of episodes of apnea are of such significance that it always needs to be treated with great caution. Prolonged failure to breathe may be an initiating factor in some cases of sudden infant death syndrome; it may also lead to neurologic injury if an infant becomes hypoxemic for a sufficient duration of time or in a highly repetitive fashion. The great problem in deciding which line of reasoning is correct, however, is underscored because convincing data to support one approach or the other have been extremely difficult to acquire. Regardless of one's philosophic thinking, however, it is generally agreed that frequent apnea that is accompanied by physiologic change (bradycardia, cyanosis, or oxygen desaturation) may need to be evaluated and treated to ensure the best possible outcome for the infant.

The Center for Research, Education, and Quality MEDNAX Services/Pediatrix Medical Group/ American Anesthesiology, 1301 Concord Terrace, Sunrise, FL 33323, USA
E-mail address: alan_spitzer@pediatrix.com

METHYLXANTHINE TREATMENT OF APNEA: HISTORICAL ASPECTS

Apnea remains the primary absolute indication for the institution of positive pressure ventilation in the NICU. Infants who fail to breathe must have their ventilation supported, especially primary apnea during resuscitation in the course of early life. Most problems with apnea clinically, however, occur when an infant is either being weaned from positive pressure support or has been removed from the common forms of ventilatory support. The infant continues to demonstrate immaturity of breathing control that results in prolonged periods of apnea. Because this issue is so common, once physicians began attempting to care for the neonate as a patient, apnea became an ongoing concern for the neonatologist.

The first NICU in the United States is generally attributed to Vanderbilt University, where Dr. Mildred Stahlman initiated such a unit in 1964. Even before NICUs started appearing, however, the issue of apnea in premature infants was recognized as a concern. In 1959, Miller and colleagues[2] wrote the following: "In spite of the frequency and serious nature of these attacks (of apnea), scant attention has been given to them in the literature." In their study, these authors defined apnea as prolonged if it lasted greater than 60 seconds, and observed that it was highly associated with mortality, especially when it occurred early during hospitalization. It seems as if respiratory insufficiency from respiratory distress syndrome was most typically operative here, an aspect of prematurity that was not as clearly appreciated as it is today. In 1964, legendary neonatologist (the term had been coined by Alexander Schaeffer in 1960) Clement Smith noted the value of oxygen administration in small volumes in abolishing the frequency and severity of AOP, although he warned against excessive use for fear of retinal changes of retinopathy of prematurity, then known as "retrolental fibroplasia."[3] Several other approaches to the treatment of apnea were suggested in this era, including hyperbaric oxygen,[4] early apnea alarm systems,[5] and apnea mattresses.[6] Finally, in 1973, Kuzemko and Paala[7] published the first report of aminophylline use (by suppository) to treat AOP, studying 10 infants with birth weights between 860 and 2200 g with positive results.

Aminophylline administration, however, especially by suppository, has had a very guarded reputation in infants, because sudden deaths in people with asthma were occasionally seen and thought to be caused by the cardiac toxicity precipitated by either irregular gastrointestinal absorption of aminophylline or excessively rapid infusion. Pediatric residents at the Children's Hospital of Philadelphia in the early 1970s were required to sit at the bedside and monitor the heart rate or electrocardiogram of every child with asthma receiving an aminophylline infusion (Spitzer AR, personal experience, 1973). Suppositories were forbidden because of their erratic absorption. Lucey,[8] however, recognized the potential benefits and risks of aminophylline to treat apnea in a very perceptive and far-sighted editorial in 1975, even suggesting that caffeine might be a preferable approach to aminophylline.

Despite these early successes (and cautions) about the use of theophylline, the introduction of a safer methylxanthine for this purpose, namely caffeine, was not that simple. Shortly after joining the faculty at the Children's Hospital of Philadelphia in 1973, William Fox proposed a trial to the institutional review board of that hospital in which caffeine would be used to treat apnea in premature infants. The study was turned down by the institutional review board as being too potentially risky and hazardous in this patient population (Fox WW, personal communication, 1982). Soon afterward, however, interest in caffeine grew and Aranda and colleagues[9] published the first paper documenting the responsiveness of AOP to caffeine therapy (**Fig. 1**). In that trial, the authors used a dose of 10 to 20 mg/kg caffeine citrate, equal to 5 to 10 mg/kg of caffeine, given

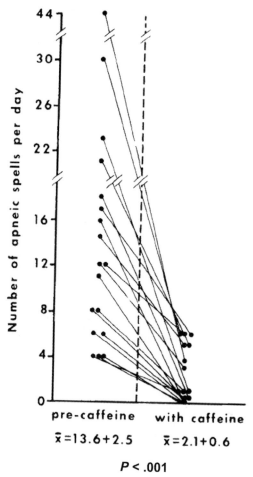

Fig. 1. Caffeine therapy study. (*From* Aranda JV, Gorman W, Bergsteinsson H, et al. Efficacy of caffeine in treatment of apnea in the low birth-weight infant. J Pediatr 1979;90:470; with permission.)

once to three times daily depending on the response. This dosing approach has not changed significantly since that time.

Caffeine Responsiveness

Although initial studies demonstrated the value of methylxanthines for the treatment of apnea, several issues remained for the neonatologist. First, the studies were somewhat limited by numbers of patients. The initial paper by Aranda[9] consisted of 18 infants, who all responded to treatment with a reduction in frequency of apnea spells. Potential toxicity in that study seemed minimal, but the sample size precluded any extensive analysis of safety, either immediate or long-term. More importantly, the actual metabolism of this drug in the neonatal period was very much unknown. In the original paper,[9] the authors did note the relatively slow elimination of caffeine on repeated doses. Given the worrisome history of aminophylline effects when certain levels of the drug were reached, the lack of pharmacokinetic data on caffeine made it a therapy that clearly needed more work before its use could be widely adopted. In addition, because the drug was recognized at least in adults as a neurostimulator, there was understandable concern about the potential for longer-term neurodevelopmental problems in treated infants.

Aranda's group at McGill University recognized these issues and followed their initial publication with a second paper delineating the effects of caffeine on their initial group of treated infants.[10] In that publication, there did not seem to be any significant differences between the treated and control groups of infants, although there was a high incidence of retrolental fibroplasia noted in the treated and control groups. The authors thought that this effect might be the result of the apnea itself, with wide fluctuations in oxygen levels during apnea spells, especially if an infant had to be treated with positive pressure oxygen. Overall complication rates, such as seizures and myopia, were also somewhat high for both groups, but that era was an early one in modern neonatal care and complications were generally more frequent than those observed today. The authors did point out that apnea was reduced with caffeine and the need for positive pressure ventilation was also lower in the caffeine-treated group. Little comment was made about acute physiologic consequences of caffeine in this paper, although the authors did note the possibility of "decreased cerebral blood flow, relaxation of the ductus arteriosus, and many complex metabolic effects."

The issue of metabolic effects of methylxanthines was further complicated by a study by Bory and colleagues,[11] which noted that in neonates given theophylline for the treatment of apnea, approximately a third of the dose was converted to caffeine. This active metabolic pathway seemed to be present only during the first months of life, and was not seen in adults. In that trial, levels of caffeine as high as 8 mg/L were noted in infants treated with theophylline, a range believed to be therapeutic for neonatal apnea. The authors were concerned that this metabolic pathway might actually lower the toxicity threshold for theophylline in the neonate and might explain the adverse cardiovascular complications (primarily tachyarrythmias) that had been noted in some infants with relatively modest theophylline levels.

These results made it problematic for investigators to define the appropriate therapeutic levels for methylxanthines in the treatment of apnea. In older children and adults, it had been known that bronchodilation in patients with asthma was achieved with a plasma theophylline concentration of 5 to 20 mg/L, with toxicity becoming more evident when levels higher than 20 were obtained. For the neonate, with a different metabolic pathway, levels of 7 to 20 mg/L were thought to be adequate for effective abolition of apnea.[12] Shannon and colleagues[13] expressed a concern that the therapeutic range for theophylline might even be narrower, observing control of apnea spells at plasma concentrations of theophylline of 6.6 mg/L, but noting cardiovascular toxicity (heart rate >180 bpm) with ranges between 13 and 32 mg/L. As a result, subsequent work by Turmen and coworkers[14] suggested that caffeine seemed to be a safer drug than theophylline, demonstrating that blood levels of caffeine as low as 3 to 4 mg/L seemed effective in abolishing apnea. Aranda also noted that caffeine, even in higher blood level ranges, did not seem to have the cardiovascular toxicity of theophylline, making it a drug more suitable for the neonate.[11] Based on all this rapidly accumulating work, the dosing schedule for caffeine was confirmed to be a loading dose of 10 mg/kg of caffeine (20 mg/kg of caffeine citrate), followed by a single daily dose of 2.5 mg/kg, aiming for a blood level between 6 and 20 mg/L. Because of the safer therapeutic range for caffeine compared with theophylline and because caffeine need only be given once daily, theophylline has nearly disappeared from use in the United States for the treatment of AOP.

The need for following caffeine levels has been questioned, however, because of the medication's relative safety profile. Leon and colleagues[15] examined this issue and found that with the dosing schedule noted previously, after stability had been reached after 14 days there was little reason to check levels unless there was a clinical change noted or signs of toxicity were observed. Natarajan and colleagues[16] similarly noted that caffeine level monitoring was not necessary in the therapeutic use of caffeine to treat AOP.

Mechanism of Action of Methylxanthines

Although methylxanthines have now been used for the treatment of AOP for more than 35 years, the precise mechanisms for their actions remain uncertain. Xanthines work in the central nervous system and peripherally. Some of the known effects of methylxanthines include an increase in minute ventilation, enhanced chemoreceptor sensitivity to carbon dioxide, increased diaphragmatic activity, reduction of periodic breathing, bronchodilation, reduction of hypoxic respiratory depression, and diuresis. Although theophylline has long been acknowledged for its bronchodilator effects, it should be noted that caffeine also possesses similar capabilities, a fact often overlooked in the NICU.[17] Many of these actions may assist the infant at risk for apnea through enhanced oxygenation and carbon dioxide responsiveness. Although the precise pharmacologic mechanisms for these effects are not clear, it is known that methylxanthines are nonspecific inhibitors of two of the four known adenosine receptors.[18] Adenosine is widely recognized as being an important regulator of sleep and arousal states, but may also increase susceptibility to seizures, and xanthines may work through these pathways. Methylxanthines also increase the metabolic rate and oxygen consumption.

Xanthines are not without serious side effects at toxic levels, with aminophylline and theophylline seeming to have a lower margin of safety than caffeine. Toxic levels of any of these agents, however, may cause tachycardia, arrhythmias, irritability and crying, feeding intolerance, and seizures. Death may occur when extreme levels (>40 mg/L) are reached, often through accidental overdose. Reports of an increased risk of necrotizing enterocolitis with methylxanthine use in premature infants have also been observed.[19] A subsequent report of 275 infants, however, from Davis and colleagues[20] was unable to substantiate any increased clinical risk of theophylline in the development of necrotizing enterocolitis, and a large randomized trial (Caffeine for Apnea of Prematurity Trial) of 2006 infants by Schmidt and colleagues[21] similarly failed to show any enhancing effect of caffeine on rates of necrotizing enterocolitis. Of particular interest in the latter trial was the important observation that the use of caffeine decreased the incidence of bronchopulmonary dysplasia and the need for treatment, either medical or surgical, of the patent ductus arteriosus (PDA). No significant short-term risks of caffeine could be demonstrated in this patient population.

The economic value of caffeine therapy was evaluated in a recently published paper.[22] In a comparison with placebo treatment, the authors noted that "the mean cost per infant was $124,466 in the caffeine group and $133,505 in the placebo group (difference: $9039 [−14,749 to −3375]; adjusted $P = .014$). Cost-effectiveness analysis showed caffeine to be a dominant or 'win-win' therapy: in >99% of 1000 bootstrap replications of the analysis, caffeine-treated infants had simultaneously better outcomes and lower mean costs. These results were robust to a 1000% increase in the individual resource items, including the price of caffeine citrate."

USES OF METHYLXANTHINES IN THE NICU
Treatment of AOP

The most common indication for initiation of methylxanthine use in the NICU is AOP. This indication has been reviewed on a recurring basis by the Cochrane Collaboration, which since 1993 has provided systematic reviews of a variety of aspects of neonatal care. The Cochrane relies on randomized controlled trials to evaluate medical practice that is based on the highest quality of available evidence. In their most recent evaluation of methylxanthine therapy, Henderson-Smart and DePaoli[23] found six trials that examined this use of methylxanthines. These trials compared the use of theophylline, caffeine, or aminophylline as treatment of apnea versus placebo or no treatment in preterm infants. The authors concluded that "methylxanthines were effective in reducing the number of apneic attacks and the use of mechanical ventilation in two to seven days after starting treatment." Caffeine was also "associated with better long-term outcomes." These improved outcomes included not only a decrease in frequency of apnea, but also a reduction in positive pressure ventilation, a reduced rate in need for PDA ligation, and a reduction in chronic lung disease at 36 weeks gestation. Several of these outcomes were primarily seen in the previously mentioned Caffeine for Apnea of Prematurity Trial, and they led to the authors' recommendation that "caffeine would be the preferred drug for the treatment of apnoea." In a further assessment of theophylline versus caffeine, it was observed that both drugs had similar short-term effects on apnea and bradycardia, but that caffeine seemed to possess some therapeutic advantages over theophylline, which had higher rates of toxicity.[24]

These same authors also examined evidence for the use of prophylactic methylxanthines for apnea prevention.[25] In that assessment, the authors found three trials that qualified for inclusion, but they could find no support for the prophylactic use of methylxanthines for apnea prevention in preterm infants at this time.

Endotracheal Extubation

Because of their effects on bronchodilation and improved minute ventilation, and central nervous system stimulation, methylxanthines have been used as an adjunct to endotracheal extubation for some time. A recent *Cochrane Review* of prophylactic use of methylxanthines for extubation found seven trials that qualified for inclusion.[26] Based on these studies, it seemed that caffeine increased the likelihood of successful extubation while improving several other outcomes, including decreased rates of bronchopulmonary dysplasia, rates of PDA ligation, cerebral palsy, and death or major disability at 18 to 21 months of age. Because of its better therapeutic margin, caffeine was believed to be the drug of choice in this clinical situation, but the authors believed that further studies based on gestational age were warranted in the future.

Alternatives to Methylxanthines

In a recent review of the impact of caffeine on neonatal morbidities, Aranda and coworkers[27] noted that "caffeine is now one of the safest, most cost-beneficial and effective therapies in the newborn." Because this therapy is so easy to use, so effective, and so inexpensive, few alternatives of note currently exist or are in use for all practical purposes. The few therapies that have been evaluated to some extent are the medication doxapram, tactile stimulation, and CO_2 inhalation.

Doxapram is a respiratory stimulant in a different class of drugs than the methylxanthines, and is most commonly used in patients with obstructive pulmonary disease, in drug-induced respiratory depression, and after anesthesia. It is not approved for use in patients less than 12 years of age, although it has been used to treat AOP off-label in a dose of 0.5 to 2.5 mg/kg/h by intravenous infusion. Because benzyl alcohol is the associated preservative, it is not recommended for use in neonates and it can also cause cardiac arrhythmias, hypoventilation, and seizures. Randomized studies comparing doxapram with methylxanthines are few, and none have been performed in recent years. In a study that compared theophylline with doxapram, Pellowski and Finer[28] noted a similar response of AOP to both drugs, which did not seem well-sustained beyond a week. Barrington and Muttitt[29] also studied doxapram for extubation, but did not find that doxapram increased the likelihood for extubation in low-birth-weight infants. At present, doxapram is rarely used in the NICU, because there are concerns about long-term effects of this drug on development.[30]

Tactile stimulation is the most common response to AOP, as any bedside nurse can readily relate. Gentle skin stimulation often terminates an episode of apnea instantaneously. Given this commonly observed response, it has only seemed natural that a process of providing repeated stimulation might well avoid apnea and the need for medication. Unfortunately, there is but a single randomized trial in the literature that has been evaluated by the *Cochrane Review*, and this trial only enrolled 20 patients.[31] My own personal experience with inflatable beds that provide stimulation on a recurring basis is that the infant gradually attenuates the stimulus, even when it is made to occur at variable times, so that the effect on apnea is gradually lost. Furthermore, the sleep disruption is substantial, making an overstimulated infant that much more fatigued.

Recently, the group in Winnipeg has evaluated the possibility of providing higher concentrations of inhaled CO_2 as a respiratory stimulus in AOP.[32] They found that CO_2 was as effective as theophylline in reducing apnea with far fewer side effects. However, some difficulties were noted with this study. Infants were older at the time of study and the practical application of CO_2 by inhalation in the NICU for long periods was not tested. In addition, theophylline, a drug now far less commonly used was chosen as the control medication rather than caffeine. Consequently, it seems unlikely that this approach will be adopted until more widespread and more convincing studies are conducted.

RECOMMENDATIONS
Treatment

Methylxanthines, especially caffeine, seem to be highly effective and safe for the treatment of AOP. Caffeine also seems to be helpful when used prophylactically for the management of endotracheal tube extubation. The standard dose for caffeine is a loading dose of caffeine citrate of 20 to 25 mg/kg (equivalent to 10–12.5 mg/kg of caffeine base) intravenously or by mouth, followed by a maintenance dose of 5 to 10 mg/kg/d. Therapeutic serum levels should be checked after approximately 48 hours of therapy, aiming for a blood level of 5 to 20 µg/mL. The dose should be adjusted based on the response to therapy, aiming for the lowest blood level that successfully abolishes apnea as the desired goal. Again, with the high therapeutic index for caffeine, the cessation of apnea with treatment and the absence of any clinical side effects may make frequent monitoring of levels unnecessary in most neonates.

For the prophylactic treatment of endotracheal tube extubation, routine use of caffeine is not necessary. The author recommends withholding this therapy until an infant has failed an attempt at extubation. In this circumstance, it is important that attention be paid to the clinical response of the infant at the time of the initial extubation. If the patient was noted to rapidly deteriorate after removal of the endotracheal tube with marked respiratory distress and evidence of upper airway obstruction from edema, it is not likely that caffeine will assist with the subsequent extubation attempt. A second attempt should not be made for several days until the infant has further stabilized. In the situation of acute postextubation obstruction, one may find that pretreatment with corticosteroids may be of more value than caffeine. If, however, the infant's respiratory deterioration after extubation was noted to be a slow, gradual failure to sustain gas exchange, caffeine may be of value in assisting a subsequent trial of extubation. In that case, a loading dose of 20 mg/kg of caffeine citrate (10 mg/kg of caffeine base) should be given 24 hours before extubation. The extubation should be performed cautiously, giving a slow, sustained, low-pressure inflation as the endotracheal tube is slowly removed from the airway to maintain lung volume. The infant should be quickly placed on nasal continuous positive airway pressure or nasal cannula with oxygen. A maintenance dose of caffeine citrate of 10 mg/kg can then be given on the day of extubation and continued for a few days, to assist in maintaining extubation.

Duration of Therapy with Methylxanthines

Few areas of neonatal practice are as controversial or as confusing as the timing of cessation of apnea therapy after treatment has been initiated in a premature infant. In making decisions regarding caffeine management, it is essential to understand that the half-life of this drug is quite long, especially in a very low-birth-weight infant. Several studies have examined caffeine pharmacokinetics in premature infants. Pearlman and colleagues[33] evaluated a group of infants at approximately 33 weeks' gestational age and found a half-life of 52 ± 24 SD hours. Ahn and colleagues[34] looked at the metabolism and half-life of theophylline and caffeine after intravenous administration of aminophylline in seven infants, using high-performance liquid chromatography. These infants weighed 1190 g and were a mean of 31.5 weeks gestation. After 6 days of therapy, mean serum concentrations were 10.4 ± 2.3 SEM μg/mL for theophylline and 2.94 ± 0.98 μg/mL for caffeine, confirming the conversion of aminophylline to theophylline and caffeine. The half-life of caffeine in this population was 95.1 ± 25.4 SEM hours. Similarly, Charles and colleagues[35] found a half-life of 101 hours in a group of premature infants at approximately 30 weeks' gestational age. In addition to the long half-life duration, they pointed out that the caffeine was completely absorbed by the gastrointestinal route, creating a favorable situation when one needs to switch from intravenous to oral therapy. What all of these studies demonstrate, however, is an exceedingly long half-life for caffeine, which makes appropriate management of cessation of treatment an important consideration.

Stopping caffeine a day before discharge, therefore, and observing the infant for only 24 hours, although a common practice, is unacceptable and represents careless thinking about the potential risks involved. Not only is the long half-life an important factor, but the fact that many infants respond to fairly low blood levels of caffeine with resolution of apnea also demands consideration. If one assumes a half-life of approximately 90 to 100 hours, or about 4 days, an infant starting with a therapeutic blood level of 15 μg/mL would still have a blood level of nearly 4 μg/mL 8 days after discontinuation of the drug. This level might still be therapeutic, so that even a week of observation off caffeine may not be sufficient to reassure that apnea will not reoccur after the drug level is subtherapeutic. These considerations must be acknowledged when managing one of these patients.

With respect to resolution of the problem, a recently published paper notes that among the 1403 infants included in the trial, 84.2% did not have an apnea event and 78.5% did not have a bradycardia event after they were otherwise ready for discharge.[36] For the entire cohort, a 95% success rate was statistically reached, with a 7-day apnea- or bradycardia-free interval. Infants with a gestational age of 30 weeks or less had a 5% to 15% lower success rate than infants with a gestational age more than 30 weeks for any given apnea- or bradycardia-free interval. The success rate was reduced by an additional 5% to 10% if the last apnea or bradycardia event occurred at a postmenstrual age of more than 36 weeks. Including only the most severe events slightly improved the success rate of a given interval.

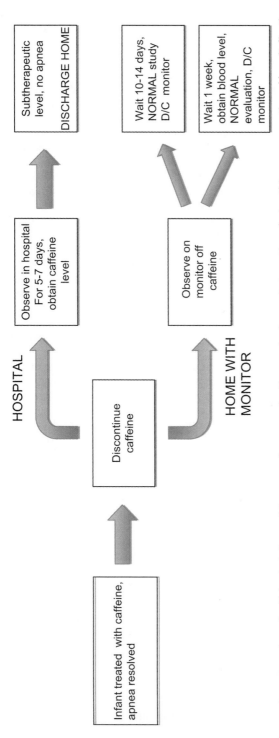

Fig. 2. Discontinuation of caffeine in infants with apnea of prematurity. If apnea is observed at any time during this process, continued hospitalization may be necessary if the apnea seems to be physiologically significant (bradycardia, oxygen desaturation) and the child is still in the hospital. If the child is home and occasional apnea is seen, therapy should be continued with the monitor and caffeine and a re-evaluation should be considered in 2 weeks. On occasion, cessation of caffeine may result in reappearance of significant apnea, which may require rehospitalization of an infant.

SUMMARY

The risk of recurrence for apnea or bradycardia differs depending on the gestational age of the infant and the postmenstrual age of the last apnea or bradycardia event. The following options are suggested for any infant treated with caffeine for AOP (**Fig. 2**). If the child is otherwise stable and ready for NICU discharge but caffeine has not yet been stopped, the infant should be sent home on caffeine and provided with a home cardiorespiratory monitor for at least the duration of time that it takes the caffeine to reach a subtherapeutic level. One could either wait approximately 10 days to 2 weeks after the caffeine has been stopped and perform a home cardiorespiratory study at that time to see if the apnea has reoccurred, or one could wait approximately 1 week and obtain a blood caffeine level. If the level is 2 μg/mL or less, caffeine is at a subtherapeutic range and a home cardiorespiratory study can be obtained. If the study is normal, monitoring can usually be safely discontinued at that point, and the caffeine need not be restarted. If apnea reappears after cessation of caffeine, caffeine should be reinstituted and the process should be repeated in approximately 2 weeks' time. If apnea becomes physiologically significant when the caffeine is stopped, as manifested by bradycardia or oxygen desaturation, consideration should be given to rehospitalizing the child and evaluating possible causes (anemia, infection, and so forth). The detailed work-up for a child with apnea is beyond the scope of this article.

An alternative approach is to anticipate the timing of hospital discharge and stop the caffeine at least 5 to 7 days before discharge. A blood caffeine level can be obtained a day before discharge and a breathing study for apnea evaluation can be performed. If normal, the child can be discharged off medication and without a home monitor. If the study reveals occasional apnea that is quickly self-terminated, the child can probably be discharged, but with caffeine and a home monitor as indicated in the previous paragraph. That approach should then be followed. If significant apnea and bradycardia appear on discontinuation of caffeine, hospitalization should continue and the child should be re-evaluated in 7 to 10 days for possible discharge. It should be noted that apnea often does not disappear in the preterm infant even at 40 weeks gestational age.[37] Consequently, caffeine therapy may need to be continued beyond the original estimated due date of the infant.

Failure to understand the long therapeutic half-life of caffeine may leave a child vulnerable to further episodes of apnea in the home environment, if caffeine is stopped and no appropriate surveillance with monitoring is undertaken.

The long-term safety of caffeine on neurodevelopmental outcome or preterm neonates has long been a concern, but recent data suggest that, if anything, caffeine has a positive influence on outcome. Doyle and colleagues[38] noted that caffeine seemed to improve the microstructure of the brain in the population of neonates treated with caffeine. Similarly, Gray and colleagues[39] observed a possible positive effect with caffeine use and stated "caffeine citrate with a dosage regimen of 20 mg/kg/day did not result in adverse outcomes for development, temperament and behavior. The borderline benefit in cognition with high-dose caffeine needs further investigation."

The introduction of methylxanthines, especially caffeine, for the treatment of AOP has been one of the most important and effective therapies in the NICU to date. A number of trials have demonstrated its effectiveness in most NICU infants. It remains a cost-effective intervention with minimal short- and long-term risks when used appropriately. Caffeine also seems to be effective for reducing the risk of bronchopulmonary dysplasia and PDA, and decreasing the need for reintubation. For the infant with apnea, there does not seem to be any more effective treatment at the present time, and caffeine is also more effective and safer than any other methylxanthine.

REFERENCES

1. Spitzer AR, Fox WW. Infant apnea: an approach to management. Clin Pediatr 1984;23:374–80.
2. Miller HC, Behrle FC, Smull NW. Severe apnea and irregular respiratory rhythms among premature infants. Pediatrics 1959;23:676–85.
3. Smith CA. Diagnosis and treatment: use and misuse of oxygen in treatment of prematures. Pediatrics 1964;33:111–2.
4. Kerr M. Hyperbaric oxygen in the treatment of apnoea neonatorum. J Obstet Gynaecol Br Commonw 1964;71:137.
5. Wick H, Schmitt H. Simple warning system for apnoea in premature infants. J Obstet Gynaecol Br Commonw 1967;71:137.
6. Lewin JE. An apnoea-alarm mattress. Lancet 1969;2(7622):667–8.
7. Kuzemko JA, Paala J. Apnoeic attacks in the newborn treated with aminophylline. Arch Dis Child 1973;48(5):404–6.
8. Lucey JE. The xanthine treatment of apnea of prematurity. Pediatrics 1975;55:584–6.
9. Aranda JV, Gorman W, Bergsteinsson H, et al. Efficacy of caffeine in treatment of apnea in the low-birth-weight infant. J Pediatr 1979;90:467–72.
10. Gunn TR, Metrakos K, Riley P, et al. Sequelae of caffeine treatment in preterm infants with apnea. J Pediatr 1979;94:106–9.
11. Bory C, Baltassat P, Porthault M, et al. Metabolism of theophylline to caffeine in premature newborn infants. J Pediatr 1979;94:988–93.
12. Aranda JV, Turmen T. Methylxanthines in apnea of prematurity. Clin Perinatol 1979;6:87–108.
13. Shannon DC, Gotay F, Stein IM, et al. Prevention of apnea and bradycardia in low birth weight infants. Pediatrics 1975;55:589–94.
14. Turmen T, Louridas TA, Aranda JV. Relationship of plasma and CSF concentrations of caffeine in neonates with apnea. J Pediatr 1979;95:644–6.
15. Leon AE, Michienzi K, Ma CX, et al. Serum caffeine concentrations in preterm neonates. Am J Perinatol 2007;24:39–47.
16. Natarajan G, Botica ML, Thomas R, et al. Therapeutic drug monitoring for caffeine in preterm neonates: an unnecessary exercise? Pediatrics 2007;119:936–40.
17. Davis JM, Stefano JL, Bhutani VK, et al. Changes in pulmonary mechanics following caffeine administration in infants with BPD. Pediatr Pulmonol 1989;6:49–52.
18. Dunwiddie TV, Masino SA. The role and regulation of adenosine in the central nervous system. Annu Rev Neurosci 2001;24:31–55.
19. Grosfeld JL, Dalsing MC, Hull M, et al. Neonatal apnea, methylxanthines, and necrotizing enterocolitis. J Pediatr Surg 1983;18:80–4.
20. Davis JM, Abbasi S, Spitzer AR, et al. Role of theophylline in pathogenesis of necrotizing enterocolitis. J Pediatr 1986;109:344–7.
21. Schmidt B, Roberts RS, Davis P, et al. Caffeine therapy for apnea of prematurity. N Engl J Med 2006;354:2112–21.
22. Dukhovny D, Lorch SA, Schmidt B, et al. Economic evaluation of caffeine for apnea of prematurity. Pediatrics 2011;127:e146–55.
23. Henderson-Smart DJ, DePaoli AG. Methyxanthine treatment for apnoea in preterm infants. Cochrane Database Syst Rev 2010;12:CD000140.
24. Henderson-Smart DJ, Steer PA. Caffeine versus theophylline for apnea in preterm infants. Cochrane Database Syst Rev 2010;1:CD000273.
25. Henderson-Smart DJ, DePaoli AG. Prophylactic methylxanthine for the prevention of apnoea in preterm infants. Cochrane Database Syst Rev 2010;12: CD000432.

26. Henderson-Smart DJ, Davis PG. Prophylactic methylxanthines for endotracheal extubation in preterm infants. Cochrane Database Syst Rev 2010;12:CD000139.
27. Aranda JV, Beharry K, Valencia GB, et al. Caffeine impact upon neonatal morbidities. J Matern Fetal Neonatal Med 2010;23(Suppl 3):20–3.
28. Pellowski A, Finer NN. A blinded, randomized, placebo-controlled trial to compare theophylline and doxapram for the treatment of apnea of prematurity. J Pediatr 1990;116:648–53.
29. Barrington KJ, Muttitt SC. Randomized, controlled, blinded trial of doxapram for extubation of the very low birth weight infant. Acta Paediatr 1998;87:191–4.
30. Lando A, Klamer A, Jonsbo F, et al. Doxapram and developmental delay at 12 months in children born extremely preterm. Acta Paediatr 2005;94:1680–1.
31. Osborn DA, Henderson-Smart DJ. Kinesthetic stimulation versus theophylline for apnea in preterm infants. Cochrane Database Syst Rev 2001;4:CD001072.
32. Al-Saif S, Alvaro R, Manfreda J, et al. A randomized controlled trial of theophylline versus CO2 inhalation for treating apnea of prematurity. J Pediatr 2008;153:513–8.
33. Pearlman SA, Duran C, Wood MA, et al. Caffeine pharmacokinetics in preterm infants older than 2 weeks. Dev Pharmacol Ther 1989;12:65–9.
34. Ahn HW, Shin WG, Park KJ, et al. Pharmacokinetics of theophylline and caffeine after intravenous administration of aminophylline to premature infants in Korea. Res Commun Mol Pathol Pharmacol 1999;105:105–13.
35. Charles BG, Townsend SR, Steer PA, et al. Caffeine citrate treatment for extremely premature infants with apnea: population pharmacokinetics, absolute bioavailability, and implications for therapeutic drug monitoring. Ther Drug Monit 2008;30:709–16.
36. Lorch SA, Srinivasan L, Escobar GJ. Epidemiology of apnea and bradycardia resolution in premature infants. Pediatr 2011;128:e366–73.
37. Eichenwald EC, Aina A, Stark AR. Apnea frequently persists beyond term gestation in infants delivered at 24 to 28 weeks. Pediatrics 1997;100:354–9.
38. Doyle LW, Cheong J, Hunt RW, et al. Caffeine and brain development in very preterm infants. Ann Neurol 2010;68:734–52.
39. Gray PH, Flenady VJ, Charles BG, et al. Caffeine citrate for very preterm infants: effects on development, temperament, and behavior. J Paediatr Child Health 2011;47:167–72.

Pulmonary Vasodilator Therapy in the NICU: Inhaled Nitric Oxide, Sildenafil, and Other Pulmonary Vasodilating Agents

Nicolas F.M. Porta, MD*, Robin H. Steinhorn, MD

KEYWORDS

- Pulmonary hypertension • Pulmonary vasculature • Vasodilator
- Phosphodiesterase • Prostacyclin

The fetal circulation uses a series of adaptive mechanisms to maximize delivery of oxygen to the most metabolically active tissues. Blood returning from the placenta through the umbilical vein has the highest oxygen content, and is directed from the right atrium through the foramen ovale into the left atrium, where it is ejected from the left ventricle into the ascending aorta, thus becoming available to the heart and brain. Blood returning from the brain and heart has the lowest oxygen content, and is directed from the right atrium into the right ventricle. High pressure is maintained in the fetal pulmonary vasculature, which serves to help direct most of the right ventricular output through the ductus arteriosus into the descending aorta and back to the placenta through the umbilical arteries.

The fetal circulatory system must also prepare for a rapid and dramatic switch to allow oxygen uptake by the lungs at birth. In preparation for this perinatal redirection of blood flow, anatomic development and growth of the lungs must occur, but separate regulation of pulmonary vascular function is required to maintain the metabolic efficiency of the fetal circulation. As a result, despite the rapid increase in the number of small pulmonary arteries,[1] high pulmonary vascular pressure is maintained by active vasoconstriction of fetal vessels.

The preparation of this manuscript was supported in part by R01HL54705 (NHLBI) and U01HL102235 (NHLBI), both to RHS.
Department of Pediatrics, Children's Memorial Hospital, Northwestern University, Chicago, IL 60614, USA
* Corresponding author.
E-mail address: n-porta@northwestern.edu

Clin Perinatol 39 (2012) 149–164
doi:10.1016/j.clp.2011.12.006
0095-5108/12/$ – see front matter © 2012 Elsevier Inc. All rights reserved.

perinatology.theclinics.com

After birth, the pulmonary vascular resistance (PVR) decreases and pulmonary vascular flow increases in response to lung expansion, increased oxygen tension, and increased pH caused by more efficient clearance of carbon dioxide. The normal perinatal physiologic changes start to occur within the first few breaths, and full pulmonary perfusion is normally achieved within minutes after birth. Pulmonary artery pressure and vascular resistance decrease more slowly, with pulmonary arterial pressure reaching its nadir approximately 2 to 3 weeks after birth.

PULMONARY HYPERTENSION

Persistent pulmonary hypertension of the newborn (PPHN) is the result of an abnormal early adaptation to the perinatal circulatory transition. PPHN is a syndrome characterized by common pathophysiologic features including sustained elevation of PVR; decreased perfusion of the lungs; and continued right-to-left shunting of blood through the fetal channels (foramen ovale and ductus arteriosus). When PVR remains high after birth, right (and sometimes left) ventricular function and cardiac output are depressed. Moderate or severe PPHN is believed to affect up to 2 to 6 per 1000 live births, and complicates the course of 10% of all infants admitted to neonatal intensive care.[2] These circulatory abnormalities are also responsible for an 8% to 10% risk of death and a 25% risk of long-term neurodevelopmental morbidity.

PPHN occurs in association with a diverse group of neonatal respiratory illnesses, but generally presents as one of three patterns: (1) a structurally normal but abnormally constricted pulmonary vasculature, which is the most common type and includes such diagnoses as meconium aspiration syndrome, respiratory distress syndrome, and sepsis; (2) a structurally abnormal vasculature that arises from antenatal remodeling, and is often termed "idiopathic PPHN"; or (3) a hypoplastic vasculature, such as is seen in congenital diaphragmatic hernia (CDH) or alveolar capillary dysplasia, a rare malformation of lung development. Although idiopathic pulmonary hypertension occurs in the minority ($\sim$20%–25%) of infants with PPHN, severe cases of meconium aspiration syndrome are almost certainly affected by parenchymal and vascular disease.

Significant pulmonary hypertension may also develop in neonates and young infants as a result of bronchopulmonary dysplasia (BPD) or cardiac disease. Pulmonary hypertension affects roughly one-third of infants with moderate-to-severe BPD,[3,4] and results in greater morbidity and mortality, poor growth and neurodevelopmental outcome, long-term mechanical ventilation support, and death caused by right heart dysfunction and multiorgan failure.[5,6] There is an increasing awareness that this association occurs frequently in high-risk populations. For instance, in a recent epidemiologic study, Slaughter and colleagues[3] reported a 37% incidence of pulmonary hypertension at 1 month of life among chronically ventilated BPD infants.

ENDOGENOUS REGULATORS OF PULMONARY VASCULAR TONE

Pulmonary vascular tone is mediated by competing vasodilatory and vasoconstrictive factors, with interrelated signaling pathways. The balance of expression and activity of intermediates in these signaling pathways determines the net pulmonary vascular tone (Figs. 1 and 2). As gestation progresses, mediators of pulmonary vasodilation become more dominant.

The postnatal stimuli that lead to pulmonary vasodilation (lung inflation with a gas, increase in oxygen tension, and decrease in carbon dioxide tension) each independently decrease PVR and increase pulmonary blood flow, but they also interact with each other synergistically. For instance, oxygen directly and indirectly stimulates the

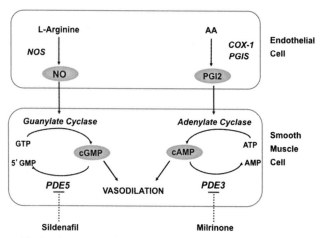

Fig. 1. Nitric oxide (NO) and prostacyclin (PGI$_2$) signaling pathways in the regulation of pulmonary vascular tone. NO is synthesized by NO synthase (NOS) from the terminal nitrogen of L-arginine. NO stimulates soluble guanylate cyclase (sGC) to increase intracellular cGMP. PGI$_2$ is an arachidonic acid (AA) metabolite formed by cyclooxygenase (COX-1) and prostacyclin synthase (PGIS) in the vascular endothelium. PGI$_2$ stimulates adenylate cyclase in vascular smooth muscle cells, which increases intracellular cAMP. Both cGMP and cAMP indirectly decrease free cytosolic calcium, resulting in smooth muscle relaxation. Specific phosphodiesterases (PDE) hydrolyze cGMP and cAMP, thus regulating the intensity and duration of their vascular effects. Inhibition of these PDE with such agents as sildenafil and milrinone may enhance pulmonary vasodilation. (*From* Steinhorn RH. Lamb models of pulmonary hypertension. Drug Discov Today Dis Models 2010;7:99–105; with permission.)

activity of endothelial nitric oxide synthase (eNOS) and cyclooxygenase (COX)-1 immediately after birth, leading to increased levels of the vasodilators, NO, and prostacyclin (PGI$_2$). Shear stress is also known to regulate the synthesis of NO in the fetal circulation. During the perinatal transition, the initial increase in pulmonary

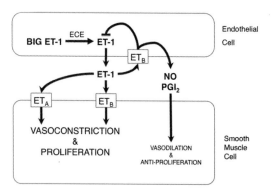

Fig. 2. Endothelin (ET)-1 signaling pathway in the regulation of pulmonary vascular tone. Big ET-1 is cleaved to ET-1 by endothelin converting enzyme (ECE) in endothelial cells. ET-1 binds its specific receptors ETA and ETB with differential effects. Binding of ET-1 to ETA or ETB on smooth muscle cells leads to vasoconstrictive and proliferative effects. ETB are transiently expressed on endothelial cells after birth; binding of ET-1 to ETB on endothelial cells leads to downregulation of ECE activity and increased production of nitric oxide (NO) and prostacyclin (PGI$_2$), which led to vasodilation and antiproliferation.

blood flow in response to ventilation or oxygenation likely leads to increased shear stress in the vasculature, which further potentiates NO production. In contrast, type-5 phosphodiesterase (PDE5) expression and activity normally fall after birth in the pulmonary vasculature,[7,8] further accentuating upstream effects leading to increased cyclic guanosine monophosphate (cGMP) and vasodilation.

Understanding the mechanisms that lead to cardiopulmonary dysfunction in PPHN is essential to selecting appropriate pharmacotherapy. Because of pathophysiologic differences among the patterns of PPHN, not all therapeutic interventions have equal effectiveness. Successful approaches in infants with lung injury may not be as successful in infants with developmental lung disorders. Understandably, many advances in PPHN therapy are derived from results of laboratory-based research. A newborn lamb created by antenatal ductal ligation is frequently used for PPHN investigations because the lambs display a phenotype that is strikingly similar to severe PPHN in human infants.[9] They have pulmonary vascular smooth muscle cell hypertrophy and require aggressive care after birth because of high mortality, severe hypoxemia and respiratory failure, and circulatory instability. Models of pulmonary hypertension caused by BPD are even more difficult to generate, but have been developed in mice, rats, and baboons exposed to hyperoxia or mechanical ventilation.

PHARMACOTHERAPY FOR PULMONARY HYPERTENSION

The primary aim of PPHN therapy is selective pulmonary vasodilatation. In all cases, treatment of pulmonary hypertension includes optimization of lung function and oxygen delivery, and support of cardiac function. Optimal lung inflation is essential because PVR is increased when the lungs are underexpanded or overexpanded, independent of lung disease. The use of lung recruitment strategies, such as high-frequency ventilation and exogenous surfactant administration, is particularly important in infants with PPHN associated with parenchymal disease, but has limited impact in infants with primary vascular disease. Correction of severe acidosis and avoidance of hypoxemia are important because both stimuli promote pulmonary vasoconstriction. Maintaining a normal hematocrit is also important to ensure adequate oxygen carrying capacity while avoiding polycythemia, because hyperviscosity can increase PVR. The focus of this article is the pharmacotherapies that specifically target pulmonary vascular tone.

Nitric Oxide

NO is the gas molecule produced endogenously by the conversion of arginine to citrulline by the enzyme NOS. Three isoforms of NOS exist, although eNOS is regarded as the most important regulator of NO production in the perinatal lung vasculature. NO generated in the endothelium readily diffuses into adjacent vascular smooth muscle cells where it stimulates soluble guanylate cyclase activity and increases cGMP, the critically important second messenger that mediates the vasodilatory pathway.

Lung eNOS mRNA and protein are present in the early fetus, but both increase toward the end of gestation, so that the lung is poised to adapt to the postnatal need for pulmonary vasodilation. This increase in lung eNOS content also explains the growing capacity of the fetal pulmonary vasculature to respond to endothelium-dependent vasodilators, such as oxygen and acetylcholine.[10] Many factors associated with pulmonary hypertension have the capacity to perturb eNOS function, even if protein levels are sufficient. Presumably, this is because the normal catalytic function of eNOS depends on numerous posttranslational modifications, including association with the chaperone protein Hsp90 and availability of essential substrates and cofactors including L-arginine, tetrahydrobiopterin (BH_4), the reduced form of nicotinamide adenine dinucleotide phosphate, and calcium–calmodulin. Depletion of Hsp90 or biopterin reduces production or bioavailability of NO, but also "uncouples" eNOS, resulting in incomplete reduction of molecular oxygen with subsequent formation of superoxide, essentially turning the enzyme into a source of oxidant stress.[11,12]

Inhaled NO (iNO) has many features of an ideal pulmonary vasodilator, including a particularly rapid onset of action, typically within minutes. Because eNOS is decreased or dysfunctional in PPHN, iNO could provide specific replacement therapy that is delivered by inhalation directly to airspaces approximating the pulmonary vascular bed. Although it is most commonly administered with mechanical ventilation, iNO can also be provided by continuous positive airway pressure or nasal cannula devices, although the concentration may need to be increased to account for the entrainment of room air.[13] It has been assumed that because NO is a small lipophilic molecule, iNO simply diffuses from alveoli through epithelial cells to gain direct access to the vasculature. However, it is now understood that NO is a free radical that can be inactivated through interaction with reactive oxygen species found in the alveolar space or alveolar lining. Others propose that NO gas gains entry into alveolar epithelium in part by forming a nitrosothiol derivative of cysteine that enters by an amino acid transporter.[14] Once in the bloodstream, NO binds avidly to hemoglobin, which is subsequently reduced by methemoglobin reductase.

The safety and efficacy of iNO for PPHN have been particularly well studied through large placebo-controlled trials. In most of these, the use of extracorporeal life support (ECMO) served as a primary endpoint in combination with mortality (**Table 1**). iNO significantly decreases the need for ECMO support in newborns with PPHN. However, it should be noted that up to 40% of infants did not improve oxygenation or maintain a response to iNO, and iNO did not reduce mortality or length of hospitalization in any study. By encompassing a range of disease severity, these studies also highlight that starting iNO for respiratory failure that is in earlier stages of evolution (for an oxygenation index of 15–25) did not decrease the incidence of ECMO or death or improve other patient outcomes (see **Table 1**), including the incidence of neurodevelopmental impairment.[15,16] However, delaying iNO initiation until respiratory failure is advanced (oxygenation index of >40) may increase length of time on oxygen.[17] In longer-term follow-up, iNO did not significantly alter the incidence of chronic lung disease or

Table 1
Summary of the large, multicenter, randomized trials of iNO in term newborns with hypoxemic respiratory failure or PPHN, showing the effect of iNO on ECMO use, mortality, and neurodevelopmental impairment

Study	N	Initial Oxygenation Index	% ECMO Control	iNO	% Mortality Control	iNO	% Neurodevelopmental Impairment Control	iNO
Neonatal Inhaled Nitric Oxide Study Group[19]	235	44	55	39*	17	14	30	35
Roberts et al[75]	58	44.4	71	40*	7	7	—	—
Clark et al[76,77]	248	39	65	48*	8	7	14	19
Davidson et al[22]	155	24.7	34	22	2	8	20	18
Konduri et al[15,16]	299	19.2	12	10	9	7	25	28

* $P<.05$; significant reduction.

neurodevelopmental impairment relative to placebo. This last observation may indicate that the underlying disease is associated with early neurologic injury that cannot be reversed by NO.

After the introduction of high-frequency ventilation, surfactant, and iNO in the early 1990s, the patient demographic of neonatal support with ECMO changed. Data from the large registry maintained by the Extracorporeal Life Support Organization indicate that the use of these therapies has increased steadily since they have become clinically available, accompanied by a greater than 40% reduction in the number of neonates cannulated for ECMO. However, because overall ECMO survival has diminished over the same time period, some physicians have speculated that these new treatment modalities may delay ECMO cannulation and negatively affect mortality and morbidity in those infants that require ECMO. In an analysis of data from the Extracorporeal Life Support Organization registry between 1996 and 2003, use of iNO, high-frequency ventilation, and surfactant was not associated with any adverse outcomes during ECMO, including increased hours on ECMO or increased time to extubation.[18] Furthermore, surfactant and iNO use were associated with lower ECMO mortality, and iNO use was associated with a decreased risk of cardiac arrest before cannulation. Because ECMO has been proved to reduce mortality for severe respiratory failure, it is reassuring that these new therapies have not had a negative impact on the most severely affected infants. More likely, the increase in ECMO mortality represents increased use in sicker infants who have failed to respond to advanced medical therapies.

The most important criterion for starting iNO is evidence for pulmonary hypertension. Clinical manifestations of PPHN include differential saturation (higher Spo_2 in the right upper extremity compared with a lower extremity in most cases), labile oxygenation, or profound hypoxemia despite optimal mechanical strategies to expand the lungs. Unfortunately, these findings are not specific for PPHN, and the accurate diagnosis of PPHN requires echocardiography to rule out congenital heart disease and rule in extrapulmonary shunting. Echocardiography also rules out left ventricular insufficiency, which could trigger pulmonary venous hypertension that would only be aggravated by a pulmonary vasodilator.

Based on the available data, iNO should be initiated at a dose of 20 ppm when there is evidence of PPHN and significant hypoxemia. Studies that adjusted the iNO dosing based on oxygenation response showed that failure to respond to 20 ppm was only rarely followed by improvement at higher doses.[19] Other studies used lower starting doses, but produced concern that inadequate early treatment could diminish the oxygenation response if escalation of the iNO dose became necessary.[20] Fineman and colleagues[21] directly measured the pulmonary artery pressure by catheterization to study the effect of delivery of iNO at 5, 20, and 40 ppm in random order. Oxygenation was improved with all three iNO doses, but a significant improvement in the ratio of pulmonary to systemic artery pressure was only seen when the iNO dose was at least 20 ppm. However, increased methemoglobinemia and nitrogen dioxide levels were reported with doses greater than 20 ppm for as little as 24 hours.[22]

Given its delivery by inhalation, the areas of the lung that are preferentially ventilated will receive more exogenous NO, resulting in improvement in ventilation–perfusion matching. The greatest improvement in oxygenation after iNO would be expected in infants with extrapulmonary right-to-left shunting but without significant pulmonary parenchymal disease. Even if the total PVR does not decrease, iNO can improve oxygenation through a "microselective" effect that reduces intrapulmonary shunting. For this reason, neonates with significant parenchymal pulmonary disease are less likely to respond to iNO unless lung expansion is optimized with high-frequency ventilation or surfactant administration.[23]

Data addressing optimal weaning procedures for iNO are more limited. After oxygenation improves, iNO usually can be weaned relatively rapidly to 5 ppm without difficulty. In the large randomized studies, most infants were treated with iNO for less than 5 days. Infants who remain hypoxemic with evidence of PPHN beyond that time are more likely to have an underlying cause of dysregulated pulmonary vascular tone, such as developmental lung abnormalities like alveolar capillary dysplasia,[24] severe pulmonary hypoplasia, or progressive lung injury. When iNO is stopped abruptly, "rebound" pulmonary hypertension sometimes develops.[25] This interesting phenomenon can occur even if no improvement in oxygenation was observed, can be life-threatening, and has raised questions about whether vascular cells respond to NO by upregulating vasoconstrictor pathways.[26,27] However, from a practical standpoint, the clinical problem can usually be overcome by weaning iNO to 1 ppm before discontinuation.

The same mechanisms that contribute to rebound pulmonary hypertension can interfere with the response to iNO. The reason some patients do not respond to iNO may be related to the severe antenatal lung vascular injury with impaired vasodilation caused by altered downstream signaling pathways, including soluble guanylate cyclase and cGMP-PDEs. For example, studies in newborn lambs indicate that iNO responsiveness is significantly blunted after even brief (30 minute) periods of ventilation with 100% O_2,[28,29] and that oxidant stress alters NO responsiveness in part through increasing expression and activity of cGMP-specific PDEs.[30] NO can also react with other radicals, such as superoxide to form peroxynitrite ($ONOO^-$), an exceptionally reactive oxidant that can aggravate lung injury; produce nonspecific nitration of proteins, such as eNOS; and cause further dysregulation of vasoactive signaling pathways.[31,32]

The use of iNO for infants with pulmonary hypertension associated with CDH is less clearly defined. The lungs of infants with CDH are characterized by parenchymal and vascular hypoplasia, and typically do not respond to lung recruitment measures. Randomized studies have not demonstrated a consistent improvement in oxygenation after early use of iNO in these infants.[33] However, the benefits of stabilizing infants and preventing cardiac arrest before ECMO suggest a potential role for iNO in some infants with CDH.[18] Worsening pulmonary hypertension after surgical repair of the diaphragmatic defect may also benefit from iNO treatment, and noninvasive delivery techniques may allow for long-term therapy.[13]

Although less well studied in humans, iNO may also have a role in the management of infants with pulmonary hypertension caused by chronic lung disease. Up to one-third of premature infants with moderate or severe BPD develop some degree of pulmonary hypertension or cor pulmonale.[3,4] Although the alterations in pulmonary vascular tone signaling are not identical to those seen in PPHN, alterations in eNOS and NO signaling seem to play a role in the vascular and lung injury.[34] Preclinical studies also indicated that prolonged NO inhalation in preterm baboons or rats with hyperoxia-induced lung injury improved lung compliance and lung growth and architecture.[35,36] Clinical trials have shown a modest benefit when iNO is used to prevent BPD,[37,38] although one large trial found that a more prolonged period of inhalation in high-risk infants led to improvements in lung function that persisted through 12 months of age.[39,40] A recent case series also indicates that iNO may reduce established BPD-associated pulmonary hypertension to a greater degree than oxygen alone.[41] However, these studies certainly highlight the complex, multifactorial nature of BPD, and further investigation is needed to understand the role of endogenous and inhaled NO for BPD prevention and therapy.

Sildenafil

cGMP is the second messenger that regulates contractility of smooth muscle through activation of cGMP-dependent kinases, PDEs, and ion channels. In vascular smooth muscle cells, NO-mediated activation of soluble guanylate cyclase is a major source of cGMP production. Because cGMP is such a central mediator of vascular contractility, it is not surprising that its concentrations are regulated within a relatively narrow range to allow fine-tuning of vascular responses to oxygen, NO, and other stimuli.

PDEs are a large family of enzymes that hydrolyze and inactivate cGMP and cAMP, thus regulating their concentrations and effects, and facilitating "cross-talk" between the two cyclic nucleotides. PDE5 is especially highly expressed in the lung, and not only uses cGMP as a substrate but also contains a specific cGMP binding domain that serves to activate its catabolic activity. As the primary enzyme responsible for regulating cGMP, PDE5 may well represent the most important regulator of NO-mediated vascular relaxation in the normal pulmonary vascular transition after birth.[42]

Fetal and neonatal lung development, along with commonly used neonatal intensive care unit therapies, seems to regulate PDE expression and activity. In developing lambs and rats, PDE5 is expressed according to specific developmental trajectories that result in a peak of expression during late fetal life, followed by an acute fall around the time of birth.[8,43] This drop in PDE5 activity would be expected to amplify the effects of NO produced by birth-related stimuli, such as oxygen and shear stress. In contrast, when pulmonary vessels of fetal lambs undergo remodeling by chronic intra-uterine pulmonary hypertension, PDE5 activity increases relative to controls.[44,45] Even more striking is that after birth, PDE5 activity does not fall in PPHN lambs, but rather increases dramatically above fetal levels, and above levels observed in spontaneously breathing or ventilated control lambs.[8,45] This abnormal increase in activity would be expected to diminish responses to endogenous and exogenous NO, and could explain the incomplete clinical efficacy of iNO in some patients.

Infants with pulmonary hypertension are commonly treated with high concentrations of oxygen to reverse hypoxemia. However, even brief exposures to hyperoxia diminish pulmonary vascular responses to endogenous and exogenous NO in healthy late-gestation lambs and lambs with pulmonary hypertension (who remain hypoxemic despite ventilation with 100% O_2). These findings suggest that lung oxidant stress exerts rapid and powerful effects on the signaling pathways that mediate vascular responses to NO. In pulmonary artery smooth muscle cells from healthy lambs, exposure to 24 hours of hyperoxia increased intracellular oxidant stress, increased PDE5 mRNA and protein expression and activity, and reduced cGMP generation in response to NO.[30] A dose-dependent effect of hyperoxia was observed, as indicated by a step-wise increase in PDE5 activity as oxygen concentration was increased from 21%, to 50%, and 95% O_2. Treatment of cells with sildenafil partially restored the cGMP response to exogenous NO, further highlighting that inhibition of PDE5 activity can counterregulate abnormal vascular cGMP responses after hyperoxia exposure.

In lambs with experimental PPHN, enteral and aerosolized sildenafil dilate the pulmonary vasculature and augment the pulmonary vascular response to iNO.[46,47] In a piglet model of meconium aspiration syndrome, intravenous sildenafil produced selective pulmonary vasodilation with efficacy equivalent to iNO, although hypotension and worsening oxygenation resulted when it was used in combination with iNO.[48] In a rat model of hyperoxia-induced BPD, chronic use of sildenafil decreased medial wall thickness and RVH and improved alveolarization.[49] Another recent study showed that antenatal administration of sildenafil to the dam reduced PDE5 activity and increased cGMP, and produced striking reductions in the vascular findings of persistent pulmonary hypertension in rat pups with experimental CDH.[50] This is the first indication that pulmonary hypertension can be treated before birth, and will likely open up a productive line of investigation in antenatal diagnosis and treatment.

The first clinical report of sildenafil use in infants was to facilitate weaning from iNO after corrective surgery for congenital heart disease.[51] In this initial case series, enteral sildenafil increased circulating cGMP and allowed two of three infants to wean from iNO without rebound pulmonary hypertension. Subsequent case series expanded these initial observations to show that enteral sildenafil may facilitate iNO discontinuation in infants with critical illness,[52] and may also reduce duration of mechanical ventilation and intensive care unit length of stay.[53] The clinical use of enteral sildenafil has also been reported in infants with PPHN, including one small, randomized controlled trial with oral sildenafil that showed a dramatic improvement in oxygenation and survival.[54]

Enteral administration of sildenafil could raise concerns about gastrointestinal absorption, particularly in conditions that may have an element of compromised intestinal perfusion. A recent open-label pilot trial demonstrated that intravenous sildenafil, delivered as a continuous infusion, improved oxygenation in a series of 36 infants with PPHN.[55] This study also showed that sildenafil clearance in neonates increases rapidly through the first week of life, likely reflecting the relative immaturity of the hepatic CYP system in the early neonatal period.[56] Hypotension was the most commonly reported adverse effect, although it was not observed when the loading dose was delivered over 3 hours or eliminated. Although most infants were treated while receiving iNO, seven infants received sildenafil without prior use of iNO, and all experienced a significant improvement in oxygenation within 4 hours after sildenafil administration (**Fig. 3**). Only one of these seven infants required iNO, and the other six infants improved and survived to hospital discharge without requiring either iNO or

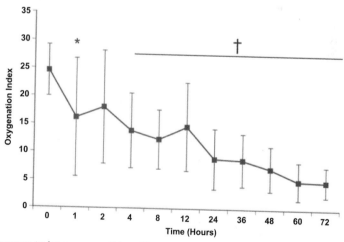

Fig. 3. Response to intravenous sildenafil. Seven infants were treated with open-label intravenous sildenafil before initiation of iNO. Oxygenation index was improved by 1 hour (24.6 ± 4.6 to 16.1 ± 9.9; *P = .0502), with significant and sustained improvement by 4 hours after initiation of sildenafil (14.7 ± 6.4; †P = .0088). Only one infant went on to require therapy with iNO. (*From* Steinhorn RH, Kinsella JP, Butrous G, et al. Open-label, multicentre, pharmacokinetic study of iv sildenafil in the treatment of neonates with persistent pulmonary hypertension of the newborn (PPHN). Circulation 2007;116:II-614; with permission.)

ECMO.[55] A randomized controlled trial is currently underway to evaluate the efficacy of intravenous sildenafil in infants with moderate PPHN (NCT01409031).

Sildenafil is also an attractive therapeutic option for infants with chronic pulmonary hypertension caused by CDH or BPD because it can be given orally, and over longer periods of time with apparent low toxicity. A recent case series examined the effect of oral sildenafil in 25 infants and children (<2 years of age) with pulmonary hypertension caused by chronic lung disease (mostly BPD). Most patients showed some improvement after a median treatment interval of 40 days, and most infants were able to wean off iNO.[57] Five patients died after initiation of sildenafil treatment, but none died from refractory pulmonary hypertension or right heart failure. A similar approach might benefit some infants with chronic pulmonary hypertension associated with lung hypoplasia.[58] These important pilot studies suggest that sildenafil is well tolerated in infants with pulmonary hypertension caused by chronic lung disease, and paves the way to further studies in this especially challenging population.

Prostacyclin

Another important vasodilatory pathway in the fetal lung is mediated by PGI_2 and cAMP (see **Fig. 1**). COX is the rate-limiting enzyme that generates prostacyclin from arachadonic acid. COX-1 is upregulated as lung development progresses in utero, leading to an increase in prostacyclin production in late gestation and early postnatal life.[59,60] Prostacyclin produced by endothelial cells initiates its signaling pathway by binding to the smooth muscle cell membrane bound receptor (IP), stimulating the associated adenylate cyclase to increase conversion of adenosine triphosphate to cAMP. Like cGMP, cAMP leads to decreased intracellular calcium ion resulting in vasodilation. In addition, PGI_2 inhibits pulmonary artery smooth muscle cell proliferation in vitro.

Systemic administration of PGI_2 is considered the most effective therapy for severe pulmonary hypertension in adults. However, rapid dosage escalation of infusions of PGI_2 may be necessary to promote acute pulmonary vasodilation. In infants, this can produce systemic hypotension, which can further compromise circulatory function. In addition, a dedicated central venous catheter is necessary for the delivery of intravenous PGI_2, with associated risks of infection and other line complications. Other systemic side effects (especially pain) also limit the use of systemic PGI_2 in the acute setting. When given as an aerosol by inhalation, PGI_2 has been shown to have vasodilator effects limited to the pulmonary circulation, making this strategy appealing when acute pulmonary vasodilation is desirable. Reports in children have been positive, but to date, there are few studies reporting the use of inhaled PGI_2 in neonates with PPHN.[61–63]

Experience suggests that inhaled PGI_2 is well tolerated and may assist in recovery without ECMO in infants with severe PPHN and inadequate response to iNO.[64] The optimal dosing of inhaled PGI_2 in critically ill mechanically ventilated infants is not known. In short-term studies of newborn lambs with pulmonary hypertension, increasing the dose of inhaled PGI_2 up to 500 ng/kg/min produced progressive improvements in pulmonary artery pressure, PVR, and pulmonary blood flow.[65] In clinical experience, the authors have used 50 to 100 ng/kg/min and have observed rapid improvement in oxygenation and limited progression to ECMO in infants with inadequate response to iNO. Concerns regarding the use of inhaled PGI_2 in critically ill infants include airway irritation from the alkaline solution needed to maintain drug stability, rebound pulmonary hypertension if the drug is abruptly discontinued, loss of medication into the circuit because of condensation, and alteration of characteristics of mechanical ventilation from the added gas flow needed for the nebulization.

Prolonged use of continuous inhaled PGI_2 may also lead to damage of mechanical ventilator valves.

Further investigations will likely focus on preparations specifically designed for inhalation, such as iloprost or treprostinil. Because these medications are more stable than PGI_2 they do not need to be dissolved in an alkaline solution, which could decrease the risk of lung injury. In addition, their longer half-lives allow for intermittent dosing using ultrasonic nebulizers, which would allow for interruption of mechanical ventilation for airway suctioning and probably interfere less with the flow patterns of mechanical ventilation. In critically ill mechanically ventilated patients, the effective dosing of inhaled prostanoids is likely to be higher and more frequent than in spontaneously breathing patients because of loss of the medication into the humidified ventilator circuit.

Although systemic hypotension may limit the use of intravenous prostanoids in the acute setting, long-term systemic prostanoids may be useful to protect the right ventricle from failing in infants with chronically progressive or severe pulmonary hypertension. This more chronic setting allows for a slower escalation of dose, which decreases the risk of side effects. However, the care of infants with severe pulmonary hypertension in the neonatal intensive care unit is often complicated by limited vascular access in older, chronically ill patients. This problem has prompted use of subcutaneous treprostinil in a small, heterogeneous cohort of infants with severe pulmonary hypertension. In three extremely premature infants with severe pulmonary hypertension associated with BPD, right ventricle size and function improved over time, and local site pain (typically a significant problem in adults) was not evident. However, the use of systemic prostanoids should be approached with caution. In particular, care must be taken to avoid excessive prostanoid therapy, which may produce severe discomfort, and could also lead to generalized vasodilation and high-output heart failure.

Milrinone

Prostacyclin–cAMP signaling operates in parallel to the NO–cGMP pathway for perinatal pulmonary vasodilation and is regulated in part by cAMP-hydrolyzing PDE isoforms, such as PDE3 and PDE4. The authors recently reported that PDE3A expression and activity in the resistance pulmonary arteries increase dramatically by 24 hours after birth.[66] These results were surprising and unexpected, because the authors would have predicted that similar to PDE5, PDE3 activity would decrease after birth to facilitate increased cAMP levels. This increase may be acting to establish cAMP-containing regulatory regions within the pulmonary vascular smooth muscle cell after birth, although it is unclear what role PDE3 has in the normal pulmonary vascular transition after birth. They also observed that addition of NO dramatically increased PDE3 levels, which suggests that milrinone might enhance the vasodilatory effects of iNO-cGMP signaling in addition to its expected effects on the cAMP pathways.[67]

The PGI_2 receptor (IP) is decreased in adult and pediatric patients with pulmonary hypertension, and animal studies point to its contribution to altered vasodilation in PPHN.[67] Bypassing these abnormalities in PGI_2 signaling by enhancing availability of cAMP may represent a useful therapeutic approach. Inhibition of PDE3 activity would be expected to increase cAMP concentration, and thus promote vasodilation. Milrinone, an inhibitor of PDE3, is frequently used in intensive care units to improve myocardial contractility and reverse diastolic dysfunction. In animal studies, milrinone has been shown to decrease pulmonary artery pressure and resistance and to act additively with iNO.[65,68] Clinical reports indicate that milrinone may decrease rebound pulmonary hypertension after iNO is stopped,[27] and may enhance pulmonary vasodilation of infants with PPHN refractory to iNO.[69] A study to better define the pharmacokinetic profile of milrinone in infants with PPHN is ongoing (NCT01088997), and should lead to clinical trials designed to test its efficacy.

Bosentan

Endothelin-1 (ET-1) is a 21–amino acid protein formed by serial enzymatic cleavage of a larger prepropeptide to the vasoactive form, and is one of the most potent vasoconstrictors described in the pulmonary vasculature (see **Fig. 2**). ET-1 is principally produced in endothelial cells in response to hypoxia, and is known to promote endothelial cell dysfunction, smooth muscle cell proliferation and remodeling, and inflammation and fibrosis.[70] ET-1 binds to two receptor subtypes, ET receptors A and B, and the binding of ET-1 to the ETA receptor on smooth muscle cells produces vasoconstriction. Increased ET-1 production and altered ET receptor activity have been consistently reported in neonatal and adult animal models of pulmonary hypertension, and lung ET-1 expression and plasma ET levels were elevated in severe pulmonary arterial hypertension in adults.[71] The use of ET-1 receptor antagonists, such as bosentan, has been shown to improve outcomes in adults with pulmonary hypertension. In PPHN, ET-1 is believed to play a role in the pathogenesis of PPHN, and ET blockade augments pulmonary vasodilation.[70] A recent prospective examination of 40 newborns with CDH and poor outcome also indicated that plasma ET-1 levels were highly correlated with the severity of pulmonary hypertension.[72] Recent case reports suggest that bosentan, an ET blocking agent, can improve oxygenation in neonates with PPHN.[73,74] A randomized controlled trial is currently underway to investigate the efficacy of bosentan in infants with severe PPHN (NCT01389856).

SUMMARY

No single therapeutic approach has been shown to be universally effective in the treatment of PPHN, and because of the complexity of the signaling pathways, this is not surprising. Although each of the therapies described in this article likely plays a role, using combinations of therapies is especially intriguing. Because the signaling pathways that regulate pulmonary vascular tone are highly interrelated, correcting only one pathway may not fully correct the vascular abnormality, and can even perturb the balance of vasodilator and vasoconstrictor production. The combination of strategies that increase cGMP and cAMP together may be more effective than either treatment alone. A thoughtful, multipronged approach may allow for more effective and efficient therapy, perhaps minimizing side effects and lung injury, especially in the most severe cases.

REFERENCES

1. Levin DL, Rudolph AM, Heymann MA, et al. Morphological development of the pulmonary vascular bed in fetal lambs. Circulation 1976;53:144–51.
2. Walsh-Sukys MC, Tyson JE, Wright LL, et al. Persistent pulmonary hypertension of the newborn in the era before nitric oxide: practice variation and outcomes. Pediatrics 2000;105:14–20.
3. Slaughter JL, Pakrashi T, Jones DE, et al. Echocardiographic detection of pulmonary hypertension in extremely low birth weight infants with bronchopulmonary dysplasia requiring prolonged positive pressure ventilation. J Perinatol 2011;31:635–40.
4. An HS, Bae EJ, Kim GB, et al. Pulmonary hypertension in preterm infants with bronchopulmonary dysplasia. Korean Circ J 2010;40:131–6.

5. Farquhar M, Fitzgerald DA. Pulmonary hypertension in chronic neonatal lung disease. Paediatr Respir Rev 2010;11:149–53.
6. Khemani E, McElhinney DB, Rhein L, et al. Pulmonary artery hypertension in formerly premature infants with bronchopulmonary dysplasia: clinical features and outcomes in the surfactant era. Pediatrics 2007;120:1260–9.
7. Sanchez LS, Del La Monte SM, Filippov G, et al. Cyclic-GMP-binding, cyclic-GMP-specific phosphodiesterase gene expression is regulated during rat pulmonary development. Pediatr Res 1998;43:163–8.
8. Farrow KN, Lakshminrusimha S, Czech L, et al. Superoxide dismutase and inhaled nitric oxide normalize phosphodiesterase 5 expression and activity in neonatal lambs with persistent pulmonary hypertension. Am J Physiol Lung Cell Mol Physiol 2010;299:L109–16.
9. Steinhorn RH. Lamb models of pulmonary hypertension. Drug Discov Today Dis Models 2010;7:99–105.
10. Tiktinsky MH, Morin FC III. Increasing oxygen tension dilates fetal pulmonary circulation via endothelium-derived relaxing factor. Am J Physiol Heart Circ Physiol 1993;265:H376–80.
11. Mata-Greenwood E, Jenkins C, Farrow KN, et al. eNOS function is developmentally regulated: uncoupling of eNOS occurs postnatally. Am J Physiol Lung Cell Mol Physiol 2006;290:L232–41.
12. Farrow KN, Lakshminrusimha S, Reda WJ, et al. Superoxide dismutase restores eNOS expression and function in resistance pulmonary arteries from neonatal lambs with persistent pulmonary hypertension. Am J Physiol Lung Cell Mol Physiol 2008;295:L979–87.
13. Kinsella JP, Parker TA, Ivy DD, et al. Noninvasive delivery of inhaled nitric oxide therapy for late pulmonary hypertension in newborn infants with congenital diaphragmatic hernia. J Pediatr 2003;142:397–401.
14. Brahmajothi MV, Mason SN, Whorton AR, et al. Transport rather than diffusion-dependent route for nitric oxide gas activity in alveolar epithelium. Free Radic Biol Med 2010;49:294–300.
15. Konduri GG, Solimani A, Sokol GM, et al. A randomized trial of early versus standard inhaled nitric oxide therapy in term and near-term newborn infants with hypoxic respiratory failure. Pediatrics 2004;113:559–64.
16. Konduri GG, Vohr B, Robertson C, et al. Early inhaled nitric oxide therapy for term and near-term newborn infants with hypoxic respiratory failure: neurodevelopmental follow-up. J Pediatr 2007;150:235–40, 240.e1.
17. Gonzalez A, Fabres J, D'Apremont I, et al. Randomized controlled trial of early compared with delayed use of inhaled nitric oxide in newborns with a moderate respiratory failure and pulmonary hypertension. J Perinatol 2010;30:420–4.
18. Fliman PJ, deRegnier RA, Kinsella JP, et al. Neonatal extracorporeal life support: impact of new therapies on survival. J Pediatr 2006;148:595–9.
19. Neonatal Inhaled Nitric Oxide Study Group. Inhaled nitric oxide in full-term and nearly full-term infants with hypoxic respiratory failure. N Engl J Med 1997;336:597–604.
20. Cornfield DN, Maynard RC, deRegnier RO, et al. Randomized, controlled trial of low-dose inhaled nitric oxide in the treatment of term and near-term infants with respiratory failure and pulmonary hypertension. Pediatrics 1999;104:1089–94.
21. Tworetzky W, Bristow J, Moore P, et al. Inhaled nitric oxide in neonates with persistent pulmonary hypertension. Lancet 2001;357:118–20.
22. Davidson D, Barefield ES, Kattwinkel J, et al. Inhaled nitric oxide for the early treatment of persistent pulmonary hypertension of the term newborn:

a randomized, double-masked, placebo-controlled, dose-response, multicenter study. Pediatrics 1998;101:325–34.

23. Kinsella JP, Truog WE, Walsh WF, et al. Randomized, multicenter trial of inhaled nitric oxide and high-frequency oscillatory ventilation in severe, persistent pulmonary hypertension of the newborn. J Pediatr 1997;131:55–62.

24. Bishop NB, Stankiewicz P, Steinhorn RH. Alveolar capillary dysplasia. Am J Respir Crit Care Med 2011;184:172–9.

25. Davidson D, Barefield ES, Kattwinkel J, et al. Safety of withdrawing inhaled nitric oxide therapy in persistent pulmonary hypertension of the newborn. Pediatrics 1999;104:231–6.

26. Black SM, Heidersbach RS, McMullan DM, et al. Inhaled nitric oxide inhibits NOS activity in lambs: potential mechanism for rebound pulmonary hypertension. Am J Physiol Heart Circ Physiol 1999;277:H1849–56.

27. Thelitz S, Oishi P, Sanchez LS, et al. Phosphodiesterase-3 inhibition prevents the increase in pulmonary vascular resistance following inhaled nitric oxide withdrawal in lambs. Pediatr Crit Care Med 2004;5:234–9.

28. Lakshminrusimha S, Russell JA, Steinhorn RH, et al. Pulmonary hemodynamics in neonatal lambs resuscitated with 21%, 50%, and 100% oxygen. Pediatr Res 2007;62:313–8.

29. Lakshminrusimha S, Swartz DD, Gugino SF, et al. Oxygen concentration and pulmonary hemodynamics in newborn lambs with pulmonary hypertension. Pediatr Res 2009;66:539–44.

30. Farrow KN, Groh BS, Schumacker PT, et al. Hyperoxia increases phosphodiesterase 5 expression and activity in ovine fetal pulmonary artery smooth muscle cells. Circ Res 2008;102:226–33.

31. Lassegue B, Griendling KK. Reactive oxygen species in hypertension: an update. Am J Hypertens 2004;17:852–60.

32. Lakshminrusimha S, Russell J, Wedgwood S, et al. Superoxide dismutase improves oxygenation and reduces oxidation in neonatal pulmonary hypertension. Am J Respir Crit Care Med 2006;174:1370–7.

33. Neonatal Inhaled Nitric Oxide Study Group. Inhaled nitric oxide and hypoxic respiratory failure in infants with congenital diaphragmatic hernia. Pediatrics 1997;99:838–45.

34. Afshar S, Gibson LL, Yuhanna IS, et al. Pulmonary NO synthase expression is attenuated in a fetal baboon model of chronic lung disease. Am J Physiol Lung Cell Mol Physiol 2003;284:L749–58.

35. McCurnin DC, Pierce RA, Chang LY, et al. Inhaled NO improves early pulmonary function and modifies lung growth and elastin deposition in a baboon model of neonatal chronic lung disease. Am J Physiol Lung Cell Mol Physiol 2005;288:L450–9.

36. Lin YJ, Markham NE, Balasubramaniam V, et al. Inhaled nitric oxide enhances distal lung growth after exposure to hyperoxia in neonatal rats. Pediatr Res 2005;58:22–9.

37. Donohue PK, Gilmore MM, Cristofalo E, et al. Inhaled nitric oxide in preterm infants: a systematic review. Pediatrics 2011;127:e414–22.

38. Steinhorn RH, Shaul PW, deRegnier RA, et al. Inhaled nitric oxide and bronchopulmonary dysplasia. Pediatrics 2011;128:e255–6 [author reply: e256–7].

39. Ballard RA, Truog WE, Cnaan A, et al. Inhaled nitric oxide in preterm infants undergoing mechanical ventilation. N Engl J Med 2006;355:343–53.

40. Hibbs AM, Walsh MC, Martin RJ, et al. One-year respiratory outcomes of preterm infants enrolled in the Nitric Oxide (to prevent) Chronic Lung Disease trial. J Pediatr 2008;153:525–9.

41. Mourani PM, Ivy DD, Gao D, et al. Pulmonary vascular effects of inhaled nitric oxide and oxygen tension in bronchopulmonary dysplasia. Am J Respir Crit Care Med 2004;170:1006–13.

42. Farrow KN, Steinhorn RH. Phosphodiesterases: emerging therapeutic targets for neonatal pulmonary hypertension. Handb Exp Pharmacol 2011;204:251–77.

43. Sanchez LS, Filippov G, Zapol WM, et al. cGMP-binding, cGMP-specific phosphodiesterase gene expression is regulated during lung development. Pediatr Res 1995;37:348A.

44. Hanson KA, Abman SH, Clarke WR. Elevation of pulmonary PDE5-specific activity in an experimental fetal ovine perinatal pulmonary hypertension model. Pediatr Res 1996;39:334A.

45. Farrow KN, Wedgwood S, Lee KJ, et al. Mitochondrial oxidant stress increases PDE5 activity in persistent pulmonary hypertension of the newborn. Respir Physiol Neurobiol 2010;174:272–81.

46. Weimann J, Ullrich R, Hromi J, et al. Sildenafil is a pulmonary vasodilator in awake lambs with acute pulmonary hypertension. Anesthesiology 2000;92:1702–12.

47. Ichinose F, Erana-Garcia J, Hromi J, et al. Nebulized sildenafil is a selective pulmonary vasodilator in lambs with acute pulmonary hypertension. Crit Care Med 2001;29:1000–5.

48. Shekerdemian L, Ravn H, Penny D. Intravenous sildenafil lowers pulmonary vascular resistance in a model of neonatal pulmonary hypertension. Am J Respir Crit Care Med 2002;165:1098–102.

49. Ladha F, Bonnet S, Eaton F, et al. Sildenafil improves alveolar growth and pulmonary hypertension in hyperoxia-induced lung injury. Am J Respir Crit Care Med 2005;172:750–6.

50. Luong C, Rey-Perra J, Vadivel A, et al. Antenatal sildenafil treatment attenuates pulmonary hypertension in experimental congenital diaphragmatic hernia. Circulation 2011;123:2120–31.

51. Atz AM, Wessel DL. Sildenafil ameliorates effects of inhaled nitric oxide withdrawal. Anesthesiology 1999;91:307–10.

52. Lee JE, Hillier SC, Knoderer CA. Use of sildenafil to facilitate weaning from inhaled nitric oxide in children with pulmonary hypertension following surgery for congenital heart disease. J Intensive Care Med 2008;23:329–34.

53. Namachivayam P, Theilen U, Butt WW, et al. Sildenafil prevents rebound pulmonary hypertension after withdrawal of nitric oxide in children. Am J Respir Crit Care Med 2006;174:1042–7.

54. Baquero H, Soliz A, Neira F, et al. Oral sildenafil in infants with persistent pulmonary hypertension of the newborn: a pilot randomized blinded study. Pediatrics 2006;117:1077–83.

55. Steinhorn RH, Kinsella JP, Pierce C, et al. Intravenous sildenafil in the treatment of neonates with persistent pulmonary hypertension. J Pediatr 2009;155:841–7.

56. Mukherjee A, Dombi T, Wittke B, et al. Population pharmacokinetics of sildenafil in term neonates: evidence of rapid maturation of metabolic clearance in the early postnatal period. Clin Pharmacol Ther 2009;85:56–63.

57. Mourani PM, Sontag MK, Ivy DD, et al. Effects of long-term sildenafil treatment for pulmonary hypertension in infants with chronic lung disease. J Pediatr 2009;154:379–84, 384,e1–2.

58. Keller RL, Moore P, Teitel D, et al. Abnormal vascular tone in infants and children with lung hypoplasia: findings from cardiac catheterization and the response to chronic therapy. Pediatr Crit Care Med 2006;7:589–94.

59. Brannon TS, MacRitchie AN, Jaramillo MA, et al. Ontogeny of cyclooxygenase-1 and cyclooxygenase-2 gene expression in ovine lung. Am J Physiol 1998;274: L66–71.
60. Brannon TS, North AJ, Wells LB, et al. Prostacyclin synthesis in ovine pulmonary artery is developmentally regulated by changes in cyclooxygenase-1 gene expression. J Clin Invest 1994;93:2230–5.
61. Bindl L, Fahnenstich H, Peukert U. Aerosolised prostacyclin for pulmonary hypertension in neonates. Arch Dis Child Fetal Neonatal Ed 1994;71:F214–6.
62. Soditt V, Aring C, Groneck P. Improvement of oxygenation induced by aerosolized prostacyclin in a preterm infant with persistent pulmonary hypertension of the newborn. Intensive Care Med 1997;23:1275–8.
63. Olmsted K, Oluola O, Parthiban A, et al. Can inhaled prostacyclin stimulate surfactant in ELBW infants? J Perinatol 2007;27:724–6.
64. Kelly LK, Porta NF, Goodman DM, et al. Inhaled prostacyclin for term infants with persistent pulmonary hypertension refractory to inhaled nitric oxide. J Pediatr 2002;141:830–2.
65. Kumar VH, Swartz DD, Rashid N, et al. Prostacyclin and milrinone by aerosolization improve pulmonary hemodynamics in newborn lambs with experimental pulmonary hypertension. J Appl Physiol 2010;109:677–84.
66. Chen B, Lakshminrusimha S, Czech L, et al. Regulation of phosphodiesterase 3 in the pulmonary arteries during the perinatal period in sheep. Pediatr Res 2009; 66:682–7.
67. Lakshminrusimha S, Porta NF, Farrow KN, et al. Milrinone enhances relaxation to prostacyclin and iloprost in pulmonary arteries isolated from lambs with persistent pulmonary hypertension of the newborn. Pediatr Crit Care Med 2009;10: 106–12.
68. Deb B, Bradford K, Pearl RG. Additive effects of inhaled nitric oxide and intravenous milrinone in experimental pulmonary hypertension. Crit Care Med 2000;28: 795–9.
69. McNamara PJ, Laique F, Muang- S, et al. Milrinone improves oxygenation in neonates with severe persistent pulmonary hypertension of the newborn. J Crit Care 2006;21:217–22.
70. Abman SH. Role of endothelin receptor antagonists in the treatment of pulmonary arterial hypertension. Annu Rev Med 2009;60:13–23.
71. Giaid A, Yanagisawa M, Lagleben D, et al. Expression of endothelin-1 in the lungs of patients with pulmonary hypertension. N Engl J Med 1993;328:1732–9.
72. Keller RL, Tacy TA, Hendricks-Munoz K, et al. Congenital diaphragmatic hernia: endothelin-1, pulmonary hypertension, and disease severity. Am J Respir Crit Care Med 2010;182:555–61.
73. Nakwan N, Choksuchat D, Saksawad R, et al. Successful treatment of persistent pulmonary hypertension of the newborn with bosentan. Acta Paediatr 2009;98: 1683–5.
74. Goissen C, Ghyselen L, Tourneux P, et al. Persistent pulmonary hypertension of the newborn with transposition of the great arteries: successful treatment with bosentan. Eur J Pediatr 2008;167:437–40.
75. Roberts JD, Fineman J, Morin FC III, et al. Inhaled nitric oxide and persistent pulmonary hypertension of the newborn. N Engl J Med 1997;336:605–10.
76. Clark RH, Huckaby JL, Kueser TJ, et al. Low-dose nitric oxide therapy for persistent pulmonary hypertension: 1-year follow-up. J Perinatol 2003;23:300–3.
77. Clark RH, Kueser TJ, Walker MW, et al. Low dose nitric oxide therapy for persistent pulmonary hypertension of the newborn. N Engl J Med 2000;342:469–74.

The Use and Misuse of Oxygen During the Neonatal Period

Máximo Vento, MD, PhD[a,b,*], Javier Escobar, PhD[b],
María Cernada, MD[b], Raquel Escrig, MD[a], Marta Aguar, MD[a]

KEYWORDS

- Oxygen • Oxidative stress • Newborn • Pulse oximetry
- Oxygen saturation • Oxygen toxicity

INTRODUCTION

Life as we know it in biologic systems depends on the ability of overcoming entropy which is the natural tendency towards molecular disorder. To overcoming entropy a great amount of energy is necessary. The present review addresses the relevance of aerobic metabolism as the most efficient means of obtaining energy from metabolic substrates rendering oxygen indispensable for life. However, as a counterpart negative aspects of oxidative metabolism will also be addressed.

AEROBIC METABOLISM

Oxygen is one of the most abundant elements in nature and also one of the most widely used drugs in neonatology (**Fig. 1**).[1] Because of its specific properties, oxygen has evolved to become indispensable to sustain life in multicellular organisms. Hence, oxygen is completely available, diffuses easily across biologic membranes, and can bind to heme in proteins, such as hemoglobin and cytochromes in mitochondria.[2] Of note, with the concourse of oxygen, cells are capable to build up sufficient ATP to meet their energy needs in the oxidative phosphorylation process. Briefly, energized electrons liberated in the tricarboxylic cycle (Krebs cycle) are transferred to the electron transport chain (ETC) by specific transporters (nicotinamide adenine dinucleotide, flavin adenine dinucleotide). This energy is used by components of the ETC to extrude protons to the intermembrane space, thus creating a mitochondrial transmembrane potential (Ψ_m). When protons are pumped back to the mitochondrial inner space,

Disclosure Statement: None of the authors of this article has any commercial or financial relation to disclose.

[a] Division of Neonatology, University & Polytechnic Hospital La Fe, Valencia, Spain
[b] Neonatal Research Unit, Health Research Institute Hospital La Fe, Valencia, Spain
* Corresponding author. Division of Neonatology, University & Polytechnic Hospital La Fe, Bulevar Sur s/n, 46026 Valencia, Spain.
E-mail address: maximo.vento@uv.es

Clin Perinatol 39 (2012) 165–176
doi:10.1016/j.clp.2011.12.014
0095-5108/12/$ – see front matter © 2012 Elsevier Inc. All rights reserved.

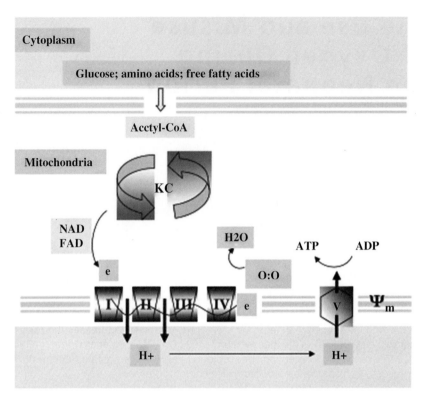

Fig. 1. Oxidative phosphorylation occurs in mitochondria, where highly energized electrons liberated in the Krebs cycle are transported to the ETC, creating a mitochondrial transmembrane potential. Extruded protons are reintroduced in the intermembrane space by the action of ATP-synthase. Energy liberated in this process is used to rebuild ATP while electrons are captured by oxygen, which becomes fully reduced.

the energy liberated in this process is used by the ATP synthase complex to rebuild ATP. Simultaneously, ground molecular dioxygen is completely reduced by 4 electrons.[3] Remarkably, aerobic metabolism (ie, with the concourse of oxygen) is 20 times more efficient than anaerobic metabolism, thus providing sufficient energy for cell growth, development, and reproduction (eg, 1 molecule of glucose forms 34 molecules of ATP through the aerobic pathway and 4 through the anaerobic). Specific cells, such as neurons, are unable to accumulate energy, however, and can survive for only a few minutes under hypoxic conditions, rendering oxygen indispensable for central nervous system survival.[1]

Oxygen Free Radicals

The oxygen molecule has 2 unpaired electrons in its outer shell that prevent it from forming new chemical bonds (**Fig. 2**). Partial reduction of oxygen with just 1 electron at a time will lead to the formation of reactive oxygen species (ROS), such as anion superoxide (O_2^-), hydroxyl radical ($OH\bullet$), and hydrogen peroxide (H_2O_2). Some of these chemicals are highly reactive species known as free radicals. In the presence of nitric oxide, oxygen free radicals will react, forming reactive nitrogen species (RNS), such as peroxynitrite ($ONOO-$). ROS and RNS are potent oxidizing and

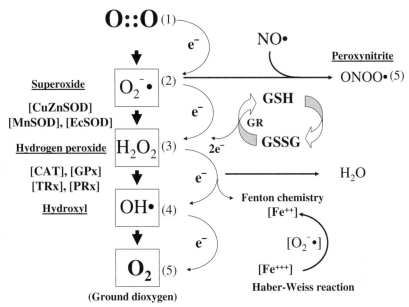

Fig. 2. Oxygen (1) is partially reduced by the action of a series of enzymatic complexes to anion superoxide (2). Anion superoxide is dismutated by superoxide dismutases (SOD) to hydrogen peroxide (3), which is turn is transformed into water and oxygen by the action of catalases (CAT) and glutathione peroxidase (GPX). In the presence of transition metals (eg, iron, copper), hydrogen peroxide can be transformed into hydroxyl radical (4). Moreover, in the presence of nitric oxide (NO), anion superoxide can also be transformed into peroxynitrite (5).

reducing agents with an extremely short half-life that will react with any nearby standing cellular structure, thereby altering their structure and function. Free radicals are atomic or molecular species capable of independent existence that contain one or more unpaired electrons in their molecular orbitals. They are able, therefore, to oxidize cellular membranes, structural proteins, enzymes, and nucleic acids.[3,4]

Antioxidant Defenses

Biologic systems using aerobic metabolism have been able to survive the deleterious effects of free radicals because a large number of enzymatic and nonenzymatic antioxidants have evolved (see **Fig. 2**). The antioxidant enzymes are represented by the family of superoxide dismutases (SOD) formed by Cu-Zn SOD or soluble SOD1 located in the cytosol, Mn-SOD or SOD2 located in the mitochondria, and extracellular, or SOD3. In addition, catalase, glutathione peroxidases, and glucose 6-phosphate dehydrogenase together constitute the most relevant enzymatic defense against free radicals. The major nonenzymatic intracellular antioxidant is glutathione (GSH), an ubiquitous tripeptide formed by γ-glutamine, L-cysteine, and glycine. GSH is able to reduce free radicals by establishing a disulfur bond with another GSH molecule, forming oxidized glutathione (GS = SG), thus providing 1 electron. Oxidized glutathione is reduced again to its reduced form (GSH) by the action of glutathione reductase (GSH-reductase) with the electrons provided by nicotinamide adenine dinucleotide phosphate (NADPH). Other relevant nonenzymatic antioxidants are proteins that bind transition metals, such as transferrin and ceruloplasmin, or molecules that quench free radicals, such as uric acid and bilirubin and certain vitamins, such as A and C.[5,6]

Oxidative Stress

The concept of oxidative stress refers to the imbalance between the formation of free radicals and the capability of the biologic system to neutralize them. To evaluate oxidative stress, different biomarkers have been used. They may directly reflect a pro-oxidant or antioxidant status, such as GSH/GSSG ratio, one of the most reliable and used oxidative stress markers. Other biomarkers may reflect direct damage to the cell structures. Hence, for lipid peroxidation, malondialdehyde or n-aldehydes (eg, 4-hydroxy-nonenal) have been widely used. Nucleic acid damage is generally reflected by guanosine base oxidation products, such as 8-oxo-dyhydroguanosine. Isoprostanes and isofurans have evolved as some of the most reliable markers of oxidative stress and reflect non–cyclo-oxygenase peroxidation of polyunsaturated fatty acids and, intriguingly, have important vasoactive properties. Oxidation of circulating amino acids can be measured by the action of free radicals on specific targets, such as phenylalanine. The oxidation of phenylalanine derived from the attack of hydroxyl radicals leads to its conversion into ortho-tyrosine (*o*-tyr) and meta-tyrosine (*met*-tyr), both highly specific markers of oxidative stress. Other markers of protein oxidation are known as carbonyl compounds (C = O), whose presence in greater amounts in the lung alveolar lavage fluid or tracheal aspiration significantly correlate with development of chronic lung disease.[4,5]

Inflammatory Response and Redox Signaling

In addition to causing oxidative damage to cell structures, ROS and RNS are capable of triggering an inflammatory response in the cells promoting the transformation of I-kB into NF-kB, a transcription factor for multiple inflammation-related genes. ROS and RNS are also capable of activating tumor necrosis factor–alpha, essential in the inflammatory response as well as in the activation of apoptosis.[5] To do so, ROS have to act on redox mechanisms that function in control of gene expression, cell proliferation, and apoptosis. Hydrogen peroxide especially, but also other ROS provide a mechanism to reversibly oxidize/reduce signaling proteins providing a means for control of protein activity, protein-protein interaction, protein trafficking, and protein-DNA interaction.[7]

FETAL TO NEONATAL TRANSITION

Fetal life develops in an environment that is relatively hypoxic compared with the extrauterine world; hence, arterial partial pressure of oxygen (p_aO_2) in utero is of 25 to 35 mm Hg in the general circulation and even less (17–19 mm Hg) in the pulmonary circulation.[8] Although seemingly isolated from the external milieu, the fetus is highly susceptible to changes in oxygenation induced in the mother. Hence, recent studies have shown that the p_aO_2 of fetuses whose mothers received oxygen supplementation during labor was significantly increased as compared with nonsupplemented controls; moreover, the former also had significantly increased concentrations of biomarkers of oxidative stress, such as malondialdehyde and F2-isoprostanes in cord blood.[9] Immediately after birth, with the initiation of spontaneous respiration and alveolar-capillary gas exchange, p_aO_2 rises to 80 to 90 mm Hg in the first 5 to 10 minutes of life. This abrupt change causes the physiologic oxidative stress necessary to trigger the expression of a number of significant genes necessary for postnatal adaptation.[10] The first studies of fetal pulse oximetry (SpO_2) during labor revealed that normal values were approximately 58% ± 10%. Studies performed in term newborn infants have shown that SpO_2 does not reach stable values of 85% or higher until 5 minutes after birth, and some healthy newborn infants need even more time, especially if they are born by cesarean section. In addition, preterm infants, especially extremely low birth weight (ELBW) infants, will not reach an SpO_2 of 85% or higher until at least 10 to 15 minutes after birth (**Fig. 3**).[11]

Arterial Oxygen Saturation Nomogram

Dawson and colleagues,[12] in 3 prospective observational studies using the same methodology, separately enrolled 468 newly born infants with gestational ages ranging from 25 to 42 weeks who did not receive oxygen at birth. Thus, arterial oxygen saturation as measured by pulse oximetry was retrieved from the first minute after birth using last-generation monitors set at maximum sensitivity attached to the right wrist to continuously measure preductal oxygen saturation until newborn infants achieved clinical stabilization. Thereafter, the 3 data sets were assembled into a graph that represents a reference range for SpO_2 for healthy babies of fewer than 42 weeks of gestation in the first 10 minutes after birth (**Fig. 4**).[12] As shown in the nomogram, it took a median of 7.9 minutes (interquartile range 5.0–10.0) to reach an SpO_2 higher than 90%, and preterm infants needed significantly more time to reach this saturation.[12] At present, Dawson and colleagues'[13] oxygen saturation nomogram represents the best estimate of the most appropriate SpO_2 targets for term but especially for preterm infants during the first minutes of life.

Oxygen Administration in the Delivery Room

In experimental and clinical studies, it has been shown that the use of room air (21% oxygen) offers substantial advantages over the use of 100% oxygen, as had been

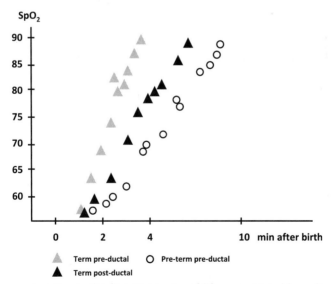

Fig. 3. Oxygen saturation in the first 10 minutes of life as measured by pulse oximetry in healthy term and preterm babies with the sensor located on the right wrist (preductal) or in term babies located on the feet (postductal). Values expressed in the graph have been retrieved from the database of the first author (M.V.) and have not been previously published.

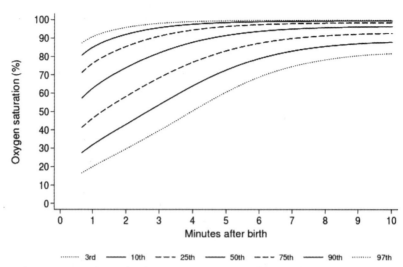

Fig. 4. Oxygen saturation reference range as measured by preductal pulse oximetry expressed in percentiles for the first 10 minutes after birth in healthy human neonates not needing resuscitation in the delivery room with gestational ages between 25 and 42 weeks. (*Data from* Dawson JA, Kamlin CO, Vento M, et al. Defining the reference range for oxygen saturation for infants after birth. Pediatrics 2010;125:e1340–7.)

traditionally recommended in the resuscitation of depressed newborn infants. Thus, a meta-analysis retrieving published evidence concluded that the use of room air significantly reduces mortality in asphyxiated neonates[14]; moreover, air-resuscitation also shortens the time needed to initiate spontaneous respiration, improves Apgar score, and reduces oxidative stress and oxidative damage to vital organs, such as myocardium and kidneys.[15,16] As a consequence, in 2010 the International Liaison Committee on Resuscitation guidelines recommended the use of air as the initial gas admixture for the depressed neonate; moreover, both pulse oximetry monitoring of SpO_2 and titration of the inspiratory fraction of oxygen (FIO_2) to avoid hyperoxic or hypoxic damage were also encouraged.[17]

Preterm babies do not generally suffer from birth asphyxia; however, they experience difficulties in adapting to the extrauterine environment because of lung and thoracic cage immaturity. Hence, a significant proportion of preterm infants will need proactive interventions in the delivery room. Positive-pressure ventilation is the cornerstone of preterm resuscitation. Initial ventilation is performed in spontaneous breathing neonates with continuous positive-pressure ventilation, applying 4 to 8 cm H_2O.[18] Randomized controlled studies have shown that it is feasible to start resuscitation even in extremely low gestational age neonates using an initial FIO_2 of 21% to 30%, as long as the inspiratory fraction of oxygen is titrated against SpO_2 and the heart rate is kept within normal limits.[19–22]

Reliable preductal readings immediately after birth can be rapidly obtained (60–90 seconds) if caregivers have been adequately trained. Data are most quickly available if the device is applied in the following order: (1) turn on the oximeter, (2) apply the sensor to the infant's right hand or wrist to reflect oxygen saturation of blood going to the brain, (3) connect the sensor to the oximeter cable to avoid erroneous calibration by the device, and (4) shield the sensor from light.[13] Once effective ventilation has been established and SpO_2 readings are available, FIO_2 should be titrated against SpO_2 readings in the pulse oximeter adjusting the air/oxygen blender to avoid hyperoxia and hypoxia. Hence, if SpO_2 is below the 10th percentile, then FIO_2 should be increased in 10% increments every 30 seconds until SpO_2 reaches the 10th to 50th percentile, always avoiding an SpO_2 greater than the 90th percentile.[13] Although recommended by experts in the field, however, this approach is not evidence-based and no randomized controlled trial to date has informed on which SpO_2 targets would be safer for preterm infants in the first minutes after birth. In this regard, the American Heart Association has defined the target ranges for 1, 2, 3, 4, 5, and 10 minutes after birth at 60% to 65%, 65% to 70%, 70% to 75%, 75% to 80%, 80% to 85%, and 85% to 90%, respectively.[17] Notwithstanding, randomized controlled studies in preterm infants have shown that the use of a lower oxygen load during resuscitation significantly decreases oxidative stress and improves clinical outcome.[20,22] Hence, until sufficiently powered studies are available, our aim should be to reduce the oxygen load during resuscitation in the first minutes of life, trying to adjust the SpO_2 to the reference charts that, at present, are our best estimate of the optimal oxygenation targets in preterm infants.

OXYGEN DURING NEONATAL CARE IN THE NICU

The conundrum regarding the establishment of upper and lower limits of oxygen saturation, especially in ELBW infants, is still open. ELBW infants are very sensitive to both hyperoxia, which may especially lead to lung and retinal damage, and to hypoxia, which may cause white matter injury.[23] Studies that have compared different limits for SpO_2 have concluded that neonatal units maintaining ELBW infants within low saturation limits (85%–95%) have a significantly lower incidence ($\sim 50\%$) of retinopathy of prematurity (ROP) and bronchopulmonary dysplasia (BPD) than those units allowing SpO_2 to rise to higher limits (>95%).[24–26] The extremely preterm (≤ 28 weeks' gestation) lung is sensitive to oxidative stress because of (1) immature antioxidant defense system; (2) lack of surfactant, which prompts the use of mechanical ventilation; (3) tendency toward infection (already in utero or manipulation in the NICU); or (4) presence of circulating free iron.[27] A connection between oxygen, oxidative stress, and later appearance of BPD has been substantiated in different studies. Thus, preterm neonates who later developed BPD exhibited elevated concentrations in blood and tracheal aspirates of carbonyl adducts, which represent by-products of the attack of oxygen free radicals on structural and functional proteins of the lung.[28–30] Similarly, elevated plasma isofurans immediately after birth from higher oxygen load and $F_{2\alpha}$ isoprostanes in the first week after birth have also been associated with later development of BPD and periventricular leukomalacia.[22,31] In addition to the acute effect of ROS, a body of evidence indicates that ROS act as triggering molecules for transcription factor activation and could be responsible for regulating cell growth, differentiation, chemotaxis, inflammatory response, or apoptosis.[7] Hence, hyperoxia exposure, especially in preterm infants, leads to the release of specific mediators, such as vascular endothelial growth factor (VEGF) and angiopoietin 2, capable of disrupting the alveolar-capillary membrane and thus leading to pulmonary edema and subsequent lung injury. Other cytokines are also released from lung cells, attracting inflammatory cells to the lung. These inflammatory cells, as well as hyperoxia per se, release ROS, which can initiate the mitochondrial-dependent cell death pathway.[32] In the Benefits of Oxygen Saturation Targeting (BOOST) trial, the effect of higher (95%–98%) versus lower (91%–94%) targeted saturations for babies at fewer than 30 weeks of gestation was compared. In the BOOST trial, the use of higher SpO_2 was associated with an increased length of oxygen therapy, a higher rate of chronic lung disease, and a greater frequency of babies discharged on home oxygen therapy. At the same time, it did not improve neurodevelopment or somatic growth.[25] In another randomized controlled trial, the STOP-ROP trial (Supplemental Therapeutic Oxygen for Pre-threshold Retinopathy of Prematurity), an SpO_2 ranging from 89% to 94% was compared with a range of 95% to 99% in preterm babies with prethreshold ROP for a minimum of 2 weeks.[33] The beneficial effect of a higher SpO_2 on the evolution of eye disease was minimal, whereas the negative effects, such as prolonged hospitalization, respiratory morbidity, and prolonged need for oxygen supplementation, were significantly higher.[33] In addition to the well-known risks of hyperoxia, recent randomized controlled trials have illustrated the risk of keeping extremely preterm infants within lower ranges of SpO_2. In this regard, in the SUPPORT trial (Surfactant Positive Airway Pressure and Pulse Oximetry Randomized Trial), it was confirmed that surviving ELBW infants randomly assigned to lower SpO_2 target ranges (85%–89%) had a lower risk of ROP (8.6% vs 17.9%; $P<.01$) than those in the higher target group (91%–95%)[34]; however, increased mortality in the low-saturation group (19.9% vs 16.2%; $P<.04$) has raised serious concerns about keeping very preterm infants at lower oxygen saturation limits.[34] In addition, the BOOST II trial performed in the United Kingdom, Australia, and New Zealand (n = 2315), in which saturation target ranges compared were also of 85% to 89% versus 91% to 95%, it was shown that with the updated calibration algorithm used in the pulse-oximeter devices used in these trials, the range groups targeted for lower saturation had significantly lower survival rates than those targeted for higher saturation limits (17.3% vs 14.4%; $P<.015$). The trial was therefore interrupted.[35] Hence, although at present there is no conclusive evidence to consider 85% an unsafe lower saturation limit, great concern relative to increased mortality, especially for infants at fewer than 28 weeks of gestation, has been expressed.[34,35] Seemingly, there is no fixed SpO_2 range or oxygen supply that safely satisfies metabolic demands of infants born at different gestational ages; moreover, even for a given gestational age, postnatal age is also a relevant factor to be taken into consideration when establishing oxygenation limits.

EVOLVING OXYGEN NEEDS IN THE FIRST WEEKS OF LIFE AND NEW METABOLIC INDICES

Recent studies have suggested that it would be possible to differentiate between 2 different periods with different oxygen limits.[36] Very preterm infants at fewer than 32 weeks of postconceptional age would theoretically benefit from lower SpO_2 limits (eg, 85%–95%). In a phase of rapid vascular growth and extreme tissue sensitivity to oxygen because of an immature antioxidant defense system, the use of higher oxygen limits would lead to oxidative stress and inflammation in the lung, intestine, or brain, leading to BPD, necrotizing enterocolitis, or intraperiventricular hemorrhage. Older neonates (>32 weeks postconceptional age) with a more mature antioxidant system and a tendency toward hyperproliferation of the vascular bed of the retina, owing to a relative hypoxia of the retinal tissue, would benefit from higher SpO_2 ranges (98%–99%), however. This latter approach has not been conclusively established.[36] **Fig. 5** summarizes what would be consistent with the available literature. Hence, in the immediate postnatal period and independently from gestational age, the target saturation in the fetal to neonatal transition, and in the first hours thereafter, SpO_2 safety limits are seemingly of 85% to 90%; however, as deduced from the SUPPORT and BOOST II trials, as the preterm baby matures, metabolic necessities increase, as does the risk for hypoxemia.[34,35] In this regard, it would be extremely useful to have at our disposal functional and noninvasive biomarkers that would allow clinicians to monitor cell aerobic metabolism and evaluate the response to intervention. Of note,

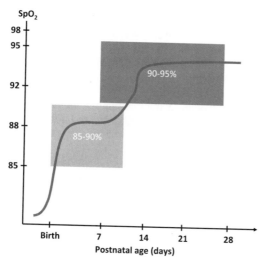

Fig. 5. Suggested SpO₂ ranges for preterm infants in the first weeks after birth, as deduced from the published literature (see text).

experimental studies performed in situations of hypoxia/reoxygenation have shown that traditional biomarkers of hypoxemia, such as lactic acid, do not significantly correlate with intensity and especially duration of hypoxia. Furthermore, glycine/branched chained amino acids (BCC) or alanine/BCC ratios are far better predictors of duration of hypoxia. In addition, if metabolites from the Krebs cycle, such as succinate and propionyl-L-carnitine, were also taken into consideration, the correlation with the duration of cell hypoxia was further increased.[37] Research performed in the experimental and clinical setting show that in the near future other biomarkers will help the clinician in assessing patients' aerobic metabolism, cell oxygen needs, and response to interventions. Hence, levels of growth factors (eg, insulinlike growth factor, VEGF, or metabolite ratios) might be used in the future to attain reliable information relative to cell oxygenation and, more importantly, to advert of the initiation of retinal vascular proliferation.[36]

GOING HOME ON OXYGEN

Chronic lung disease and prolonged oxygen needs among extremely preterm infants (≤28 weeks' gestation) is still a matter of concern. Of note, a relevant number of these babies are still being discharged home from the hospital on supplemental oxygen.[38] The goal of home oxygen therapy is to prevent the effects of chronic hypoxemia, which include pulmonary vasoconstriction leading to pulmonary hypertension, bronchial constriction leading to airway obstruction, and changes in growth of pulmonary and ocular vasculature. Hence, improved oxygenation may lead to improved lung growth and repair, better nutritional status, and somatic growth.[39] Although there is a great variation among institutions regarding indications for home oxygen use, in a recent retrospective study including 8167 preterm infants between 23 and 31 weeks of gestation born in 280 NICUs in the United States, home use of oxygen was recorded in 59% of infants of 23 to 24 weeks of gestation and in 8% of infants of 29 to 31 weeks of gestation.[40] Moreover, the authors underscored that gestational age was by far the most significant risk factor for being discharged on oxygen; however, other relevant factors included small for gestational age, congenital anomalies, need for mechanical ventilation or for FiO_2 higher than 40% in the first 72 hours after birth, and patent ductus arteriosus.[40] Remarkably, many of these infants are going to experience acute life-threatening events at home with high risk for their physical and especially neurologic integrity.[41] As a safety measure, air tests can be performed before discharge. The purpose of this approach is to determine the nadir of SpO_2 reached in room air after supplemental oxygen has been suppressed. In most units, a minimum SpO_2 of higher than 80% should be maintained in air for 30 minutes before discharge, and after discharge, clinical signs, such as respiratory rate and growth, are combined with continuous overnight oximetry (or polysomnography) where available.[39]

To date, with our present knowledge of oxygen needs and oxygen-derived complications secondary to hyperoxia and/or hypoxia, babies with chronic neonatal lung disease should be targeted for SpO_2 range of 93% to 95%.

REFERENCES

1. Maltepe E, Saugstad OD. Oxygen in health and disease. Pediatr Res 2009;65: 261–8.
2. Buonocore G, Perrone S, Tataranno ML. Oxygen toxicity: chemistry and biology of reactive oxygen species. Semin Fetal Neonatal Med 2010;15:186–90.
3. Brunelle JK, Chandel NS. Oxygen deprivation induced cell death: an update. Apoptosis 2002;7:475–82.
4. Halliwell B. Biochemistry of oxidative stress. Biochem Soc Trans 2007;35:1147–50.
5. Davis JM, Auten RL. Maturation of the antioxidant system and the effects on preterm birth. Semin Fetal Neonatal Med 2010;15:191–5.
6. Lu SC. Regulation of glutathione synthesis. Mol Aspects Med 2009;30:42–59.
7. Jones DP, Go YM, Anderson CL, et al. Cysteine/cystine couple is a newly recognized node in the circuitry for biologic redox signaling and control. FASEB J 2004; 18:1246–8.
8. Gao Y, Raj JU. Regulation of pulmonary circulation in the fetus and newborn. Physiol Rev 2010;90:1291–335.
9. Khaw KS, Ngan Kee WD, Chu CY, et al. Effect of different inspired oxygen fractions on lipid peroxidation during general anaesthesia for elective Caesarean section. Br J Anaesth 2010;105:355–60.
10. Vento M, Aguar M, Escobar J, et al. Antenatal steroids and antioxidant enzyme activity in preterm infants: influence of gender and timing. Antioxid Redox Signal 2009;11:2945–55.
11. Vento M, Saugstad OD. Role of management in the delivery room and beyond in the evolution of bronchopulmonary dysplasia. In: Abman SH, editor. Bronchopulmonary Dysplasia. 1st edition. New York: Informa Healthcare USA Inc; 2010. p. 292–313.
12. Dawson JA, Kamlin CO, Vento M, et al. Defining the reference range for oxygen saturation for infants after birth. Pediatrics 2010;125:e1340–7.
13. Dawson JA, Vento M, Finer NN, et al. Managing oxygen therapy during delivery room stabilization of preterm infants. J Pediatr 2012;160:158–61.
14. Saugstad OD, Ramji S, Soll RF, et al. Resuscitation of newborn infants with 21% or 100% oxygen: an updated systematic meta-analysis. Neonatology 2008;94:176–82.
15. Saugstad OD. Resuscitation of newborn infants: from oxygen to air. Lancet 2010; 376:1970–1.
16. Vento M, Saugstad OD. Oxygen supplementation in the delivery room: updated information. J Pediatr 2011;158:e5–7.

17. Perlman JM, Wyllie J, Kattwinkel J, et al. Part 11: Neonatal Resuscitation: 2010 International consensus on cardiopulmonary resuscitation and emergency cardiovascular care science with treatment recommendations. Circulation 2010; 122:S516–38.

18. Vento M, Cheung PY, Aguar M. The first golden minutes of the extremely low gestational age neonate: a gentle approach. Neonatology 2009;95:286–98.

19. Rabi Y. Oxygen in the delivery room. Neoreviews 2010;11:e130–8.

20. Escrig R, Arruza L, Izquierdo I, et al. Achievement of targeted saturation values in extremely low gestational age neonates resuscitated with low or high oxygen concentrations: a prospective, randomized trial. Pediatrics 2008;121:875–81.

21. Wang CL, Anderson C, Leone TA, et al. Resuscitation of preterm neonates by using room air or 100% oxygen. Pediatrics 2008;121:1083–9.

22. Vento M, Moro M, Escrig R, et al. Preterm resuscitation with low oxygen causes less oxidative stress, inflammation and chronic lung disease. Pediatrics 2009; 124:439–49.

23. Saugstad OD. Optimal oxygenation at birth and in the neonatal period. Neonatology 2007;91:319–22.

24. Tin W, Milligan DW, Pennefather P, et al. Pulse oximetry, severe retinopathy, and outcome at one year in babies of less than 28 weeks gestation. Arch Dis Child Fetal Neonatal Ed 2001;84:F106–10.

25. Askie LM, Henderson-Smart DJ, Irwig L, et al. Oxygen-saturation targets and outcomes in extremely preterm infants. N Engl J Med 2003;349:959–67.

26. Sola A. Avoiding hyperoxia in infants < or = 1,250 g is associated with improved short- and long-term outcomes. J Perinatol 2006;26:700–5.

27. Saugstad OD. Oxygen and oxidative stress in bronchopulmonary dysplasia. J Perinat Med 2010;28:1–7.

28. Ellis RM. Reactive carbonyls and oxidative stress: potential for therapeutic interventions. Pharmacol Ther 2007;115:13–24.

29. Winterbourn CC, Chan T, Buss IH, et al. Protein carbonyls and lipid peroxidation products as oxidation markers in preterm infant plasma: associations with chronic lung disease and retinopathy and effects of selenium supplementation. Pediatr Res 2000;48:84–90.

30. Ballard PL, Truog WE, Merrill JD, et al. Plasma biomarkers of oxidative stress: relationship to lung disease and inhaled nitric oxide therapy in premature infants. Pediatrics 2008;121:555–61.

31. Ahola T, Fellman V, Kjellmer I, et al. Plasma 8-isoprostane is increased in preterm infants who develop bronchopulmonary dysplasia or periventricular leukomalacia. Pediatr Res 2004;56:88–93.

32. Bhandari V. Hyperoxia-derived lung damage in preterm infants. Semin Fetal Neonatal Med 2010;15:223–9.

33. The STOP-ROP Multicenter Study Group. Supplemental therapeutic oxygen for pre-threshold retinopathy of prematurity (STOP-ROP), a randomized controlled trial: I primary outcomes. Pediatrics 2000;105:295–310.

34. Carlo WA, Finer NN, Walsh MC, et al. Target ranges of oxygen saturation in extremely preterm infants. N Engl J Med 2010;362:1959–69.

35. Stenson B, Brocklehurst P, Tarnow-Mordi W. Increased 36-week survival with high oxygen saturation target in extremely preterm. N Engl J Med 2011;364:1680–2.

36. Saugstad OD, Aune D. In search of the optimal saturation for extremely low birth weight infants: a systematic review and meta-analysis. Neonatology 2011;100:1–8.

37. Solberg R, Enot D, Deigner HP, et al. Metabolomic analyses of plasma reveals new insights into asphyxia and resuscitation in pigs. PLoS One 2010;5:e9606.

38. Saletti A, Stick S, Doherty D, et al. Home oxygen therapy after preterm birth in Western Australia. J Paediatr Child Health 2004;40:519–23.

39. Fitzgerald DA, Massie RJH, Nixon GM, et al. Infants with chronic neonatal lung disease: recommendations for the use of home oxygen therapy. Med J Aust 2008;189:578–82.

40. Lagatta J, Clark R, Spitzer A. Clinical predictors and institutional variation in home oxygen use in preterm. J Pediatr 2011. [Epub ahead of print].

41. Harrison G, Beresford M, Shaw N. Acute life threatening events among infants on home oxygen. Paediatr Nurs 2006;18:27–9.

Hematological Interventions in NICU Care: the Use of rEpo, IVIG, and rG-CSF

Robert D. Christensen, MD[a,b]

KEYWORDS

• rEPO • IVIG • rG-CSF • NICU

This article focuses on the use of rEpo, IVIG, and rG-CSF in the NICU. It discusses the most recent studies and the most definitive and clinically relevant evidence, rather than summarizing all published studies. The last section was written for NICU practice groups that choose to use any of these medications and are seeking a consistent approach for doing so. The section provides the author's approach to the use of rEpo, IVIG, and rG-CSF, revealing personal preferences, interpretations, and experiences, and is based on the dictum, "if you are going to use it, use it the same way each time."

Many of the medications reviewed in this issue of *Clinics in Perinatology* are used almost every day in a busy neonatal intensive care unit (NICU). That is not the case with the 3 medications reviewed in this article. Erythropoietin (or the long-acting analog darbepoetin) is primarily used by neonatologists in an attempt to avoid red blood cell (RBC) transfusions, although its use as a neuroprotectant is capturing attention and stimulating important clinical investigation. After promising animal and preclinical studies, it is now clear that the effect size of intravenous immunoglobulin (IVIG) in preventing neonatal nosocomial infection is too small to be of practical value, and its use as adjunctive treatment for suspected or proven infection does not improve mortality rate or major disability rate at the age of 2 years, nor does it reduce the incidence of subsequent sepsis episodes. The use of IVIG in alloimmune cytopenias has decreased with the application of more specific and effective therapies. The role of recombinant granulocyte colony-stimulating factor (rG-CSF) in neonatology is important, but limited to the rare cases of severe congenital neutropenia.

This article is organized into 4 sections. The first 3 sections focus respectively on the use of recombinant erythropoietin (rEpo), IVIG, and rG-CSF in the NICU. These 3 sections primarily deal with the most recent studies and (in the author's opinion) the

[a] The Women and Newborns Program, Intermountain Healthcare, 36 South State Street, Salt Lake City, UT 84111, USA
[b] NICU, McKay-Dee Hospital Center, 4th Floor, 4401 Harrison Boulevard, Ogden, UT 84403, USA
E-mail address: Robert.christensen@imail.org

Clin Perinatol 39 (2012) 177–190
doi:10.1016/j.clp.2011.12.005
0095-5108/12/$ – see front matter © 2012 Elsevier Inc. All rights reserved.
perinatology.theclinics.com

most definitive and clinically relevant evidence, rather than attempting to summarize all published studies. This approach gives added weight to the refining-effect of the accumulating body of information on which the most recent studies were designed. Indeed, with growing evidence, each of these 3 medications is settling into a rather limited "niche use" in neonatology. Perhaps each NICU practice group will wish to determine whether it is in the best interest of their patients to employ these niche uses.

The fourth section of this article was written for NICU practice groups that choose to use any of these medications and are seeking a consistent approach for doing so. Adopting a consistent approach can facilitate interpretable outcomes analyses. Even if the approach adopted is flawed and destined to be replaced when a better approach is discovered, it is generally much better than having no consistency. Thus, the fourth section was intended to provide the author's approach to the use of rEpo, IVIG, and rG-CSF, revealing personal preferences, interpretations, and experiences. This section is based on the dictum, "if you are going to use it, use it the same way each time."

RECOMBINANT ERYTHROPOIETIN

Intended uses of rEpo in the NICU have included (1) preventing or reducing "early RBC transfusions" (those given during the first days to weeks after birth, primarily to treat the anemia resulting from repeated phlebotomy), (2) preventing or reducing "late RBC transfusions" (those given after the first weeks, primarily to treat the hyporegenerative, normocytic, normochromic "anemia of prematurity"), and (3) as a neuroprotectant. Many studies conducted worldwide over a period of 20 years have focused on the first 2 uses. A few recent studies, and some currently under way and in the planning stages, are taking advantage of Epo's neuroprotectant properties.

Darbepoetin, a long-acting Epo analog, has 2 additional glycosylation sites on the rEPO molecule (**Fig. 1**). This modification gives a longer half-life and thereby enables less frequent dosing.[1,2] Some articles reported that switching patients from rEpo to darbepoetin resulted in lower costs and greater patient satisfaction.[3–5] This was the case at Intermountain Healthcare (see the last section of this article).

"Early" RBC Transfusions

In the 2006 Cochrane analysis of early rEpo usage, Ohlsson and Aher[6] included 23 studies involving 2074 preterm infants in 18 countries. The various reports included in the analysis were heterogeneous, using different rEpo doses, dosing schedules, routes of administration, and concomitant hematinics (vitamin E, folate, iron); however, in sum, they show a modest reduction in number of early RBC transfusions.[6]

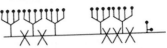

ERYTHROPOIETIN

- 3 N-linked CHO chains
- ≤14 sialic acid residues
- 30,400 daltons
- 40% carbohydrate

DARBEPOETIN

- 5 N-linked CHO chains
- ≤22 sialic acid residues
- 38,500 daltons
- 52% carbohydrate

Fig. 1. Schematic representations of erythropoietin and darbepoetin illustrating the 2 additional glycosylation sites in the latter, responsible for the longer half-life and need for less frequent dosing.

One argument raised against the early use of rEpo involves the questionable clinical significance of a small reduction in number of early transfusions; however, this benefit should be considered in light of the association between early transfusion and the subsequent development of severe intraventricular hemorrhage (IVH).[7–9] The banking process results in loss of RBC nitric oxide synthase and thus transfused banked RBCs are unable to dilate small capillary beds; moreover, banked RBCs become less flexible. These changes, part of the "storage lesion," can occlude capillaries and paradoxically lead to a temporary reduction in flow through partly occluded capillaries.[10,11] Capillaries in the periventricular and germinal matrix areas of extremely low birth weight neonates lack pericytes, which are mesenchymal cells that surround and strengthen capillaries.[12] Transfusion of banked donor RBCs into very low birth weight (VLBW) neonates in the first days after birth has the potential to temporarily occlude such capillaries, leading to upstream capillary rupture.[7–9]

In addition, early RBC transfusions suppress endogenous Epo production, thereby lowering serum Epo levels at a critical time in neurodevelopment.[13] It is possible that the poor neurodevelopmental outcome observed in neonates given RBC transfusions according to "liberal" guidelines is on the mechanistic basis of transfusion-induced Epo suppression.[14,15] Tempera and colleagues[16] recently reported early rEpo (300 U/k per dose 3 times per week subcutaneously) not only reduced RBC transfusion but also reduced broncho pulmonary dysplasia (BPD) rates, possibly on the basis of the anti-inflammatory and antioxidative actions of Epo.

"Late" RBC Transfusions

In the 2006 Cochrane analysis of late rEpo usage, Aher and Ohlsson[17] included 28 studies enrolling 1302 preterm infants in 21 countries. As with the analysis of early rEpo usage, the studies were heterogeneous and generally small. Their meta-analysis showed a significant effect of rEpo on reducing transfusions (typical relative risk [RR] 0.66, 95% confidence interval [CI] 0.59, 0.74; typical risk difference [RD] −0.21, 95% CI −0.26, −0.16); typical number needed to treat to benefit [NNTB] of 5, 95% CI 4, 6). As with the interpretation of the studies on early rEpo use, however, the question is raised of the value and clinical significance of 1 or 2 fewer late RBC transfusions.

An issue to consider regarding late transfusions involves the association between these and the subsequent development of necrotizing enterocolitis (NEC).[18–23] About one-third of NEC cases follow a banked donor RBC transfusion, generally by 6 to 24 hours. Thus, perhaps reducing late RBC transfusions has the potential to eliminate one-third of NEC cases. Although the mechanism by which late RBC transfusions associate with NEC is not clear, hypotheses involve temporary occlusion of mesenteric capillaries by donor RBC compromised by the "storage lesion," and immunologic interactions similar to transfusion-related lung injury reaction in the lung.[18,21,23]

Late RBC transfusions, like early RBC transfusions, suppress Epo production and thereby reduce erythropoiesis and predispose to the need for a subsequent RBC transfusion a week or so later.[24] As shown in **Fig. 2** administering rEpo simultaneously with a late transfusion stimulates, rather than reduces, erythropoiesis, thereby potentially lowering the odds that the patient will subsequently qualify for yet another RBC transfusion[24]

Neuroprotectant

Intact and functional Epo receptors are expressed on the surface of neurons. This was first reported convincingly by Li and colleagues[25] using human fetal spinal cord tissue, and then with a wide variety of human fetal neural tissue.[26–29] Epo is produced in the

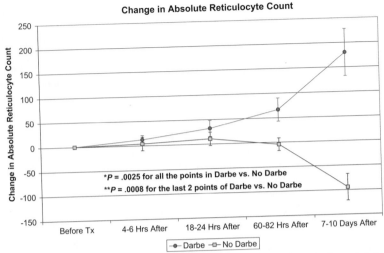

Fig. 2. Serial absolute reticulocyte counts performed on VLBW infants before and at various intervals after receiving a "late" RBC transfusion. Half received a single dose of darbepoetin (10 μg/kg subcutaneously) along with the transfusion and half were randomized not to receive darbepoetin (controls). Values shown are the changes from the baseline (before transfusion) in reticulocytes × 10^3/μL blood (mean ± SEM). Darbe, darbepoetin. (*From* Warwood TL, Lambert DK, Henry E, et al. Very low birth weight infants qualifying for a 'late' erythrocyte transfusion: does giving darbepoetin along with the transfusion counteract the transfusion's erythropoietic suppression? J Perinatol 2011;31(Suppl 1):S17–21; with permission.)

central nervous system by microglia in response to reduced oxygen tension. The process is mediated by hypoxia-inducible factor-1,[30] and acts in a paracrine fashion to reduce apoptosis in neurons otherwise marked for posthypoxic apoptosis.[30–36] Thus, in addition to its erythropoietic actions, Epo is a natural and potent neuroprotectant. Administration of rEpo in animal models of hypoxic-ischemic encephalopathy (HIE) results in reduced inflammation, reduced oxidative and glutamate-induced toxicity, better neuronal and morphologic recovery, and better neurodevelopmental outcomes.[30,32,34–36] For details on the in vitro and animal studies demonstrating the benefits of rEpo in models of neonatal HIE, readers are referred to reviews by McPherson and Juul[34] and Sola and colleagues.[35] For more information on the potential use of rEpo for neuroprotection outside the setting of HIE, readers are referred to the studies by Dr Ohls and her group.[37–41]

Retrospective studies implicated rEpo as a risk factor for retinopathy of prematurity (ROP),[6] but prospective randomized studies have not found this association. It has been suggested that perhaps excessive supplemental iron administration to rEpo-treated neonates raises the risk of ROP.[42] Readers are referred to the recent additional studies by Juul and her group[43,44] regarding lack of an association between rEpo and ROP.

INTRAVENOUS IMMUNOGLOBULIN

Proposed uses of IVIG in neonatology have included (1) preventing nosocomial infections, (2) treating suspected or proven infections, and (3) shortening the time to recovery of neonatal immune cytopenias.

ophylaxis Against Infection

though based on sound rationale, and supported by encouraging animal investiga-
on, IVIG has only a very small effect-size in preventing infection among VLBW
eonates; so small that it cannot be recommended for this purpose. Many clinical
als, involving more than 5000 neonates, tested this potential use. Summary statistics
these studies are confounded by the substantial differences in individual studies.
nlsson and Lacy[45] quantified the between-study heterogeneity (P = .0006) and noted
o statistically significant differences for mortality from all causes, mortality from infec-
on, incidence of NEC, BPD, and IVH or length of hospital stay. No major adverse
fects of IVIG were reported in any of the studies. IVIG administration was associated
th a 3% reduction in sepsis and a 4% reduction in any serious infection. From a clin-
al perspective, a 3% to 4% reduction without a reduction in mortality or other impor-
nt clinical outcomes is of questionable value. Ohlsson and Lacey[45] concluded that
ere is no justification for further randomized clinical trials testing the efficacy of previ-
usly studied IVIG preparations to reduce nosocomial infections in preterm and/or
3W infants and other avenues should be pursued for preventing nosocomial infec-
ons. One such avenue has been to test antistaphylococcal antibody. Polyclonal prep-
ations have thus far not been sufficiently successful to warrant endorsement, but
me monoclonal preparations performed well in phase II studies.[46–49]

eatment of Suspected or Proven Infection

ne most recent Cochrane review of this potential use of IVIG gives modest support to
e use of IVIG as an adjunct to antibiotics for neonates with infections,[50] but the
cent International Neonatal Immunotherapy Study (INIS) does not.[51] In 7 studies
fore the INIS trial, the mortality rate in neonates with *suspected infection* was lower
llowing IVIG treatment (n = 378), with typical RR of 0.58 (95% CI 0.38, 0.89) and
mber needed to treat of 10 (95% CI 6, 33). In cases of *proven infection* (n = 262),
e mortality rate was reduced, with a similar typical RR of 0.55 (95% CI 0.31, 0.98).
The INIS trial enrolled almost 10 times more neonates than the sum of all previous
IG treatment studies (n = 3493), recruiting subjects from October 2001 through
eptember 2007 from 9 countries.[51] Study subjects were receiving antibiotics for
oven or suspected serious infection and had at least one of the following: birth
eight less than 1500 g; respiratory support using an endotracheal tube; or evidence
infection in blood culture, cerebrospinal fluid, or usually sterile body fluid. Qualifying
tients were randomized to receive 2 doses of IVIG of 500 mg/kg each or a matching
acebo. The IVIG treatment had no effect on the outcomes of death or major disability
: 2 years) or on the rate of subsequent sepsis.

The field of neonatology owes a great debt of gratitude to Dr Brocklehurst and his
any associates for conducting this trial, spanning almost 10 years from first enrolment
final publication. It is an outstanding example of how a "negative finding" in a large
d well-done study can have a large impact on clinical practice. As this article's author
as one who conducted some of the early neonatal animal studies, and observed first-
nd the marked benefit of IVIG in preventing and treating experimental group B strep-
coccal (GBS) and *E coli* sepsis in those models,[52–56] the INIS results were certainly
sappointing. Moreover, seeing firsthand that in a small randomized placebo-
ntrolled trial, IVIG administration shortened the duration of neutropenia and provided
ti-GBS opsonins,[57,58] gave biologic plausibility to the hypothesis that IVIG would
ovide value to infected neonates. Animal studies and clinical trials based only on
provements in laboratory surrogates (neutropenia) are clearly not sufficient to
arrant wide clinical use, however; therefore, as listed in the accompanying Consistent

Approach to IVIG usage (**Fig. 3**), the authors do not advocate IVIG administration either as a means of preventing infection among VLBW neonates or as an adjunctive treatment for suspected or confirmed neonatal infection.

Immune-mediated Neonatal Cytopenias

IVIG can reduce the odds of qualifying for and receiving an exchange transfusion when administered to neonates with Coombs-positive hemolytic jaundice. This is the case for Rh and ABO alloimmunization.[59] The authors know of no evidence that IVIG provides value for hemolytic anemia attributable to other mechanisms. The value of IVIG in shortening the period of jaundice must be weighed, in each case, against the risk of NEC.[59] It should be noted that in the INIS trial, NEC was not more common among those randomized to receive IVIG than in those randomized to receive placebo; thus, the actual risk of NEC after IVIG administration is questionable.

IVIG administration can shorten the duration of neutropenia in neonates with alloimmune neutropenia[60,61]; however, the authors do not use it for this purpose, because authors find that severe and prolonged cases of alloimmune neonatal neutropenia are easier to manage using rG-CSF. IVIG can shorten the duration of neonatal immune-mediated thrombocytopenia and can be used for cases where maternal apheresed platelets or typed (usually HPA-lb) platelets are not available for a neonate with severe alloimmune thrombocytopenia. Severe thrombocytopenic hemorrhage is rare in neonates whose mothers have autoimmune thrombocytopenia (such as idiopathic thrombocytopenic purpura), but if the thrombocytopenia is particularly severe or accompanied by hemorrhage, IVIG administration can be useful along with random donor platelet transfusions.[62]

RECOMBINANT GRANULOCYTE COLONY-STIMULATING FACTOR

G-CSF and granulocyte-macrophage colony-stimulating factor (GM-CSF) are naturally occurring proteins involved in proliferation and differentiation of myeloid

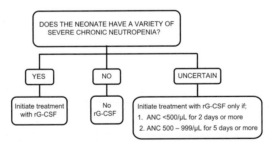

Fig. 3. A consistent approach to rG-CSF administration in the NICU. Background: The US Food and Drug Administration approved rG-CSF for use in children with severe chronic neutropenia, and for children receiving myelosuppressive chemotherapy for marrow transplantation. The rG-CSF generally used in the United States is produced by Amgen (Thousand Oaks, CA, USA) and has a molecular weight slightly lower than natural G-CSF, because it is produced in *Escherichia coli* and is not glycosylated. It has an amino acid sequence identical to that of natural G-CSF, except for the addition of an N-terminal methionine, which is necessary for its expression in *E coli*. Severe chronic neutropenia includes Kostmann syndrome, Shwachman-Diamond syndrome, cyclic neutropenia, Bart syndrome, severe and prolonged alloimmune neonatal neutropenia, or any syndrome or condition where severe and chronic neutropenia are a consistent finding. G-CSF administration is not recommended for neonates with neutropenia of a nonsevere, or a nonchronic nature, such as the neutropenia associated with pregnancy-induced hypertension, sepsis, or chronic idiopathic (mild) neutropenia.

precursors. The genes for both have been cloned and the purified recombinant factors are commercially available in pharmacologic quantities.[63,64] These factors have been widely used in adult and pediatric medicine primarily to treat severe congenital neutropenia and bone marrow failure syndromes. They can shorten the duration of neutropenia after chemotherapy for leukemia and solid tumors and after bone marrow transplantation. G-CSF is used in patients undergoing peripheral blood hematopoietic stem cell collection.

Target cells for these factors differ. G-CSF is lineage specific for the committed progenitors of neutrophils.[65] It stimulates proliferation and differentiation, expanding the available pool of neutrophil precursors and shortening their transit time through the marrow. It has been reported that G-CSF enhances several functions of mature neutrophils, but this has been questioned. GM-CSF acts on multilineage progenitors and on those of monocyte and neutrophil lineage and enhances bactericidal activities of mature phagocytes.

Patients with severe congenital neutropenia generally derive considerable benefit from rG-CSF administration. Almost all respond to dosages of 5 to 10 µg/kg administered at intervals ranging from every day to once per week to achieve neutrophil concentrations higher than 500 to 1000/µL.[65,66]

Explanted blood monocytes and mononuclear cells from human neonates produce G-CSF and GM-CSF poorly, compared with cells from adults; moreover, cells from preterm infants produce these proteins more poorly than do cells from term infants.[67,68] Plasma concentrations of G-CSF are relatively low in newborn infants with neutropenia and in infants with presumed sepsis, and progenitor cells of neonates

---

Box 1

A consistent approach to darbepoetin therapy in the NICU

Background: As used in our system, darbepoetin can be a cost-effective way to reduce the number of RBC transfusions administered in the NICU. RBC transfusions suppress endogenous Epo production. Because Epo is an important neurotrophic and neuroprotective factor, suppressing the production of Epo during critical periods of development may have adverse neurodevelopmental consequences. Some evidence now correlates early Epo administration among extremely low birth weight neonates with better neurodevelopmental outcome.

Two uses of darbepoetin in the NICU:

1. Accompanying RBC transfusions: A single dose of darbepoetin can be given along with an RBC transfusion (limited to 1 dose of darbepoetin per week even if more than 1 transfusion is given per week). This strategy can prevent the transfusion-induced hypoerythropoietinemia and the consequent suppression of RBC production that normally follows RBC transfusion. This practice has the potential to reduce the need for additional RBC transfusions and reduce costs.

2. As a means of avoiding "late" RBC transfusions: Sometimes at the nadir of the anemia of prematurity (3–5 weeks) the hemoglobin falls low enough to qualify the neonate for an RBC transfusion. A second use of darbepoetin in the NICU can be to prevent the need for "late" transfusions. Late transfusions have been associated with NEC in about one-third of NEC cases. Late transfusions can generally be avoided completely by targeting preterm neonates before their qualifying for a late transfusion, and intervening with darbepoetin. In general, these will be growing preterm neonates with a hemoglobin lower than 8 to 10 g/dL and falling but not yet qualifying for transfusion.

Dose: For both uses, Calhoun and colleagues recommend a dose of 10 µg/kg subcutaneously (or intravenously [IV]). The tested method for IV administration is in 4-mL sterile saline and given at a rate of 1 mL/h for 4 h (an IV bolus results in spillage of drug into the urine). When given accompanying a transfusion, our consistent approach is to give 1 dose. When given as a means of avoiding a "late" transfusion authors suggest 2 doses 1 week apart.

are as responsive as adult bone marrow progenitors to the actions of G-CSF and GM-CSF in culture. The rapid neutrophil response to infection is impaired in the murine model of *E coli* sepsis.[69] Cairo and colleagues[70,71] clearly demonstrated, in animal studies, that during experimental bacterial sepsis neonatal subjects generate G-CSF poorly compared with adults, and that G-CSF or GM-CSF administration in these models significantly improves survival.

Following these promising studies in vitro and in animal models, early trials of rG-CSF and GM-CSF in human neonates with presumed or proven sepsis were encouraging, demonstrating higher blood neutrophil count among the recipients.[72,73] However, larger subsequent trials by Cairo and colleagues,[74] Carr and colleagues,[75] and Kuhn and colleagues[76] showed that higher counts did not indicate more meaningful improvements, such as lower mortality rates. The systematic reviews by Carr and colleagues[77,78] of G-CSF or GM-CSF administration to newborns for treatment of suspected or proven systemic infection, identified no substantial evidence that these are of value.

It is not clear why rG-CSF treatment was so promising in the neonatal animal studies but failed to reduce mortality in the large clinical trials. In this respect, it is similar to the very favorable early studies with IVIG, also failing to reduce mortality in large trials. Obviously, animal experiments can be controlled much more precisely than a clinical

---

Box 2
A consistent approach to IVIG administration in the NICU

Prevention of Infection. In general, IVIG is not useful as prophylaxis against nosocomial infections among VLBW neonates. This is the case regardless of dose; manufacturer; or titers toward *Staphylococcus epidermidis*, other coagulase-negative staphylococci, or *Candida* species. Therefore, Calhoun and colleagues do not recommend IVIG administration as a means of preventing hospital-acquired infections.

Treatment of Suspected or Proven Infection. Neonates with sepsis, shock, and acidosis have a poor prognosis for survival. Some studies reported better outcomes when IVIG was administered to these patients; however a large international study (International Neonatal Immunotherapy Study) failed to show any significant benefit. For that reason, Calhoun and colleagues do not recommend IVIG as an adjunctive treatment for neonates with suspected or proven infection.

Immune-Mediated Neutropenia or Thrombocytopenia. For neonates with severe and prolonged immune-mediated neutropenia, Calhoun and colleagues find rG-CSF to be more effective in raising the neutrophil count, and more conducive to titrating the dosage so as to keep the neutrophil count above 1000/μL. Therefore, Calhoun and colleagues do not use IVIG as a treatment for immune-mediated neutropenia. For immune-mediated thrombocytopenia, IVIG can sometimes be helpful. Specifically, IVIG can be used for alloimmune cases where Calhoun and colleagues do not have maternal aphereshed platelets or typed (usually HPA-Ib) platelets to transfuse to a neonate with severe thrombocytopenic hemorrhage. Severe thrombocytopenic hemorrhage is rare in neonates whose mothers have autoimmune thrombocytopenia (such as idiopathic thrombocytopenic purpura), but in such cases IVIG administration can be useful, along with random donor platelet transfusions.

Immune-Mediated Hemolytic Anemia. IVIG can reduce the rate of hemolysis of antibody-coated erythrocytes. Thus, neonates with immune-mediated hemolytic jaundice might be spared an exchange transfusion, or the number of exchange transfusions might be reduced, if IVIG is administered early during the course of hemolytic jaundice while the serum bilirubin concentration is rising.

Other Potential Uses. Calhoun and colleagues know of no evidence that IVIG is useful for Coombs-negative hemolytic jaundice, nonimmune cytopenias including pregnancy-induced hypertension, or chronic benign neutropenia. Therefore, Calhoun and colleagues do not recommend IVIG administration for any of these conditions.

trial, particularly with regard to the relative uniformity of the hosts, and the timing of administration of the bacterial agent and the growth factors. This level of control cannot exist in clinical trials. Thus, the role of rG-CSF in neonatology does not include prevention of infection or treatment of suspected or proven infection, but does include the important usage in cases of severe chronic neutropenia, where rG-CSF can be very helpful or even life-saving[79,80] (see the following section).

A "CONSISTENT APPROACH" TO THE USE OF rEPO, IVIG, AND rG-CSF IN THE NICU

A few years ago, a group interested in neonatal hematology proposed a schema regarding consistency in the approach to neonatal transfusion medicine and hematology, including the issues of rEpo, IVIG, and rG-CSF.[81] That publication was intended as a rough guide, to serve as a voluntary means of consistency to all who were interested, until sufficient data accumulated to warrant a yet better treatment approach.

An updated version of the Consistent Approach documents, in use at the author's NICU, are listed in this section as **Boxes 1** and **2**; (see **Fig. 3**). Unlike the former document,[81] Calhoun and colleagues changed from rEpo to darbepoetin, largely for economic reasons but also for the advantage of less frequent dosing. The updated document regarding IVIG considers recently published studies, particularly the INIS study. The final Consistent Approach involves the use of rG-CSF in the NICU (**Fig. 3**). Briefly, if neutropenia is discovered to be one of the rare varieties of severe congenital neutropenia (SCN), the patient should be enrolled in the SCN International Registry and treatment with rG-CSF initiated. Enrollment in the SCN International Registry can be accomplished at the Web site http://depts.washington.edu/registry/. The authors propose beginning treatment with a dosage of 10 μg/kg subcutaneously, once per day for 3 consecutive days. Thereafter, doses are given as needed to titrate the absolute neutrophil count (ANC) to about 1000/μL. The authors propose if a neonatal patient has neutropenia, and the variety of neutropenia is known, and that variety is NOT one of the varieties of SCN, rG-CSF treatment should not be used. If the variety of neutropenia is NOT known (and therefore might be an SCN variety), while evaluating the variety of neutropenia, rG-CSF treatment could be instituted if the ANC was lower than 500/μL for 2 days or more, or lower than 1000/μL for 5 to 7 days or more.

REFERENCES

1. Testa U. Erythropoietic stimulating agents. Expert Opin Emerg Drugs 2010;15: 119–38.
2. Song S, Long SR, Marder WE, et al. The impact of methodological approach on cost findings in comparison of epoetin alfa with darbepoetin alfa. Ann Pharmacother 2009;43:1203–10.
3. Warwood TL, Ohls RK, Lambert DK, et al. Intravenous administration of darbepoetin to NICU patients. J Perinatol 2006;26:296–300.
4. Warwood TL, Ohls RK, Lambert DK, et al. Urinary excretion of darbepoetin after intravenous vs. subcutaneous administration to preterm neonates. J Perinatol 2006;26:636–9.
5. Warwood TL, Ohls RD, Wiedmeier SE, et al. Single-dose darbepoetin administration to anemic preterm neonates. J Perinatol 2008;25:725–30.
6. Ohlsson A, Aher SM. Early erythropoietin for preventing red blood cell transfusion in preterm and/or low birth weight infants. Cochrane Database Syst Rev 2006;3: CD004863.

7. Baer VL, Lambert DK, Henry E, et al. Among very-low-birth-weight neonates is red blood cell transfusion an independent risk factor for subsequently developing a severe intraventricular hemorrhage? Transfusion 2011;51:1170–8.

8. Baer VL, Lambert DK, Henry E, et al. Red blood cell transfusion of preterm neonates with a Grade 1 intraventricular hemorrhage is associated with extension to a Grade 3 or 4 hemorrhage. Transfusion 2011;51:1933–9.

9. Christensen RD, Lambert DK, Baer VL, et al. Postponing or eliminating red blood cell transfusions of very low birth weight neonates by obtaining all baseline laboratory blood tests from otherwise discarded fetal blood in the placenta. Transfusion 2011;51:253–8.

10. Donadee C, Raat NJ, Kanias T, et al. Nitric oxide scavenging by red blood cell microparticles and cell-free hemoglobin as a mechanism for the red cell storage lesion. Circulation 2011;124:465–76.

11. Reynolds JD, Ahearn GS, Angelo M, et al. S-nitrosohemoglobin deficiency: a mechanism for loss of physiological activity in banked blood. Proc Natl Acad Sci U S A 2007;104:17058–62.

12. Ballabh P. Intraventricular hemorrhage in premature infants: mechanism of disease. Pediatr Res 2010;67:1–8.

13. Bell EF, Strauss RG, Widness JA, et al. Randomized trial of liberal versus restrictive guidelines for red blood cell transfusion in preterm infants. Pediatrics 2005; 115:1685–91.

14. McCoy TE, Conrad AL, Richman LC, et al. Neurocognitive profiles of preterm infants randomly assigned to lower or higher hematocrit thresholds for transfusion. Child Neuropsychol 2011;17:347–67.

15. Nopoulos PC, Conrad AL, Bell EF, et al. Long-term outcome of brain structure in premature infants: effects of liberal vs restricted red blood cell transfusions. Arch Pediatr Adolesc Med 2011;165:443–50.

16. Tempera A, Stival E, Piastra M, et al. Early erythropoietin influences both transfusion and ventilation need in very low birth weight infants. J Matern Fetal Neonatal Med 2011;24:1060–4.

17. Aher S, Ohlsson A. Late erythropoietin for preventing red blood cell transfusion in preterm and/or low birth weight infants. Cochrane Database Syst Rev 2006;3: CD004868.

18. Christensen RD. Association between red blood cell transfusions and necrotizing enterocolitis. J Pediatr 2011;158:349–50.

19. Christensen RD, Lambert DK, Henry E, et al. Is "transfusion-associated necrotizing enterocolitis" an authentic pathogenic entity? Transfusion 2010;50: 1106–12.

20. Josephson CD, Wesolowski A, Bao G, et al. Do red cell transfusions increase the risk of necrotizing enterocolitis in premature infants? J Pediatr 2010;157:972–8, e1–3.

21. Blau J, Calo JM, Dozor D, et al. Transfusion related acute gut injury: necrotizing enterocolitis in very low birth weight neonates following packed red blood cell transfusion. J Pediatr 2011;158:403–9.

22. El-Dib M, Narang S, Lee E, et al. Red blood cell transfusion, feeding and necrotizing enterocolitis in preterm infants. J Perinatol 2011;31:183–7.

23. Gordon PV. What progress looks like in NEC research. J Perinatol 2011;31(3):149.

24. Warwood TL, Lambert DK, Henry E, et al. Very low birth weight infants qualifying for a 'late' erythrocyte transfusion: does giving darbepoetin along with the transfusion counteract the transfusion's erythropoietic suppression? J Perinatol 2011; 31(Suppl 1):S17–21.

25. Li Y, Juul SE, Morris-Wiman JA, et al. Erythropoietin receptors are expressed in the central nervous system of mid-trimester human fetuses. Pediatr Res 1996; 40:376–80.

26. Juul SE, Harcum J, Li Y, et al. Erythropoietin is present in the cerebrospinal fluid of neonates. J Pediatr 1997;130:428–30.

27. Juul SE, Anderson DK, Li Y, et al. Erythropoietin and erythropoietin receptor in the developing human central nervous system. Pediatr Res 1998;43:40–9.

28. Juul SE, Yachnis AT, Christensen RD. Tissue distribution of erythropoietin and erythropoietin receptor in the developing human fetus. Early Hum Dev 1998;52: 235–49.

29. Juul SE, Yachnis AT, Rojiani AM, et al. Immunohistochemical localization of erythropoietin and its receptor in the developing human brain. Pediatr Dev Pathol 1999;2:148–58.

30. Sola A, Rogido M, Lee BH, et al. Erythropoietin after focal cerebral ischemia activates the Janus kinase-signal transducer and activator of transcription signaling pathway and improves brain injury in postnatal day 7 rats. Pediatr Res 2005;57: 481–7.

31. Juul SE, Beyer RP, Bammler TK, et al. Microarray analysis of high-dose recombinant erythropoietin treatment of unilateral brain injury in neonatal mouse hippocampus. Pediatr Res 2009;65:485–92.

32. Juul SE, McPherson RJ, Bauer LA, et al. A phase I/II trial of high-dose erythropoietin in extremely low birth weight infants: pharmacokinetics and safety. Pediatrics 2008;122:383–91.

33. Juul SE, McPherson RJ, Bammler TK, et al. Recombinant erythropoietin is neuroprotective in a novel mouse oxidative injury model. Dev Neurosci 2008;30: 231–42.

34. McPherson RJ, Juul SE. Recent trends in erythropoietin-mediated neuroprotection. Int J Dev Neurosci 2008;26:103–11.

35. Sola A, Peng H, Rogido M, et al. Animal models of neonatal stroke and response to erythropoietin and cardiotrophin-1. Int J Dev Neurosci 2008;26:27–35.

36. Sola A, Wen TC, Hamrick SE, et al. Potential for protection and repair following injury to the developing brain: a role for erythropoietin? Pediatr Res 2005; 57(5 Pt 2):110R–7R.

37. Bierer R, Roohi M, Peceny C, et al. Erythropoietin increases reticulocyte counts and maintains hematocrit in neonates requiring surgery. J Pediatr Surg 2009; 44:1540–5.

38. Bishara N, Ohls RK. Current controversies in the management of the anemia of prematurity. Semin Perinatol 2009;33:29–34.

39. Bierer R, Peceny MC, Hartenberger CH, et al. Erythropoietin concentrations and neurodevelopmental outcome in preterm infants. Pediatrics 2006;118:e635–40.

40. Ohls RK, Ehrenkranz RA, Das A, et al, National Institute of Child Health and Human Development Neonatal Research Network. Neurodevelopmental outcome and growth at 18 to 22 months' corrected age in extremely low birth weight infants treated with early erythropoietin and iron. Pediatrics 2004;114:1287–91.

41. Ohls RK, Dai A. Long-acting erythropoietin: clinical studies and potential uses in neonates. Clin Perinatol 2004;31:77–89.

42. Inder TE, Clemett RS, Austin NC, et al. High iron status in very low birth weight infants is associated with an increased risk of retinopathy of prematurity. J Pediatr 1997;131:541–4.

43. Slusarski JD, McPherson RJ, Wallace GN, et al. High-dose erythropoietin does not exacerbate retinopathy of prematurity in rats. Pediatr Res 2009;66:625–30.

44. McPherson RJ, Juul SE. Erythropoietin for infants with hypoxic-ischemic encephalopathy. Curr Opin Pediatr 2010;22:139–45.

45. Ohlsson A, Lacy JB. Intravenous immunoglobulin for preventing infection in preterm and/or low-birth-weight infants. Cochrane Database Syst Rev 2004;1: CD000361.

46. Shah PS, Kaufman DA. Antistaphylococcal immunoglobulins to prevent staphylococcal infection in very low birth weight infants. Cochrane Database Syst Rev 2009;2:CD006449.

47. Figueras-Aloy J, Rodríguez-Miguélez JM, Iriondo-Sanz M, et al. Intravenous immunoglobulin and necrotizing enterocolitis in newborns with hemolytic disease. Pediatrics 2010;125:139–44.

48. DeJonge M, Burchfield D, Bloom B, et al. Clinical trial of safety and efficacy of INH-A21 for the prevention of nosocomial staphylococcal bloodstream infection in premature infants. J Pediatr 2007;151:260–5.

49. Weisman LE, Thackray HM, Steinhorn RH, et al. A randomized study of a monoclonal antibody (pagibaximab) to prevent staphylococcal sepsis. Pediatrics 2011;128:271–9.

50. Ohlsson A, Lacy J. Intravenous immunoglobulin for suspected or subsequently proven infection in neonates. Cochrane Database Syst Rev 2010;3:CD001239.

51. Brocklehurst P, INIS Collaborative Group. Treatment of neonatal sepsis with intravenous immune globulin. N Engl J Med 2011;365:1201–11.

52. Christensen RD, Brown MS, Hall DS, et al. Effect on neutrophil kinetics and serum opsonic capacity of intravenous administration of immune globulin to neonates with clinical signs of early-onset sepsis. J Pediatr 1991;118:606–14.

53. Harper TE, Christensen RD, Rothstein G, et al. Effect of intravenous immunoglobulin G on neutrophil kinetics during experimental group B streptococcal infection in neonatal rats. Rev Infect Dis 1986;8(Suppl 4):S401–8.

54. Harper TE, Christensen RD, Rothstein G. The effect of administration of immunoglobulin to newborn rats with *Escherichia coli* sepsis and meningitis. Pediatr Res 1987;22:455–60.

55. Lassiter HA, Christensen RD, Parker CJ. Immunologic regulation of *E. coli* K1 by serum from neonatal rats is enhanced following intraperitoneal administration of human IgG. J Infect Dis 1989;159:518–25.

56. Redd H, Christensen RD, Fischer GW. Circulating and storage neutrophils in septic neonatal rats treated with immune globulin. J Infect Dis 1988;157: 705–12.

57. Lassiter HA, Christensen RD, Parker C, et al. Neutrophil-mediated killing, opsonization, and serum-mediated killing of *Escherichia coli* K1 by neonatal rats. Biol Neonate 1988;53:156–62.

58. Lassiter HA, Robinson TW, Brown MS, et al. Effect of intravenous immunoglobulin G on the deposition of immunoglobulin G and C3 onto type III group B streptococcus and *Escherichia coli* K1. J Perinatol 1996;16:346–51.

59. Alcock GS, Liley H. Immunoglobulin infusion for isoimmune haemolytic jaundice in neonates. Cochrane Database Syst Rev 2002;3:CD003313.

60. Maheshwari A, Christensen RD, Calhoun DA. Immune-mediated neutropenia in the neonate. Acta Paediatr Suppl 2002;91(438):98–103.

61. Desenfants A, Jeziorski E, Plan O, et al. Intravenous immunoglobulins for neonatal alloimmune neutropenia refractory to recombinant human granulocyte colony-stimulating factor. Am J Perinatol 2011;28:461–6.

62. Rayment R, Brunskill SJ, Soothill PW, et al. Antenatal interventions for fetomaternal alloimmune thrombocytopenia. Cochrane Database Syst Rev 2011;5:CD004226.

63. Crawford J, Armitage J, Balducci L, et al, National Comprehensive Cancer Network. Myeloid growth factors. J Natl Compr Canc Netw 2009;7:64–83.
64. Satwani P, Morris E, van de Ven C, et al. Dysregulation of expression of immuno-regulatory and cytokine genes and its association with the immaturity in neonatal phagocytic and cellular immunity. Biol Neonate 2005;88:214–27.
65. Dale DC, Bonilla MA, Davis MW, et al. A randomized, controlled phase III trial of recombinant human granulocyte colony-stimulating factor (filgrastim) for treatment of severe chronic neutropenia. Blood 1993;81:2496–502.
66. Bonilla MA, Gillio AP, Ruggeiro M, et al. Effects of recombinant human granulocyte colony-stimulating factor on neutropenia in patients with congenital agranulocytosis. N Engl J Med 1989;320:1574–80.
67. Cairo M, Suen Y, Knoppel E, et al. Decreased G-CSF and IL-3 production and gene expression from mononuclear cells of newborn infants. Pediatr Res 1992;31:574–8.
68. Schibler K, Leichty K, White W, et al. Production of granulocyte colony-stimulating factor in vitro by monocytes from-preterm and term neonates. Blood 1993;82:2479–84.
69. Leichty K, Schibler K, Ohls R, et al. The failure of newborn mice infected with *Escherichia coli* to accelerate neutrophil production correlates with their failure to increase transcripts for granulocyte colony-stimulating factor and interleukin-6. Biol Neonate 1993;64:331–40.
70. Cairo M, Plunkett J, Mauss D, et al. Seven-day administration of recombinant granulocyte colony-stimulating factor to newborn rats: modulation of neonatal neutrophilia, myelopoiesis, and group B streptococcal sepsis. Blood 1990;76:1788–94.
71. Cairo MS, van de Ven C, Mauss D, et al. Modulation of neonatal rat myeloid kinetics resulting in peripheral neutrophilia by single pulse administration of Rh granulocyte-macrophage colony-stimulating factor and Rh granulocyte colony-stimulating factor. Biol Neonate 1991;59:13–21.
72. Gillan ER, Christensen RD, Suen Y, et al. A randomized, placebo-controlled trial of recombinant human granulocyte colony-stimulating factor administration in newborn infants with presumed sepsis: significant induction of peripheral and bone marrow neutrophilia. Blood 1994;84:1427–33.
73. Cairo MS, Christensen RD, Sender LS, et al. Results of a phase I/II trial of recombinant human granulocyte-macrophage colony-stimulating factor in very low birthweight neonates: significant induction of circulatory neutrophils, monocytes, platelets, and bone marrow neutrophils. Blood 1995;86:2509–15.
74. Cairo MS, Agosti J, Ellis R, et al. A randomized, double-blind, placebo-controlled trial of prophylactic recombinant human granulocyte-macrophage colony-stimulating factor to reduce nosocomial infections in very low birth weight neonates. J Pediatr 1999;134:64–70.
75. Carr R, Brocklehurst P, Dore C, et al. Granulocyte-macrophage colony stimulating factor administered as prophylaxis for reduction of sepsis in extremely preterm, small for gestational age neonates (the PROGRAMS trial): a single-blind, multi-centre, randomized controlled trial. Lancet 2009;373:226–33.
76. Kuhn P, Messer J, Paupe A, et al. A multicentre, randomized, placebo-controlled trial of prophylactic recombinant granulocyte colony stimulating factor in preterm neonates with neutropenia. J Pediatr 2009;155:324–30.
77. Carr R. Is there a role for GM- or G-CSF and immunoglobulins in the prevention and treatment of neonatal sepsis? Neonatology 2011;100:338 (A).
78. Carr R, Modi N, Dore C. G-CSF and GM-CSF for treating or preventing neonatal infections. Cochrane Database Syst Rev 2003;3:CD003066.

79. Walkovich K, Boxer LA. Congenital neutropenia in a newborn. J Perinatol 2011; 31(Suppl 1):S22–3.
80. Dale DC, Welte K. Cyclic and chronic neutropenia. Cancer Treat Res 2011;157: 97–108.
81. Calhoun DA, Christensen RD, Edstrom CS, et al. Consistent approaches to procedures and practices in neonatal hematology. Clin Perinatol 2000;27:733–53.

Management of Neonatal Thrombosis

Matthew A. Saxonhouse, MD

KEYWORDS

• Neonatal thrombosis • Thromboembolism • Vasospasm
• Venous thrombosis • Arterial thrombosis
• Prothrombotic disorder

THE NEONATAL HEMOSTATIC SYSTEM

The incidence of neonatal thromboembolic (TE) events varies and is dependent on how aggressively centers screen for thromboses. Ranges of neonatal TE events have varied from 2.4 clinically apparent events (excluding stroke) per 1000 neonatal ICU (NICU) admissions[1] to 5.1 events per 100,000 live births.[2] A more recent review of 4734 neonates reported an incidence of 6.8 per 1000 NICU admissions.[3] Neonatal thromboses occur in both preterm and term infants and affect male and female infants equally.[1–3]

The neonatal coagulation (anticoagulation and fibrinolytic systems included) system differs from those of children and adults (**Table 1**).[4] These differences place a neonate in a relative prothrombotic state, but are usually balanced by other factors that prevent a well term or relatively well premature infant from experiencing spontaneous thromboses.[5] Any disruption of this balance can place a neonate at risk for developing thromboses.[6–9] Age-appropriate reference ranges have been published by Andrew and colleagues[6–8] and should be referred to when interpreting diagnostic testing in preterm and term neonates.

TYPES OF NEONATAL THROMBOSES

The main locations of neonatal thromboses and the imaging modalities recommended for how to properly identify them are listed in **Table 2**. Common signs and symptoms for each type of thromboses (described later) are listed in **Table 3**.

Arterial Thromboses

Ischemic perinatal

An important cause of infant morbidity and neurodevelopmental disability,[10,11] ischemic perinatal stroke (IPS), occurs within 2 days surrounding birth and can extend to the 28th postnatal day.[12] With an estimated incidence of 1 in 2300 live births,[10] IPS

Pediatrix Medical Group, Jeff Gordon Children's Hospital, 920 Church Street North, CMC-NE, Concord, NC 28025, USA
E-mail address: Matthew_saxonhouse@pediatrix.com

Clin Perinatol 39 (2012) 191–208
doi:10.1016/j.clp.2011.12.018   **perinatology.theclinics.com**
0095-5108/12/$ – see front matter © 2012 Elsevier Inc. All rights reserved.

Table 1
Comparison of anticoagulant and procoagulant protein levels between neonates and adults

Neonatal Level Compared with Adults	Procoagulant Proteins	Anticoagulant Proteins
Increased	Factor VIII von Willebrand factor activity	
Decreased	Factors II, VII, IX, X, XI, and XII	Protein S Protein C Antithrombin Heparin cofactor II

Data from Refs.[6–9] and Manco-Johnson MJ. Controversies in neonatal thrombotic disorders. In: Ohls R, Yoder MC, editors. Hematology, immunology, and infectious disease: neonatology questions and controversies, vol. 1. Philadelphia: Saunders Elsevier; 2008. p. 58–74.

mainly occurs in the left hemisphere within the distribution of the middle cerebral artery, with anterior and posterior cerebral artery lesions less common.[13,14] Rarely, multifocal cerebral infarctions can occur and are usually embolic in origin.[13]

Many potential risk factors have been implicated in the etiology of IPS (**Table 4**).[10] A recent review of 5 neonates with AIS found that all cases had multiple risk factors involved, with placenta pathology a contributing factor.[10] The presence of 3 or more of these risk factors may be associated with a 25-fold increase risk of perinatal stroke.[15] Prothrombotic disorders may play a significant contributory role in the pathogenesis of IPS, especially if placental pathology is included.

Although no randomized clinical trial has addressed the management of neonates with IPS, current guidelines from the American College of Chest Physicians recommend treatment with unfractionated heparin (UFH) or low-molecular-weight heparin (LMWH) only for neonates with proved cardioembolic stroke or recurrent ischemic perinatal stroke.[16]

Iatrogenic/spontaneous arterial thromboses

Iatrogenic arterial thromboses are mainly related to complications from umbilical arterial catheters (UACs), peripheral arterial catheters (PALs), and femoral arterial catheters.[17] The most frequent complication of both PAL and UAC use is episodes of

Table 2
Types, locations, and recommended imaging modalities for neonatal thromboses

Vessel	Type/Location	Imaging Modality
Arterial	Ischemic perinatal stroke	Diffusion-weighted MRI/magnetic resonance angiography
	Iatrogenic or spontaneous	Doppler ultrasound
Venous	IVC, abdominal veins, lower extremities	
	Renal vein	
	Portal venous	
	Cerebral sinovenous	Diffusion-weighted MRI with venography
	Right atrium and SVC	Echocardiography

Data from Monagle P, Chalmers E, Chan A, et al. Antithrombotic therapy in neonates and children: American College of Chest Physicians Evidence-Based Clinical Practice Guidelines (8th Edition). Chest 2008;133(Suppl 6):887S–968S.

Table 3
Signs and symptoms of neonatal thromboses

		Presenting Signs and/or Symptoms
Arterial	Ischemic perinatal stroke	Seizures,[a] lethargy, hypotonia, apnea, poor feeding
	Iatrogenic[b]	Line dysfunction, extremity blanching and/or cyanosis, persistent thrombocytopenia, sepsis
	Spontaneous	Symptoms depend on location[c]
Venous	Iatrogenic[b]	Line dysfunction, persistent thrombocytopenia, persistent infection
	Intracardiac	Pericardial tamponade, symptoms of right heart failure
	RVTs	Macroscopic hematuria, palpable abdominal mass, thrombocytopenia, acute hypertension
	PVTs	Liver dysfunction, portal hypertension
	CSVT	Seizures, fever, apnea, lethargy

[a] Most common.
[b] Catheter related.
[c] See **Box 1** for most common locations.
Data from Refs.[13,53,95,96]

blanching and cyanosis of the extremities.[18] Reports of UAC use in NICUs have been as high as 64.4% of all admissions.[19] Potential complications of UACs include thrombosis in the abdominal aorta, renal failure, tissue necrosis, hypertension, septicemia, and death.[20] High UAC positioning has been associated with fewer clinical complications,[16,21] and low-dose continuous heparin infusion at 1 U/mL has been found to prolong catheter patency without reducing the risk of thrombosis.[21,22]

The probability of developing an aortic thrombus in situ with a UAC increases proportionally to the duration of placement, with an incidence reaching 80% within 21 days.[20] Suspicion or confirmation of an arterial thrombosis due to catheter placement

Table 4
Risk factors for the development of neonatal thromboembolism

Maternal Risk Factors	Delivery Risk Factors	Neonatal Risk Factors
Infertility	Emergent	Central catheters
Oligohydramnios	cesarean section	Congenital heart disease
Prothrombotic disorder	Fetal heart rate	Sepsis
Preeclampsia	abnormalities	Birth asphyxia
Diabetes	Instrumentation	Respiratory distress syndrome
Intrauterine growth		Dehydration
restriction		Congenital nephritic/nephrotic syndrome
Chorioamnionitis		Necrotizing enterocolitis
Prolonged rupture of		Polycythemia
membranes		Pulmonary hypertension
Autoimmune disorders		Prothrombotic disorders (see **Table 4**)
		Surgery
		Extracorporeal membrane oxygenation
		Medications (steroids, heparin)

Data from Saxonhouse MA, Manco-Johnson MJ. The evaluation and management of neonatal coagulation disorders. Semin Perinatol 2008;33:52–65; and *Data from* Refs.[2,13,15,44,45,51,53,58–61,64,67,93,95,97–99]

should warrant prompt removal of the arterial catheter. Thrombus imaging, however, should be performed before catheter removal and careful consideration should be given to whether local instillation of recombinant tissue plasminogen activator (rtPA) into the thrombus via the catheter may be indicated.[16]

Spontaneous arterial thromboses are rare but usually involve the aorta or other large vessels (**Box 1**). Treatment of arterial thromboses depends on the clinical symptoms and location of the thrombus. The ultimate goal is restoration of blood flow if there is evidence of limb or organ ischemia. Treatment modalities and management of arterial vasospasm are discussed later.

Venous Thrombosis

Catheter related, noncardiac

Umbilical venous catheters (UVCs) and peripherally inserted central venous catheters are routinely used in NICUs although thrombus formation remains a significant complication. A recent study found that 21.4% of 28 babies with UVCs had thrombus formation, 4 of which were in the inferior vena cava (IVC) and 2 in the portal vein.[27] Autopsies have estimated that 20% to 65% of infants who die with a UVC in situ have microscopic evidence of TE.[28–30] The Centers for Disease Control and Prevention currently recommend that the use of UVCs be limited to 14 days.[31] Long-term complications of venous TE include chronic venous obstruction with cutaneous collateral circulation, chylothorax, portal hypertension, and post-thrombotic syndrome.[11,32–34]

Suspicion or confirmation of a venous thrombus warrants prompt catheter removal, however, due to the risk for emboli; current recommendations are to delay central venous catheter removal if a thrombus has been detected until 3 to 5 days after anticoagulant therapy has been given, although no clinical studies exist to support this practice.[16]

Intracardiac thromboses and thromboses in infants with complex congenital heart disease

Right atrial catheter placement in neonates remains controversial due to the risk of either pericardial tamponade and/or intracardiac thrombi development.[35,36] Intracardiac (mainly right atrial thrombi) thromboses is a life-threatening complication due to the risk for dissemination of emboli into the lungs or obstruction of the right pulmonary artery.[37,38] Several case reports exist describing thrombolysis, mainly using rTPA, of catheter-related atrial thromboses in neonates.[37–41] rTPA has also been used in the management of premature infants with infective endocarditis.[42] Caution must be used, however, when administering thrombolytics to premature infants only for infective endocarditis due to the high incidence of intracranial hemorrhage. Thromboses, especially of the superior vena cava (SVC), have also become a common complication in infants undergoing repair of complex congenital heart disease.[43]

Box 1
Potential locations for spontaneous arterial thromboses in neonates

Iliac artery

Left pulmonary artery

Aortic arch

Descending aorta

Data from Refs.[23–26]

Renal vein thrombosis

A review of 271 neonatal cases of renal vein thromboses (RVTs) demonstrated that 70% of cases were unilateral (with 64% of these involving the left kidney), and that male infants were more frequently affected.[44] Acute complications of RVT include adrenal hemorrhage, extension of the clot into the IVC, renal failure, hypertension, and death.[44] Chronically, most infants with RVT suffer complete, cortical, or segmental infarction of the affected kidney(s) and/or hypertension.

Genetic prothrombotic risk factors have been found in 43% to 67% of patients with RVT.[44–47] Ultrasonographic features suggestive of RVT include enlarged, echogenic kidneys with attenuation or loss of corticomedullary differentiation. Color flow Doppler shows absence of flow in the main or arcuate renal veins. The treatment of RVT is controversial because there are no large randomized clinical trials addressing specific treatment options. Current recommendations for both unilateral and bilateral RVT are presented in **Table 5**.

Portal vein thrombosis

Risk factors for the development of portal vein thrombosis (PVT) include sepsis/oomphalitis, exchange transfusion, or umbilical catheterization.[48] Neonates tend to remain asymptomatic during the neonatal period. Spontaneous resolution of asymptomatic PVT is common (30%–70% of the time) and can take from days to months.[48] The detection of PVT, however, even in asymptomatic patients, warrants close observation for signs of portal hypertension. This problem may manifest itself up to 10 years after the neonatal period.[11] A recent review of 70 children with documented PVTs during the neonatal period who were re-evaluated at a mean age of 5 years demonstrated that 28% had asymptomatic left lobar atrophy of the liver, 7% had progressive splenomegaly, and 3% required portacaval shunting due to portal hypertension.[49] Currently, there is no evidence that anticoagulation improves time to resolution or decreases the likelihood of portal hypertension.[48]

Cerebral sinovenous thrombosis

The majority of neonates with cerebral sinovenous thrombosis (CSVT) present on the day of birth or within the first week of life.[50] A large majority of neonates with CSVT have either maternal and/or neonatal predisposing risk factors (see **Table 4**; **Table 6**), demonstrating that the pathogenesis of CSVT is multifactorial.[53–56]

Table 5
Management options for neonates with renal vein thrombosis

	Unilateral RVT	Bilateral RVT
Absence of renal impairment or extension into the IVC	Supportive care with monitoring of the RVT for extension or anticoagulation for up to 3 months	Supportive care with monitoring of the RVT for extension or anticoagulation for up to 3 months
Extension into the IVC	Anticoagulation[a]	Anticoagulation[a]
Renal failure	N/A	Initial thrombolytic[b] therapy with rTPA, followed by anticoagulation

[a] See **Tables 7–9** for dosing options.
[b] See **Tables 7** and **11** for dosing options and appropriate monitoring.
Data from Refs.[16,44–47]

Table 6 Laboratory evaluation for suspected prothrombotic disorder	
Initial Laboratory Testing[a]	**Collection Tube**
Antiphospholipid antibody panel, anticardiolipin, and lupus anticoagulant (IgG, IgM)	Citrated plasma
Fibrinogen[b]	Citrated plasma
Protein C activity[b] Protein S activity[b] Antithrombin (activity assay)[b]	Citrated plasma
Factor V Leiden[c] Prothrombin G[c] MTHFR[c]	EDTA
Homocysteine[b] Lipoprotein a[b]	Citrated plasma
Additional Laboratory Testing[d]	
Factor VIII activity[b] Factor XII activity[b] Plasminogen activity[b] Heparin cofactor II[b]	Citrated Plasma

Abbreviation: MTHFR, methylenetetrahydrofolate reductase.

A possible limitation to this laboratory evaluation is the amount blood required for adequate testing, especially when evaluating a premature or anemic infant. The evaluation should, therefore, take place at an experienced tertiary referral center that has either a reference laboratory or a reliable referral center limiting blood volumes to 4–6 mL for an entire evaluation.

[a] The following is performed if other acquired risk factors (see **Table 4**) are present.

[b] Protein-based assays are affected by the acute TE event and must be repeated at 3 to 6 months of life, before a definitive diagnosis can be made.[51,52] If anticoagulation is administered, then these assays should be obtained 14 to 30 days after discontinuing the anticoagulant.

[c] DNA-based assays.

[d] The following is performed if other acquired risk factors (see **Table 4**) are not present.

Data from Saxonhouse MA, Manco-Johnson MJ. The evaluation and management of neonatal coagulation disorders. Semin Perinatol 2008;33:52–65; and Manco-Johnson MJ, Grabowski EF, Hellgreen M, et al. Laboratory testing for thrombophilia in pediatric patients. On behalf of the Subcommittee for Perinatal and Pediatric Thrombosis of the Scientific and Standardization Committee of the International Society of Thrombosis and Haemostasis (ISTH). Thromb Haemost 2002;88(1):155–6.

The most frequently involved sites are the superior sagittal sinus and transverse (lateral) sinuses of the superficial venous system and the straight sinus of the deep system.[57] After CSVT, venous pressure escalates and hemorrhagic infarction develops and can be present in up to 50% to 60% of newborns on first imaging.[57] Spontaneous intraventricular or thalamic hemorrhages in full-term infants warrant evaluation for CSVT.

The primary goal in the management of CSVT is to treat the underlying cause that may have predisposed the infant to develop CSVT.[57] Current recommendations for antithrombotic therapy for neonatal CSVT are listed in **Fig. 1**. Mortality from CSVT ranges from 2% to 24%.[57] Rate of disabilities, such as epilepsy, cerebral palsy, and cognitive impairments, range from 10% to 80% of patients.[57]

RISK FACTORS FOR NEONATAL TE, INCLUDING APPROPRIATE LABORATORY EVALUATION
Acquired Risk Factors

Central venous and arterial catheters constitute the greatest acquired risks for the development of TE in neonates.[1–3,58,59] In a retrospective review of 32 neonates

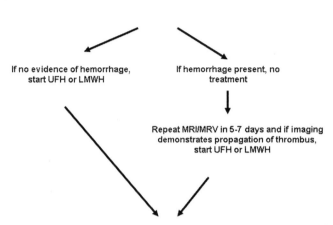

Confirmed diagnosis of CSVT by MRI/MRV

If no evidence of hemorrhage, start UFH or LMWH

If hemorrhage present, no treatment

Repeat MRI/MRV in 5-7 days and if imaging demonstrates propagation of thrombus, start UFH or LMWH

Repeat MRI/MRV in 6-weeks for vessel recanalization. If complete, stop therapy. If not, consider additional 6-weeks of treatment

Fig. 1. Management of neonatal CSVT.[57] The figure displayed represents the current recommendations for appropriate evaluation, management, and follow-up of neonates diagnosed with CSVT. If either UFH or LMWH is provided, dosing guidelines are provided in **Tables 7** and **8**, respectively. MRI, magnetic resonance imaging; MRV, magnetic resonance venography.

diagnosed with thrombosis, 97% had either an umbilical catheter or peripherally inserted central venous catheter line before or at the detection of the thrombotic event.[3] Other risk factors implicated in the pathogenesis of neonatal thromboses are listed in **Tables 4** and **6**.

Genetic Risk Factors

A deficiency/dysfunction of an inhibitor of hemostasis, an overproduction of a procoagulant protein (see **Table 1**), a deficiency/dysfunction of fibrinolysis, and/or endothelial damage (eg, hyperhomocysteinemia or antiphospholipid antibodies) may lead to a prothrombotic phenotype in neonates. The prevalence rates of some of the more common genetic prothrombotic risk factors are presented in **Table 7**.

Homozygous or compound heterozygous disorders, such as severe protein C deficiency, protein S deficiency, or antithrombin III deficiency, usually present in newborns with severe clinical manifestations (purpura fulminans).[16] Although the exact role of thrombophilia in the pathogenesis of neonatal TE events remains uncertain, registry data and case series have demonstrated that the majority of symptomatic neonatal TE events are associated with either multiple hemostatic prothrombotic defects or a combination of prothrombotic defects and environmental/clinical risk factors (see **Tables 4** and **6**).[1,2,44–46,51,58,60,62–73] The Subcommittee for Perinatal and Pediatric Thrombosis of the Scientific and Standardization Committee of the International Society on Thrombosis and Hemostasis recommends that pediatric patients with thrombosis (regardless of risk factors) be tested for a full panel of genetic prothrombotic traits.[61]

Table 7	
Prevalence of certain prothrombotic risk factors	
Mutation	Prevalence
Factor V Leiden mutation	4%–6% of whites[60–63]
Prothrombin 20210G>A mutation	1%–2% of whites (heterozygous)[51,64–66]
MTHFR667	African Americans[63,67,68] 1%–2% (homozygous) 18%–21.6% (heterozygous) Whites[63,67,68] 9.6%–11% (homozygous) 41%–43.5% (heterozygous)
MTHFR1298	African Americans[63,67,68] 2%–4% (homozygous) 27%–30% (heterozygous) Whites[63,67,68] 9%–12.6% (homozygous) 43.6%–47% (heterozygous)
Increased plasma factor VIII activity	10% of whites[36]

From Saxonhouse MA, Burchfield DJ. The evaluation and management of postnatal thromboses. J Perinatol 2009;33:52–65; with permission.

Laboratory Evaluation

Proposed laboratory evaluations, based on the presence of other risk factors, are presented in **Table 6**.

MANAGEMENT OF THROMBOSIS

Management options in neonatal TE events include expectant management (observation only), nitroglycerin ointment (vasospasm), thrombolytic and/or anticoagulant therapy, and surgery. In a recent review of 32 neonates with thromboses, 7 were managed expectantly with 6 neonates experiencing complete clot resolution.[3] Expectant management is a reasonable alternative considering that recommendations and dosing regimens for anticoagulant/thrombolytic therapy in neonates are based on uncontrolled studies, extrapolation from adult and pediatric data, small case series, cohort studies, and/or expert opinion.[16] There are severe cases, however, where limb, organ, and/or a neonate's life is at risk and antithrombotic treatment is warranted. Although no randomized clinical trials exist demonstrating the effectiveness of rTPA in a limb/life-threatening neonatal TE event, it is reasonable to assume that one may never be performed due to the effectiveness of rTPA in neonates that has already been demonstrated in case series. The risk of withholding such treatment may far outweigh the benefit of a controlled trial. The potential for serious complications (intracranial hemorrhage) must be considered in any neonate before initiating antithrombotic therapy.

Antithrombotic treatment must occur in a tertiary care center that has adequate laboratory, neonatal, hematology, transfusion medicine, and pediatric surgical support and should use consultation from pediatric coagulation.[5] Clinicians may also use the service 1-800-NO CLOTS (1-800-662-5687) to receive up-to-date management guidance from expert consultants over the phone. Absolute and relative contraindications for thrombolytic and anticoagulant therapy in neonates are listed in **Table 8**.

Table 8
Absolute and relative contraindications for initiating thrombolytic/anticoagulant therapy in neonates

Absolute	Relative
1. CNS surgery or ischemia (including birth asphyxia) within 10 d	1. Platelet count <50 × 10⁴/μL (100 × 10⁴/μL for ill neonates)
2. Active bleeding	2. Fibrinogen concentration <100 mg/dL
3. Invasive procedures within 3 d	3. International normalized ratio >2
4. Seizures within 48 h	4. Severe coagulation deficiency
	5. Hypertension

Data from Manco-Johnson MJ. Controversies in neonatal thrombotic disorders. In: Ohls R, Yoder MC, editors. Hematology, immunology and infectious disease: neonatology questions and controversies, vol. 1. Philadelphia: Saunders Elsevier; 2008. p. 58–74; and *Data from* Refs.[11,16,17,52,59]

Nitroglycerin

Peripheral vasospasm observed during UAC and/or PAL use may be managed with just reflex vasodilatation of the contralateral hand or leg.[74] If symptoms do not improve or get worse after 15 minutes, however, the catheter should be removed. In rare cases, perfusion of the extremity may remain poor even after catheter removal and may be attributed to persistent vasospasm or small emboli in distal end arteries. Case reports (total of 6 cases) in which local application of 2% nitroglycerin ointment at a dose of 4 mm/kg exist, with all demonstrating improvement of perfusion with few (short-lived systemic hypotension) or no side effects.[74–77]

Nitroglycerin is a nitric oxide donor that may have a direct effect on vascular smooth muscle producing vasodilatation of veins and arteries.[78–80] Resultant increased blood flow, due to this acute dilatation, may overcome the vasospasm allowing flow around microthrombi and/or improve collateral circulation to the affected areas.[78–80]

Unfractionated Heparin

UFH should be limited to clinically significant thromboses with the goal of preventing clot expansion or embolism. Traditional and current dosing guidelines for UFH therapy in neonates as well as proper monitoring guidelines are listed in **Table 9**. Therapy is usually continued for 5 to 30 days,[16] but data to support this recommendation are lacking. Due to low levels of antithrombin and an increased rate of heparin clearance, neonates tend to require higher doses to achieve therapeutic levels.[80]

Bleeding is the major complication of UFH therapy in neonates, with one registry reporting a 2% major hemorrhage rate.[2] Due to UFH's short half-life, cessation of the infusion usually resolves any experienced bleeding. If this maneuver does not control hemorrhage, however, a full coagulation assessment should be performed and hemostatic deficiencies replaced as indicated. If the anti-factor Xa activity is greater than 0.8 U/mL in the face of active bleeding, then protamine may be considered. One unit of protamine neutralizes 100 units of UFH. The plasma heparin burden can be estimated by multiplying estimated plasma volume by anti-Xa concentration.[5] Protamine dosing should be conservative and one-half the calculated dose is

Table 9
Clinical indications and recommended dosing guidelines for UFH therapy in neonates

Clinical Indication	Traditional Dosing	Current Recommended Dosing	Appropriate Monitoring (Applied to All Dosing Regimens)
Asymptomatic or symptomatic thrombus but non–limb threatening	Bolus dose: 75 U/kg IV over 10 min Maintenance dose: 28 U/kg/h	**<28 wk GA** Bolus dose: 25 U/kg IV over 10 min Maintenance dose: 15 U/kg/h **28–37 wk GA** Bolus dose: 50 U/kg over 10 min Maintenance dose: 15 U/kg/h **>37 wk GA** Bolus dose: 100 U/kg over 10 min Maintenance dose: 28 U/kg/h	Maintain anti–factor Xa level of 0.03–0.7 U/mL (PTT 60–85 s) Check anti–factor Xa level 4 h after loading dose and 4 h after each change in infusion rate Complete blood count, platelet count, and coagulation screening (including APTT, PT and fibrinogen) should be performed before starting UFH therapy Platelet count and fibrinogen levels should be repeated daily for 2–3 d once therapeutic levels are achieved and at least twice weekly thereafter

Abbreviations: APTT, activated partial thromboplastin time; GA, gestational age; IV, intravenous; PT, prothrombin time.

Data from Manco-Johnson MJ. Controversies in neonatal thrombotic disorders. In: Ohls R, Yoder MC, editors. Hematology, immunology and infectious disease: neonatology questions and controversies, vol. 1. Philadelphia: Saunders Elsevier; 2008. p. 58–74; and *Data from* Refs.[16,52,83]

generally given initially because excess protamine is also an anticoagulant. Heparin-induced thrombocytopenia rarely occurs in neonates[81,82]; a drop in the platelet count by 50% or persistent platelet counts less than 70/mm^3 to 100,000/mm^3 occurring 5 to 10 days after the first exposure to heparin should alert the clinician to the possibility of heparin-induced thrombocytopenia.

Low-Molecular-Weight Heparin

Since the 1990s, despite limited evidence on the safety and efficacy of anticoagulant treatment in preterm neonates, LMWH (specifically enoxaparin) has become the neonatal anticoagulant of choice.[3,83–88] Reasons for its appeal include its more predictable dose response, lack of requirement for venous access, and reduced monitoring requirements.[17] LMWH has predominant anti–factor Xa activity with less anti–factor IIa (thrombin) activity. Current dosing recommendations for LMWH use in neonates are listed in **Table 10**. LMWH may be administered either by subcutaneous injection or through an indwelling subcutaneous catheter (Insuflon [Unomedical, Birkerod, Denmark]).[52,83–88]

Table 10
Clinical indications and recommended dosing guidelines for LMWH therapy in neonates

Clinical Situation	Traditional Dosing	Current Dosing	Appropriate Monitoring
Asymptomatic or symptomatic thrombus but non–limb threatening	1.5 mg/kg SQ[a] q 12 h	Term neonates: 1.7 mg/kg SQ q 12 h Preterm neonates: 2.0 mg/kg SQ q 12 h	Goal of anti–factor Xa levels of 0.5–1.0 U/mL Check level 4 hours after second dose and then q wk If infants with high hemorrhagic profile, use dosing regimen of 1 mg/kg SQ q 12 h Guidelines for adjusting LMWH therapy are published in other sources.

Abbreviation: SQ, subcutaneous.
[a] Same dose applies if Insuflon catheter is used.
Data from Manco-Johnson MJ. Controversies in neonatal thrombotic disorders. In: Ohls R, Yoder MC, editors. Hematology, immunology and infectious disease: neonatology questions and controversies, vol. 1. Philadelphia: Saunders Elsevier; 2008. p. 58–74; and *Data from* Refs.[16,83,86]

Although adverse effects from LMWH are considered rare, several major complications have been described.[84,88–90] Neonatal experiences with LMWH have varied and the most recent reports are displayed in **Table 11**. Overall, LMWH therapy has been effective in the NICU setting, and centers have reported partial or complete resolution of TEs in 59% to 100% of cases.[84–86,88]

Table 11
Adverse effects of low-molecular-weight heparin therapy in neonates

Study	No. of Infants Treated	Minor Events	Major Events/Description
Van Elteren et al,[3] 2011	25	Not reported	3 (12%) Severe hematoma at site of Insuflon catheter Large abscess at site of Insuflon catheter Grade II IVH and thalamic hemorrhage
Malowany et al,[88] 2007	16	9 (56%)	5 (31%) Scleral hemorrhage Gastrointestinal bleeding Infected hematoma
Streif et al,[84] 2003	62	4 (6%)	4 (6%) 2 Major hematomas at site of injection 1 Intracerebral hemorrhage
Michaels et al,[85] 2004	10	3 (30%)	None

Data from Manco-Johnson MJ. Controversies in neonatal thrombotic disorders. In: Ohls R, Yoder MC, editors. Hematology, immunology and infectious disease: neonatology questions and controversies, vol. 1. Philadelphia: Saunders Elsevier; 2008. p. 58–74.

Table 12
Clinical indications and recommended dosing guidelines for rTPA therapy in neonates

Clinical Situation	Recommended Dosing	Appropriate Monitoring
Limb/life-threatening thrombus	0.06 mg/kg/h UFH at 10 U/kg/h	Dose escalation up to 0.24 mg/kg/h can be considered but has to be done slowly with continuing monitoring of the patient (see **Table 13**). Because rTPA does not inhibit clot propagation or directly affect hypercoagulability, simultaneous infusion of UFH is recommended.[16,40] Supplementation with plasminogen before commencing therapy is recommended to ensure adequate thrombolysis[16]

Data from Manco-Johnson MJ. Controversies in neonatal thrombotic disorders. In: Ohls R, Yoder MC, editors. Hematology, immunology and infectious disease: neonatology questions and controversies, vol. 1. Philadelphia: Saunders Elsevier; 2008. p. 58–74; and *Data from* Refs.[40,52]

Thrombolysis

Thrombolytic therapy, mainly rTPA, for use in neonates, should be reserved for limb, organ, and/or life-threatening thromboses, including right atrial thromboses.[16,17,40,91,92] The safety and efficacy of rTPA treatment in neonates has only been demonstrated in case reports, case series, and cohort studies. The majority of

Table 13
Monitoring recommendations for thrombolytic therapy in neonates

Testing	When Performed	Levels Desired (If Applicable)[a]
Imaging of thrombosis	Before initiation of treatment Every 12–24 h during treatment	
Fibrinogen level	Before initiation of treatment 4–6 h after starting treatment Every 12–24 h	Minimum of 100 mg/dL[10] Supplement with cryoprecipitate
Platelet count	Before initiation of treatment 4–6 h after starting treatment Every 12–24 h	Minimum of $50–100 \times 10^4/\mu L$,[93] dependent on bleeding risk
Cranial imaging	Before initiation of treatment Daily	
Coagulation testing	Before initiation of treatment 4–6 h after starting treatment Every 12–24 h	
Plasminogen	Before initiation of treatment 4–6 h after starting treatment Every 12–24 h	Adequate to achieve thrombolysis Supplementation with plasminogen before commencing therapy is recommended to ensure adequate thrombolysis[16,40]

[a] Levels should be obtained before the initiation of treatment, 4–6 hours after starting treatment, and every 12–24 hours during treatment.
   Data from Saxonhouse MA, Manco-Johnson MJ. The evaluation and management of neonatal coagulation disorders. Semin Perinatol 2008;33:52–65; and *Data from* Refs.[17,40,91]

these reports have shown either complete or partial clot lysis.[40,52,91,92] Dosing recommendations (although based on a few studies) are listed in **Table 12**, and appropriate monitoring for thrombolytic therapy is presented in **Table 13**.

Surgery

The use of microsurgical techniques combined with thrombolytic regimens has the potential to rapidly restore blood flow and avoid tissue loss without major bleeding complications, especially in patients with peripheral arterial occlusion.[94] One center's experience of 11 patients with arterial vascular access-associated thrombosis secondary to peripheral arterial line complications described 5 patients who required arteriotomy, embolectomy, and subsequent microvascular reconstruction.[94] When faced with a significant thrombosis from a peripheral arterial line or if a life/limb-threatening arterial or venous thrombosis and antithrombotic therapy is contraindicated, surgery should be considered as a viable option.

SUMMARY

The lack of randomized clinical trials addressing the management of neonatal TE emergencies forces neonatologists to base their medical decisions on limited evidence. The ultimate goal is to treat effectively without causing additional harm. This can be difficult when treatment of thromboses has significant risks. Although randomized clinical trials investigating treatment options for neonatal thromboses are critically needed, current guidelines have been presented in order for those caring for neonates to make the best-educated medical decisions. It is likely that these guidelines will be continuously updated as new therapies that are approved for use in neonates emerge or more evidence is collected on appropriate management of neonatal TE emergencies. Therefore, neonatologists and others caring for high-risk infants should continuously refer to the literature as new guidelines are recommended.

REFERENCES

1. Schmidt B, Andrew M. Neonatal thrombosis: report of a prospective Canadian and international registry. Pediatrics 1995;96:939–43.
2. Nowak-Gottl U, von Kries R, Gobel U. Neonatal symptomatic thromboembolism in Germany: two year survey. Arch Dis Child Fetal Neonatal Ed 1997;76:F163–7.
3. van Elteren HA, Veldt HS, te Pas AB, et al. Management and outcome in 32 neonates with thrombotic events. Int J Pediatr 2011;1–5.
4. Ries M. Molecular and functional properties of fetal plasminogen and its possible influence on clot lysis in the neonatal period. Semin Thromb Hemost 1997;23: 247–52.
5. Saxonhouse MA, Manco-Johnson MJ. The evaluation and management of neonatal coagulation disorders. Semin Perinatol 2008;33:52–65.
6. Andrew M, Paes B, Milner R, et al. Development of the human coagulation system in the full-term infant. Blood 1987;70:165–72.
7. Andrew M, Paes B, Milner R, et al. Development of the human coagulation system in the healthy premature infant. Blood 1988;72:1651–7.
8. Andrew M, Paes B, Johnston M. Development of the hemostatic system in the neonate and young infant. Am J Pediatr Hematol Oncol 1990;12:95–104.
9. Manco-Johnson MJ. Development of hemostasis in the fetus. Thromb Res 2005; 115:55–63.

10. Elber J, Viero S, MacGregor D, et al. Placental pathology in neonatal stroke. Pediatrics 2011;127:e722–9.
11. Greenway A, Massicotte MP, Monagle P. Neonatal thrombosis and its treatment. Blood Rev 2004;18:75–84.
12. Raju TN, Nelson KB, Ferriero D, et al. Ischemic perinatal stroke: summary of a workshop sponsored by the National Institute of Child Health and Human Development and the National Institute of Neurological Disorders and Stroke. Pediatrics 2007;120:609–16.
13. Chalmers EA. Perinatal stroke—risk factors and management. Br J Haematol 2005;130:333–43.
14. Hunt RW, Inder TE. Perinatal and neonatal ischaemic stroke: a review. Thromb Res 2006;118:39–48.
15. Lee J, Croen LA, Backstrand KH, et al. Maternal and infant characteristics associated with perinatal arterial stroke in the infant. JAMA 2005;293:723–9.
16. Monagle P, Chalmers E, Chan A, et al. Antithrombotic therapy in neonates and children: American College of Chest Physicians Evidence-Based Clinical Practice Guidelines (8th Edition). Chest 2008;133(Suppl 6):887S–968S.
17. Thornburg C, Pipe S. Neonatal thromboembolic emergencies. Semin Fetal Neonatal Med 2006;11:198–206.
18. Mokrohisky ST, Levine RL, Blumhagen JD, et al. Low positioning of umbilical-artery catheters increases associated complications in newborn infants. N Engl J Med 1978;299:561–4.
19. Bryant BG. Drug, fluid, and blood products administered through the umbilical artery catheter:complication experiences from one NICU. Neonatal Netw 1990; 9:27–32, 43–6.
20. McAdams RM, Winter VT, McCurnin DC, et al. Complications of umbilical artery catherization a model of extreme prematurity. J Perinatol 2009;29:685–92.
21. Barrington K. Umbilical artery catheters in the newborn: effects of position of the catheter tip. Cochrane Database Syst Rev 1999;1:CD000505.
22. Barrington KJ. Umbilical artery catheters in the newborn: effects of heparin. Cochrane Database Syst Rev 2000;2:CD000507.
23. Sharathkumar AA, Lamear N, Pipe S, et al. Management of neonatal aortic arch thrombosis with low-molecular weight heparin: a case series. J Pediatr Hematol Oncol 2009;31:516–21.
24. Nagel K, Tuckuviene R, Paes B, et al. Neonatal aortic thrombosis: a comprehensive review. Klin Padiatr 2010;222:134–9.
25. Tridapalli E, Stella M, Capretti M, et al. Neonatal arterial iliac thrombosis in type-I protein C deficiency: a case report. Ital J Pediatr 2010;36:23.
26. ElHassan NO, Sproles C, Sachdeva R, et al. A neonate with left pulmonary artery thrombosis and left lung hypoplasia: a case report. J Med Case Reports 2010;4: 1–5.
27. Turebylu R, Salis R, Erbe R, et al. Genetic prothrombotic mutations are common in neonates but are not associated with umbilical catheter-associated thrombosis. J Perinatol 2007;27(8):490–5.
28. Tanke RB, van Megen R, Daniels O. Thrombus detection on central venous catheters in the neonatal intensive care unit. Angiology 1994;45(6):477–80.
29. Schmidt B, Zipursky A. Thrombotic disease in newborn infants. Clin Perinatol 1984;11(2):461–88.
30. Khilnani P, Goldstein B, Todres ID. Double lumen umbilical venous catheters in critically ill neonates: a randomized prospective study. Crit Care Med 1991; 19(11):1348–51.

31. O'Grady NP, Alexander M, Dellinger EP, et al. Guidelines for the prevention of intravascular catheter-related infections. The Hospital Infection Control Practices Advisory Committee, Center for Disese Control and Prevention, U.S. Pediatrics 2002;110(5):e51.
32. Le Coultre C, Oberhansli I, Mossaz A, et al. Postoperative chylothorax in children: differences between vascular and traumatic origin. J Pediatr Surg 1991;26(5): 519–23.
33. Barnes C, Newall F, Monagle P. Post-thrombotic syndrome. Arch Dis Child 2002; 86(3):212–4.
34. Siu SL, Yang JY, Hui JP, et al. Chylothorax secondary to catheter related thrombosis successfully treated with heparin. J Paediatr Child Health 2011.
35. Cartwright DW. Central venous lines in neonates: a study of 2186 catheters. Arch Dis Child Fetal Neonatal Ed 2004;89(6):F504–8.
36. Cartwright DW. Placement of neonatal central venous catheter tips: is the right atrium so dangerous? Arch Dis Child Fetal Neonatal Ed 2002;87(2):F155 [discussion: F155–6].
37. Torres-Valdivieso MJ, Cobas J, Barrio C, et al. Successful use of tissue plasminogen activator in catheter-related intracardiac thrombus of a premature infant. Am J Perinatol 2003;20(2):91–6.
38. Bose J, Clarke P. Use of tissue plasminogen activator to treat intracardiac thrombosis in extremely low-birth-weight infants. Pediatr Crit Care Med 2011;12(6): e407–9.
39. Mondi V, Di Paolo A, Fabiano A, et al. Combined thrombolytic therapy for atrial thrombus in a preterm infant. Minerva Pediatr 2011;63:115–8.
40. Wang M, Hays T, Balasa V, et al. Low-dose tissue plasminogen activator thrombolysis in children. J Pediatr Hematol Oncol 2003;25(5):379–86.
41. Tardin FA, Avanza AC Jr, Andiao MR, et al. Combined rTPA and aspirin therapy for intracardiac thrombosis in neonates. Arq Bras Cardiol 2007; 88(5):e121–3.
42. Marks KA, Zucker N, Kapelushnik J, et al. Infective endocarditis successfully treated in extremely low birth weight infants with recombinant tissue plasminogen activator. Pediatrics 2002;109(1):153–8.
43. Cholette JM, Rubenstein JS, Alfieris GM, et al. Elevated risk of thrombosis in neonates undergoing initial palliative cardiac surgery. Ann Thorac Surg 2007; 84(4):1320–5.
44. Lau KK, Stoffman JM, Williams S, et al. Neonatal renal vein thrombosis: review of the English-language literature between 1992 and 2006. Pediatrics 2007;120(5): e1278–84.
45. Kosch A, Kuwertz-Broking E, Heller C, et al. Renal venous thrombosis in neonates: prothrombotic risk factors and long-term follow-up. Blood 2004; 104(5):1356–60.
46. Marks SD, Massicotte MP, Steele BT, et al. Neonatal renal venous thrombosis: clinical outcomes and prevalence of prothrombotic disorders. J Pediatr 2005; 146(6):811–6.
47. Messinger Y, Sheaffer JW, Mrozek J, et al. Renal outcome of neonatal renal venous thrombosis: review of 28 patients and effectiveness of fibrinolytics and heparin in 10 patients. Pediatrics 2006;118(5):e1478–84.
48. Williams S, Chan AK. Neonatal portal vein thrombosis: diagnosis and management. Semin Fetal Neonatal Med 2011;16:329–39.
49. Moraq L, Shah PS, Epelman M, et al. Childhood outcomes of neonates diagnosed with portal vein thrombosis. J Paediatr Child Health 2011;47:356–60.

50. Fitzgerald KC, Williams LS, Garg BP, et al. Cerebral sinovenous thrombosis in the neonate. Arch Neurol 2006;63:405–9.
51. Nowak-Gottl U, Duering C, Kempf-Bielack B, et al. Thromboembolic diseases in neonates and children. Pathophysiol Haemost Thromb 2004;33(5-6):269–74.
52. Manco-Johnson MJ. How I treat venous thrombosis in children. Blood 2006; 107(1):21–9.
53. Wasay M, Dai AI, Ansari M, et al. Cerebral venous sinus thrombosis in children: a multicenter cohort from the United States. J Child Neurol 2008;23(1):26–31.
54. Heller C, Heinecke A, Junker R, et al. Childhood stroke study group. Cerebral venous thrombosis in children: a multifactorial origin. Circulation 2003;108:1362–7.
55. Sebire G, Tabarki B, Saunders DE, et al. Cerebral venous sinus thrombossi in children:risk factors, presentation, diagnosis, and outcome. Brain 2005;128:477–89.
56. deVeber G, Andrew M, Adams C, et al. Cerebral sinovenous thrombosis in children. N Engl J Med 2001;345(6):417–23.
57. Yang JY, Chan AK, Callen DJ, et al. Neonatal cerebral sinovenous thrombosis: sifting the evidence for a diagnostic plan and treatment strategy. Pediatrics 2010;126:e693–700.
58. van Ommen CH, Heijboer H, Buller HR, et al. Venous thromboembolism in childhood: a prospective two-year registry in The Netherlands. J Pediatr 2001;139:676–81.
59. Beardsley DS. Venous thromboembolism in the neonatal period. Semin Perinatol 2007;31(4):250–3.
60. Boffa MC, Lachassinne E. Infant perinatal thrombosis and antiphospholipid antibodies: a review. Lupus 2007;16(8):634–41.
61. Manco-Johnson MJ, Grabowski EF, Hellgreen M, et al. Laboratory testing for thrombophilia in pediatric patients. On behalf of the Subcommittee for Perinatal and Pediatric Thrombosis of the Scientific and Standardization Committee of the International Society of Thrombosis and Haemostasis (ISTH). Thromb Haemost 2002;88(1):155–6.
62. Ridker PM, Miletich JP, Hennekens CH, et al. Ethnic distribution of factor V Leiden in 4047 men and women. Implications for venous thromboembolism screening. JAMA 1997;16:1305–7.
63. Nowak-Gottl U, Strater R, Heinecke A, et al. Lipoprotein (a) and genetic polymorphisms of clotting factor V, prothrombin, and methylenetetrahydrofolate reductase are risk factors of spontaneous ischemic stroke in childhood. Blood 1999; 94(11):3678–82.
64. Kenet G, Nowak-Gottl U. Fetal and neonatal thrombophilia. Obstet Gynecol Clin North Am 2006;33(3):457–66.
65. Nowak-Gottl U, Dubbers A, Kececioglu D, et al. Factor V Leiden, protein C, and lipoprotein (a) in catheter-related thrombosis in childhood: a prospective study. J Pediatr 1997;131(4):608–12.
66. Bucciarelli P, Rosendaal FR, Tripodi A, et al. Risk of venous thromboembolism and clinical manifestations in carriers of antithrombin, protein C, protein S deficiency, or activated protein C resistance: a multicenter collaborative family study. Arterioscler Thromb Vasc Biol 1999;19(4):1026–33.
67. Alioglu B, Ozyurek E, Tarcan A, et al. Heterozygous methylenetetrahydrofolate reductase 677C-T gene mutation with mild hyperhomocysteinemia associated with intrauterine iliofemoral artery thrombosis. Blood Coagul Fibrinolysis 2006;17(6):495–8.
68. Rosendaal FR. Venous thrombosis: the role of genes, environment, and behavior. Hematology Am Soc Hematol Educ Program 2005;1–12.
69. Dahlback B, Hillarp A, Rosen S, et al. Resistance to activated protein C, the FV: Q506 allele, and venous thrombosis. Ann Hematol 1996;72(4):166–76.

. Saxonhouse MA, Burchfield DJ. The evaluation and management of postnatal thromboses. J Perinatol 2009;33:52–65.

. Nowak-Gottl U, Junker R, Kreuz W, et al. Risk of recurrent venous thrombosis in children with combined prothrombotic risk factors. Blood 2001;97(4):858–62.

. Nowak-Gottl U, Junker R, Hartmeier M, et al. Increased lipoprotein(a) is an important risk factor for venous thromboembolism in childhood. Circulation 1999; 100(7):743–8.

. Brenner B. Thrombophilia and adverse pregnancy outcome. Obstet Gynecol Clin North Am 2006;33(3):443–56, ix.

. Denker KA, Cohen BE. Reversal of dopamine extravasation injury with topical nitroglycerin ointiment. Plast Reconstr Surg 1989;84:811–3.

. Baserga MC, Puri A, Sola A. The use of topical nitroglycerin ointment to treat peripheral tissue ischemia secondary to arterial line complications in neonates. J Perinatol 2002;22(5):416–9.

. Wong AF, McCulloch LM, Sola A. Treatment of peripheral tissue ischemia with topical nitroglycerin ointment in neonates. J Pediatr 1992;121:980–3.

. Varughese M, Koh TH. Successful use of topical nitroglycerin in ischaemia associated with umbilical arterial line in a neonate. J Perinatol 2001;21:556–8.

. Abrams J. Glyceryl trinitrate (nitroglycerine) and the organic nitrates. Choosing the method of administration. Drugs 1987;34:391–403.

. Bogaert MG. Clinical pharmacokinetics of glyceryl trinitrate following the use of systemic and topical preparations. Clin Pharmacokinet 1987;12:1–11.

. Male C, Johnston M, Sparling C, et al. The influence of developmental haemostasis on the laboratory diagnosis and management of haemostatic disorders during infancy and childhood. Clin Lab Med 1999;19(1):39–69.

. Spadone D. Heparin induced thrombocytopenia in the newborn. J Vasc Surg 1996;15:306–12.

. Martchenke J, Boshkov L. Heparin-induced thrombocytopenia in neonates. Neonatal Netw 2005;24(5):33–7.

. NEOFAX. Thomson Reuters; 2011. p. 172–4, 184–6.

. Streif W, Goebel G, Chan AK, et al. Use of low molecular mass heparin (enoxaparin) in newborn infants: a prospective cohort study of 62 patients. Arch Dis Child Fetal Neonatal Ed 2003;88(5):F365–70.

. Michaels LA, Gurian M, Hegyi T, et al. Low molecular weight heparin in the treatment of venous and arterial thromboses in the premature infant. Pediatrics 2004; 114(3):703–7.

. Malowany JI, Monagle P, Knoppert DC, et al. Enoxaparin for neonatal thrombosis: a call for a higher dose for neonates. Thromb Res 2008;122(6):826–30.

. Ramasethu J. Management of vascular thrombosis and spasm in the Newborn. Neoreviews 2005;6(6):e298–311.

. Malowany JI, Knoppert DC, Chan AK, et al. Enoxaparin use in the neonatal intensive care unit: experience over 8 years. Pharmacotherapy 2007;27(9):1263–71.

. Obaid L, Byrne PJ, Cheung PY. Compartment syndrome in an ELBW infant receiving low-molecular weight heparins. J Pediatr 2004;144:549.

. van Elteren HA, Te Pas AB, Kollen WJ, et al. Severe hemorrhage after low-molecular-weight heparin treatment in a preterm neonate. Neonatology 2010;99:247–9.

. Nowak-Gottl U, Auberger K, Halimeh S, et al. Thrombolysis in newborns and infants. Thromb Haemost 1999;82(Suppl 1):112–6.

. Caner I, Olgun H, Buyukavci M, et al. A giant thrombus in the right ventricle of a newborn with Down syndrome: successful treatment with rt-PA. J Pediatr Hematol Oncol 2006;28(3):120–2.

93. Manco-Johnson MJ. Controversies in neonatal thrombotic disorders. In: Ohls R, Yoder MC, editors. Hematology, immunology and infectious disease: neonatology questions and controversies, vol. 1. Philadelphia: Saunders Elsevier; 2008. p. 58–74.

94. Coombs CJ, Richardson PW, Dowling GJ, et al. Brachial artery thrombosis in infants: an algorithm for limb salvage. Plast Reconstr Surg 2006;117(5):1481–8.

95. Nelson KB. Perinatal ischemic stroke. Stroke 2007;38:742–5.

96. Kenny D, Tsai-Goodman B. Neonatal arterial thrombus mimicking congenital heart disease. Arch Dis Child Fetal Neonatal Ed 2007;92(1):F59–61.

97. Golomb MR, Dick PT, MacGregor DL, et al. Neonatal arterial ischemic stroke and cerebral sinovenous thrombosis are more commonly diagnosed in boys. J Child Neurol 2004;19:493–7.

98. de Veber G. Canadian paediatric ischaemic stroke registry: analysis of children with arterial ischaemic stroke. The Canadian Pediatric Stroke Study Group. Ann Neurol 2000;526a.

99. Wu YW, Lynch JK, Nelson KB. Perinatal arterial stroke: understanding mechanisms and outcomes. Semin Neurol 2005;25(4):424–34.

Neonatal Diuretic Therapy: Furosemide, Thiazides, and Spironolactone

Jeffrey L. Segar, MD

KEYWORDS

- Bronchopulmonary dysplasia • Diuretic • Neonate
- Prematurity • Sodium

Diuretics are one of the most frequently prescribed medications in the neonatal intensive care unit (NICU). In a study using the Pediatrix Medical Group data warehouse, Clark and colleagues[1] reported that furosemide was the seventh most commonly reported medication in the NICU, with more than 8% of all NICU patients being exposed to the agent. This high usage rate exists despite a relative paucity of studies supporting routine use in this population. Because of this lack of data, furosemide, metolazone, a thiazidelike diuretic, hydrochlorothiazide, and spironolactone have at various times, in response to the Best Pharmaceuticals for Children Act, been placed on US Food and Drug Administration and National Institutes of Health lists of drugs for which pediatric studies are needed.

Rational use of diuretics requires an understanding of developmental renal physiology and function in the neonate, knowledge of the mechanisms of action of various diuretic agents as well as the limitations and potential adverse effects. Randomized trials of diuretics for the prevention and treatment of lung disease, including respiratory distress syndrome (RDS) and bronchopulmonary dysplasia (BPD), have been performed, providing the practitioner with some guidance regarding the use of these drugs. However, these trials primarily took place before routine use of antenatal steroids and surfactant replacement therapy. Extrapolation of these data to infants with the new BPD may not be logical or justified.[2]

FUNCTIONAL DEVELOPMENT OF THE KIDNEY

The human renal excretory system passes through 3 stages of morphogenic development. The first stage is characterized by the emergence of paired tubules to form the nonfunctional pronephros. The second stage is the development of the mesanephros,

Division of Neonatology, Department of Pediatrics, University of Iowa Children's Hospital, 200 Hawkins Drive, Iowa City, IA 52242, USA
E-mail address: jeffrey-segar@uiowa.edu

Clin Perinatol 39 (2012) 209–220
doi:10.1016/j.clp.2011.12.007   perinatology.theclinics.com

consisting of approximately 20 pairs of glomeruli and tubules, which are able to form urine. The mesanephros degenerates by the 12th week of gestation and is followed by the appearance of the metanephros, the development of which is dependent on interaction between the ureteric bud and the undifferentiated mesenchyme containing the nephrogenic blastema. After the formation of the metanephric nephron, the first evidence of renal tubular function appears between 9 and 12 weeks of gestation. New nephrons continue to form up to the 36th week of gestation in the human fetus. Nephrogenesis is complete at birth in full-term infants, but continues after birth in preterm infants.[3,4]

During the last trimester of gestation, the fetal kidneys receive only 2% to 4% of the combined ventricular blood output. After birth, there is a decrease in renal vascular resistance associated with an increase in arterial pressure, both contributing to the increase in renal blood flow during the weeks after birth such that the newborn kidney receives 8% to 10% of cardiac output at the end of the first week of life and 15% to 18% by a few months of age. In comparison, 25% of cardiac output is distributed to the kidneys in the normal adult. In addition to an increase in renal blood blow, there is a redistribution of blood flow to the superficial cortex, a process that continues with maturation. The mechanisms regulating these developmental changes in renal blood flow include anatomic, hemodynamic, and neurohumoral factors. Studies performed in animals, primarily the sheep fetus and newborn rabbits and piglets, provide evidence for important roles of the renin-angiotensin system, prostaglandins, nitric oxide and renal sympathetic nerves, and adrenergic function.[5]

Accompanying postnatal changes in blood flow are marked increases in glomerular filtration rate (GFR) and renal sodium reabsorption. It is estimated that GFR increases at least 50% during the first day of life in the term infant and doubles by 2 weeks of age. In premature infants, GFR, measured as clearance of inulin or creatinine correlates closely with gestational age, increasing from ~ 5 mL/min/m^2 at 28 weeks' gestation to ~ 12 mL/min/m^2 at term.[6] Developmental changes in renal sodium excretion also occur during the perinatal period. Fractional excretion of sodium (FENa), or urinary sodium excretion as a percentage of the amount of sodium filtered at the glomerulus, is widely used to estimate the excretory capacity of sodium by the kidney. In utero, urinary sodium excretion is high, averaging 10% to 15%. In the full-term infant, FENa decreases to 2% to 4% in the first few hours of life and to even lower values in the subsequent 48 hours. In the first few days of life, urine sodium excretion typically exceeds dietary sodium intake, resulting in a state of negative sodium balance coincident with loss of body weight. As urinary sodium losses decrease further (FENa ~ 0.2–0.3%) and sodium intake increases, a state of positive weight and water gain occurs. In premature infants, FENa during the first few days of life is proportionate to gestational age and decreases with maturation. By 36 weeks' postconceptional age, FENa is typically less than 1%.

SODIUM AND CHLORIDE REABSORPTION IN THE KIDNEY

Sodium and chloride reabsorption normally occur at 4 major sites in the nephron: the proximal tubule (50%–70%), the loop of Henle (25%–30%), the distal tubule (5%), and the collecting duct (3%). The proximal tubule and thick ascending loop of Henle are responsible for the reabsorption of a large amount of filtered sodium to maintain constancy of total body sodium, whereas the distal tubule and collecting duct are responsible for fine regulation of sodium balance. Within the proximal tubule, active transport of sodium by the sodium-potassium-adenosine triphosphatase (Na$^+$K$^+$-ATPase) system drives passive transport of chloride and water. Because the process is highly interdependent, inhibition of sodium and chloride reabsorption also affects water reabsorption. In the thick ascending loop of Henle, sodium and chloride are actively transported via the $Na^+K^+\text{-}2Cl^-$ membrane carrier from the tubular lumen into the tubular cell. The electrochemical gradient required for the carrier to function is maintained by the transport of Na^+ out of the tubular cell into the peritubular capillary by the Na^+K^+-ATPase pump. In the distal convoluted tubule, sodium is actively transported against an electrochemical gradient by the $Na^+\text{-}Cl^-$ cotransporter. Some sodium is reabsorbed from the lumen of the collecting duct by the epithelial sodium channel on principal cells and an Na^+-dependent Cl^-/HCO_3 exchanger on the intercalated cells. Different classes of diuretics, described later, target these different, apically located transporters to block sodium, chloride, and ultimately water reabsorption in the kidney, leading to various degrees of natriuresis, chloruresis, and diuresis.

DIURETICS: CLASSES AND MECHANISMS OF ACTION

Diuretics can be classified by type, mechanisms of action, and chemical structure. Several types of diuretics have limited use in the neonatal population and are not discussed in detail. Mannitol is an osmotic diuretic that mainly acts in the proximal tubule. The agent is filtered by the glomerulus and is not reabsorbed, thus increasing osmolality of tubular fluid, with resultant decrease in water and salt reabsorption. Carbonic anhydrase inhibitors, such as acetazolamide, block bicarbonate absorption by inhibiting the reaction: ($CO_2 + H_2O \leftrightharpoons H_2CO_3 \leftrightharpoons H^+ + HCO_3^-$), leading to decreased sodium reuptake and a mild diuresis. Although previously suggested as a therapy for posthemorrhagic hydrocephalus, randomized trials showed a lack of efficacy in decreasing the rate of shunt placement and an association with increased neurologic morbidity.[7] Use of the agent may also lead to a hyperchloremic metabolic acidosis. Amiloride directly blocks the epithelial sodium channel in collecting ducts of the kidney, promoting sodium and water loss and sparing potassium. Aside from its potential use in patients with Liddle syndrome or pseudohypoaldosteronism, amiloride has no role as a diuretic in the neonatal population.

LOOP DIURETICS

The loop diuretics furosemide and bumetanide have their principal action on the thick ascending loop of Henle and are characterized by a prompt onset of action and short duration of diuresis. Because of the limited clinical use of bumetanide, only furosemide is discussed in this review. Furosemide is highly protein bound and thus not readily filtered at the glomerulus. To be functional, loop diuretics require secretion into the proximal tubular lumen via organic acid transporters (OAT1 and OAT 3). They act in the thick ascending loop of Henle to block the site of chloride in the $Na^+K^+\text{-}2Cl^-$ membrane carrier, thereby inhibiting sodium, chloride, and potassium reabsorption. Furosemide is primarily eliminated in the urine as unchanged drug. Plasma clearance is low, the volume of distribution greater, and the half-life prolonged in preterm and term infants compared with adults, likely related to decreased binding of the drug to plasma proteins and low rate of tubular secretion.[8] Mirochnick and colleagues[9] reported that plasma half-life frequently exceeded 24 hours in infants less than 31 weeks' postconceptional age. As postconceptional age approached term, the half-life declined to approximately 4 hours, similar to that of term newborn infants.

Repeated administration of loop diuretics produces pharmacologic tolerance, resulting in a significant reduction in its diuretic and natriuretic efficacy.[9,10] The mechanisms related to this response likely result from a decrease in extracellular fluid volume, leading to a compensatory increase in water and sodium absorption in the proximal and distal renal tubule. In addition, decreased sodium reabsorption in the thick ascending loop of Henle leads to increased sodium delivery to the distal and collecting tubules, resulting in a compensatory increase is sodium reabsorption in this part of the tubule. In preterm infants with chronic lung disease, coadministration of metolazone, a thiazidelike diuretic, with furosemide enhances diuresis, natriuresis, and chloruresis and overcomes the development of tolerance to furosemide.[11] This effect seems to result from metolazone blocking the renal compensatory mechanisms in the distal tubule, the primary site of action for thiazide diuretics. Similar findings using combined diuretic therapies have been reported in pediatric patients with chronic renal failure and furosemide-resistant edema.[12,13]

Prompt diuresis often results after initial doses of furosemide, potentially resulting in hypotension from decreased plasma volume. This effect may be of particular concern in infants with BPD who may already be significantly fluid restricted. To address this issue, O'Donovan and Bell[14] examined changes in body water compartments in infants with BPD after a single dose of furosemide. Four hours after furosemide dosing, total body water, extracellular water, and interstitial water were significantly decreased compared with predose measurements, without an accompanying change in plasma volume. These investigators postulated that mobilization of water from the interstitial space of the lung may account, in part, for the acute effects of furosemide on lung function (described later). Repetitive dosing of furosemide with or without combined administration of metolazone over 4 days also resulted in a significant decrease in extracellular water without effects of plasma volume.[15] However, not all water mobilized from the interstitial compartment seems to be excreted, and a transfer of water from the extracellular to the intercellular spaces likely results from a diuretic-induced decrease in extracellular sodium concentration and production of a gradient favoring the movement of water into the intracellular space.[14,15]

ADVERSE EFFECTS OF FUROSEMIDE

Careful attention to fluid and electrolyte status is necessary, particularly when first initiating diuretic therapy. Because of the effects on charge across the apical membrane, passive reabsorption of potassium, calcium, and magnesium is inhibited. Therefore, patients receiving furosemide should be monitored for hypochloremic metabolic alkalosis, hyponatremia, hypokalemia, hypomagnesemia, and hypocalcemia.

Because significant amounts of divalent cations such as Ca^{2+} are reabsorbed in the loop of Henle by passive mechanisms that depend on the active transport of sodium chloride, administration of furosemide may result in hypercalciuria, bone demineralization, and renal calcifications.[16-18] Exposure to furosemide more than 10 mg/kg body weight cumulative dose has recently been shown by multivariate analysis to be the strongest independent risk factor for nephrocalcinosis (odds ratio [OR] confidence interval [CI] 4.0–585, $P<.01$).[19]

Although rare, ototoxicity remains a risk, particularly in preterm infants with impaired clearance and with concomitant administration of other ototoxic drugs or agents or conditions that impair furosemide clearance. In a study of survivors of the Canadian arm of the Neonatal Inhaled Nitric Oxide Study, cumulative dosage and duration of loop diuretic use was linked to sensorineural hearing loss.[20]

FUROSEMIDE AND PATENT DUCTUS ARTERIOSUS

The renal side effects of indomethacin therapy are well known, with an increase in renal vascular resistance and decrease in renal blood flow being related to inhibition of the prostaglandin system. Because furosemide stimulates renal prostaglandin E_2 production,[21,22] it has been proposed that administration of furosemide during indomethacin therapy could ameliorate indomethacin-related renal toxicity. No large, randomized trial has been conducted to examine this question, and the results of several smaller studies are contradictory and nonconclusive. A 2001 Cochrane review found insufficient evidence to support the administration of furosemide to premature infants treated with indomethacin for patent ductus arteriosus (PDA).[23] This meta-analysis, involving 70 patients enrolled in 3 trials, failed to show any reduction in toxicity of indomethacin therapy in PDA or increase in treatment failure (relative risk [RR] = 1.25; 95% CI 0.62–2.52). In recent studies conducted after publication of this Cochrane review, the incidence of acute kidney injury (AKI) (serum creatinine >1.6 mg/dL) or changes in serum creatinine concentrations were significantly increased in the furosemide-exposed group.[24,25] Thus, the use of furosemide to decrease the renal side effects of indomethacin cannot be supported.

Concern regarding the use of furosemide in the preterm infant is also raised because of the potential to induce prostaglandin-regulated dilation of the ductus arteriosus. In neonatal rats, postnatal furosemide treatment delays ductal closure and dilates the constricted ductus arteriosus in a dose-dependent manner.[26] In premature infants randomized to receive either furosemide or chlorothiazide for treatment of RDS, Green and colleagues[27] found the incidence of PDA significantly greater in the furosemide group. Several other studies, not specifically designed to address this question, failed to show a relationship between early furosemide use in preterm infants and increased incidence of PDA.[28,29]

FUROSEMIDE AND RESPIRATORY DISEASE
RDS

Several trials have evaluated the use of furosemide in treating RDS and lessening the need for mechanical ventilator support. The rationale for these trials was derived from observations that RDS is associated with fluid in the alveolar and interstitial spaces, thus impairing gas exchange and lowering lung compliance, and tissue water mobilization and spontaneous diuresis often precedes improvement in infants with RDS.[30] In newborn lambs, Bland and colleagues[31] reported that furosemide decreased transvascular filtration of fluid in the lung, whereas in 1-week-old preterm infants with RDS a single dose of furosemide resulted in acute improvement in lung compliance and $Pao_2 - Pao_2$ before any significant diuresis, both findings suggesting a direct effect of furosemide on lung fluid dynamics.[32] Green and colleagues[33] randomized 99 infants with RDS (mean gestational age ~30 weeks) to receive either furosemide or chlorothiazide in an unblinded fashion, beginning the second to fourth day of life if a diuretic was deemed necessary. Infants not deemed to require diuretics were also included in the study. Only a single dose was prescribed by the study; additional dosing was at the discretion of the neonatologist. Furosemide use was positively correlated with increased survival as well as development of PDA. In a later blinded, prospective study, this same group found prophylactic administration of furosemide (1 mg/kg × 4 doses beginning at 24 hours) resulted in adverse cardiovascular effects compared with the as-needed group without any differences in pulmonary severity indices.[34] In a separate randomized trial, Yeh and colleagues[28] found that early furosemide therapy enhanced urine output and sodium excretion in infants with RDS. Mean airway pressure but not Fio_2 or $Pao_2 - Pao_2$ was significantly lower at 48 to 72 hours in the furosemide group, although no differences in long-term morbidity or mortality were identified. A recent Cochrane review, which included 7 studies, concluded that there are no data to support the routine administration of furosemide in preterm infants with RDS.[35] Six studies involving a total of 124 patients were included in the analysis of mortality of infants receiving furosemide compared with placebo, no diuretic or as-needed diuretic administration. Diuretic therapy showed a trend toward increased mortality, with a RR of 1.35 (95% CI 0.71–2.56) and did not significantly change BPD or long-term outcome. There are no data to support the routine administration of furosemide in preterm infants with RDS.

BPD

Several studies have examined the short-term and long-term effects of furosemide in infants with BPD. In an early study, Kao and colleagues[36] examined pulmonary mechanics in 11-week-old infants with who had developed stage 3 or 4 BPD by 1 month of age. After furosemide (1 mg/kg intravenously [IV]), airway resistance, airway conductance, and pulmonary compliance all improved within 1 hour, although no significant effect of furosemide was detected on multiple measurements between 1 and 24 hours after administration. In 10 infants with stage III to IV BPD who received 2 doses of furosemide 24 hours apart, Patel and colleagues[37] found only transient improvement in arterial $PaCo_2$ and no improvement in alveolar-arterial oxygen gradient. Engelhardt and colleagues[38] found that chronic intravenous administration of furosemide (6–10 days) to spontaneously breathing infants with BPD improved mechanical lung properties but had limited effect on gas exchange. Steward and Brion[39] have recently updated a meta-analysis of treatment effects of loop diuretics on infants with BPD. Only 6 studies met criteria for inclusion in the analysis, and because of heterogeneity in study design, conclusions were limited. In patients older than 3 weeks, pulmonary mechanics and oxygenation improved after a week of furosemide. However, data on relevant long-term clinical outcomes are lacking, and routine use of loop diuretics in this population cannot be recommended.

Aerosolized delivery of furosemide has also been evaluated in infants with BPD because the agent seems to inhibit induced bronchoconstriction. In examining 9 ventilator-dependent infants with BPD in a randomized, double-blind crossover study, Kugelman[40] found no improvement in pulmonary mechanics in response to inhaled furosemide (1 mg/kg). A Cochrane review that assessed aerosolized furosemide for preterm infants with (or developing) chronic lung disease found a single dose may transiently improve lung mechanics, although not enough information is available to assess the effect of chronic administration on oxygenation and pulmonary mechanics.[41]

FUROSEMIDE AND FLUID OVERLOAD

Diuretics are used in the neonatal population for treatment of several fluid retention states, including renal dysfunction, postoperative management, and during treatment with extracorporeal membrane oxygenation (ECMO). Because of concern for acute fluctuations in intravascular volume associated with bolus administration of loop diuretics, the use of continuous intravenous administration has been proposed. In adults with congestive heart failure, there is no significant increase in total urine output of sodium excretion associated with continuous infusion of furosemide compared with bolus dosing.[42] Studies in a young pediatric population, particularly neonates, are limited. In cardiac postoperative patients less than 6 months of age, urinary output per dose of drug was significantly greater in a group receiving continuous (0.1 mg/kg/h) furosemide compared with intermittent dosing (1 mg/kg IV every 4 hours), whereas the need for fluid replacement was decreased.[43] In contrast, using an adjustable dosing of furosemide based on clinical parameters, Klinge and colleagues[44] found urine production was greater (per mg of drug) in the intermittent compared with continuous group and required a significantly smaller total daily dose of the drug. In neonates treated with ECMO, there was no observed benefit of continuous compared with intermittent furosemide administration, although in this study dosing regimes were not standardized and varied widely.[45]

FUROSEMIDE AND AKI

Early use of furosemide has been proposed to prevent the progression of AKI (also known as acute renal failure). A meta-analysis of furosemide to prevent or treat acute renal failure in adults found no significant clinical benefit, although the risk for ototoxicity may have been increased.[46] In the neonate, most causes of AKI involve prerenal mechanisms, such as hypovolemia, hypotension, and hypoxemia that contribute to renal arteriole vasoconstriction, reduced renal blood flow and GFR, and oliguria. The pathophysiologic basis for use of furosemide includes: (1) reduction of energy requirements of tubular cells because of blockade of cotransporter activity, (2) preservation of renal blood flow via prostaglandin-mediated vasodilation, and (3) clearing of tubular debris by maintaining luminal salt and water and thus urine flow.[47] However, clinical data from controlled trials to support this approach are lacking, and given the risk of ototoxicity from increased plasma levels of furosemide, use in this setting cannot be recommended.

THIAZIDE DIURETICS

Thiazide diuretics are sulfonamide derivatives that differ from loop diuretics with respect to mechanism and sites of action, efficacy, and side effects.[48] Similar to loop diuretics, thiazide diuretics reach the lumen of the proximal tubules via OAT1 and OAT3, reaching the distal tubules, where they exert their effects on the potassium-independent Na^+/Cl^- transporter. Although the exact mechanism is unclear, it seems that thiazides bind to the Cl^- site on the transporter, thus inhibiting Na^+/Cl^- cotransport. Because less sodium is typically reabsorbed in this region of the tubule compared with the ascending loop of Henle, thiazides show only moderate potency as diuretics. Thiazides also have an indirect effect on potassium secretion, leading to increased intracellular K^+ and thus, a cell-to-lumen gradient that favors increased potassium secretion.[49] As opposed to loop diuretics, thiazides do not increase urinary calcium or magnesium loss and may increase distal tubule calcium reabsorption. The hypocalciuric effect is lost when sodium supplementation is provided because increased luminal sodium concentration impairs calcium reuptake.[50] Thiazides also show activity against carbonic anhydrase, preventing some sodium reabsorption in the proximal tubules and increasing sodium presentation to the distal convoluted tubule. Increased sodium concentration in this part of the kidney enhances binding of the diuretic to the Cl^- site on the Na^+/Cl^- cotransporter, increasing efficacy of the drug.

Similar to furosemide, thiazide diuretics have been studied in the setting of neonatal lung disease, and are commonly used in infants with BPD. In a double-blind, crossover design trial allocating nonventilated infants with BPD to either diuretics or placebo for 1 week, Kao and colleagues[51] found the combination of chlorothiazide (20 mg/kg/ dose and spironolactone 1.5 mg/kg/dose, both given twice a day) resulted in significant decreases in airway resistance, and dynamic compliance compared with placebo. Diuretic therapy was also associated with increased urine output and potassium and phosphorus excretion. In a randomized, double-blind, controlled trial on long-term diuretic therapy on ventilated infants requiring 30% or more Fio_2 and greater than 30 days of age, Albersheim and colleagues[52] reported no statistical difference in hospital or ventilator days in infants receiving hydrochlorothiazide and spironolactone. After 4 weeks of therapy, respiratory compliance was significantly higher in the treatment compared with control group. Survival to discharge was significantly increased (84%) in the treatment compared with placebo (47%). In a study of 43 infants with oxygen-dependent lung disease randomized to either chlorothiazide and spironolactone or placebo until no longer requiring supplemental oxygen, Kao and colleagues[53] found diuretics improved lung function but did not decrease the total number of days requiring supplemental oxygen. A 2011 Cochrane review found 6 studies in which preterm infants with or developing chronic lung disease and at least 5 days of age were randomly allocated to receive a thiazidelike diuretic.[54] Most studies failed to assess important clinical outcomes. Because of the paucity of randomized controlled trials and numbers of patients studied, the investigators concluded there is no strong evidence of benefit from the routine use of distal diuretics in preterm infants with chronic lung disease. The investigators further stated that studies are needed to assess (1) whether thiazide administration improves mortality, duration of O_2 dependency, duration of ventilator-dependency, length of hospital stay, and long-term outcome in patients exposed to current therapy and (2) whether adding spironolactone to thiazides or adding metolazone to furosemide modifies the risks and benefits.

SPIRONOLACTONE

Spironolactone is a synthetic steroid that acts as a competitive aldosterone receptor antagonist. Aldosterone, which is secreted by the adrenal gland in response to intravascular volume depletion, acts on the distal tubule and collecting duct to increase reabsorption of sodium in exchange for potassium and hydrogen ions. By inhibiting aldosterone, spironolactone attenuates sodium reabsorption and spares potassium loss. Because little of the filtered sodium load reaches the distal tubule, spironolactone is a weak diuretic. Rather, it is primarily prescribed in the neonatal population for its potassium-sparing effects, typically in conjunction with a thiazide diuretic. However, in comparing outcomes of infants treated with the combination of chlorothiazide and spironolactone or chlorothiazide alone, Hoffman and colleagues[55] found no difference in the need for electrolyte supplementation. Spironolactone also exerts antiandrogen activity by competitive binding to the androgen receptor and inhibition of formation of the receptor complex.[56] Concern has been raised regarding its long-term use in the neonatal population. However, it is unknown whether these effects occur at the doses commonly prescribed to infants.

SUMMARY

Despite limited data regarding efficacy, diuretics are commonly used in preterm infants to optimize urine output, improve respiratory status, and treat edematous states. A recently conducted survey of US neonatologists involving hypothetical clinical scenarios suggests diuretic therapy for very low birth weight infants in the first 28 days of life is commonly used, despite limited evidence of benefit from randomized trials.[57] Most respondents expected sustained improvements in pulmonary mechanics, decreased days on mechanical ventilation and decreased length of stay, despite lack of evidence in current literature. Although the list of potential complications from diuretic therapy is extensive, including electrolyte abnormalities, bone demineralization, PDA and hearing loss, these appear to have limited influence on the decision-making process.

Although data on the long-term benefits of chronic diuretic therapy in infants with lung disease are lacking, most practitioners can identify infants who clinically benefited for variable lengths of time after the initiation of diuretic therapy. If diuretics are to be used, a rational and individualized approach needs to be developed. Such an approach needs to recognize and monitor for potential side effects, and the practitioner needs to be cognizant of the risk-benefit balance before initiating diuretic therapy. Clinical use of diuretics in patients with chronic lung disease may be considered in infants with BPD displaying deterioration in pulmonary status or infants whose progress of resolution of lung injury has ceased. If the decision to initiate diuretic therapy is made, the clinician should decide a priori the duration of the initial course of diuretics and the degree of expected improvement in lung function for which the decision may be made to continue diuretic therapy. Dosing regimens need to consider the developmental state of the kidney, taking into account postnatal changes in renal blood flow and nephrogenesis. After initial clinical improvement, should it occur, the practitioner should consider stopping diuretics, allowing time to evaluate whether continued therapy is clinically beneficial and thus indicated. One approach in the hospitalized patient is to reevaluate the necessity for diuretic therapy every 7 to 10 days, with a therapeutic trial off diuretics to see if the patient's clinical condition changes. Careful monitoring of potential side effects, including electrolyte and mineral imbalance and development of nephrocalcinosis, is necessary.

REFERENCES

1. Clark RH, Bloom BT, Spitzer AR, et al. Reported medication use in the neonatal intensive care unit: data from a large national data set. Pediatrics 2006;117(6): 1979–87.
2. Jobe AJ. The new BPD: an arrest of lung development. Pediatr Res 1999;46(6): 641–3.
3. Brophy PD, Robillard JE. Functional development of the kidney in utero. In: Polin RA, Fox WW, Abman SH, editors. Fetal and neonatal physiology. 3rd edition. Philadelphia: WB Saunders; 2004. p. 1229–41.
4. Sweeney WE Jr, Avner ED. Embryogenesis and anatomic development of the kidney. In: Polin RA, Fox WW, Abman SH, editors. Fetal and neonatal physiology. 3rd edition. Philadelphia: WB Saunders; 2004. p. 1223–9.
5. Solhaug MJ, Jose PA. Postnatal maturation of renal blood flow. In: Polin RA, Fox WW, Abman SH, editors. Fetal and neonatal physiology. 3rd edition. Philadelphia: WB Saunders; 2004. p. 1242–9.
6. Guignard JP. Postnatal development of glomerular filtration rate in neonates. In: Polin RA, Fox WW, Abman SH, editors. Fetal and neonatal physiology. 3rd edition. Philadelphia: WB Saunders; 2004. p. 1256–66.
7. Kennedy CR, Ayers S, Campbell MJ, et al. Randomized, controlled trial of acetazolamide and furosemide in posthemorrhagic ventricular dilation in infancy: follow-up at 1 year. Pediatrics 2001;108(3):597–607.
8. Aranda JV, Perez J, Sitar DS, et al. Pharmacokinetic disposition and protein binding of furosemide in newborn infants. J Pediatr 1978;93(3):507–11.
9. Mirochnick MH, Miceli JJ, Kramer PA, et al. Renal response to furosemide in very low birth weight infants during chronic administration. Dev Pharmacol Ther 1990; 15(1):1–7.
10. Chemtob S, Doray JL, Laudignon N, et al. Alternating sequential dosing with furosemide and ethacrynic acid in drug tolerance in the newborn. Am J Dis Child 1989;143(7):850–4.

11. Segar JL, Robillard JE, Johnson KJ, et al. Addition of metolazone to overcome tolerance to furosemide in infants with bronchopulmonary dysplasia. J Pediatr 1992;120(6):966–73.

12. Arnold WC. Efficacy of metolazone and furosemide in children with furosemide-resistant edema. Pediatrics 1984;74(5):872–5.

13. Garin EH. A comparison of combinations of diuretics in nephrotic edema. Am J Dis Child 1987;141(7):769–71.

14. O'Donovan BH, Bell EF. Effects of furosemide on body water compartments in infants with bronchopulmonary dysplasia. Pediatr Res 1989;26(2):121–4.

15. Segar JL, Chemtob S, Bell EF. Changes in body water compartments with diuretic therapy in infants with chronic lung disease. Early Hum Dev 1997;48(1-2):99–107.

16. Chang HY, Hsu CH, Tsai JD, et al. Renal calcification in very low birth weight infants. Pediatr Neonatol 2011;52:145–9.

17. Atkinson SA, Shah JK, McGee C, et al. Mineral excretion in premature infants receiving various diuretic therapies. J Pediatr 1988;113(3):540–5.

18. Venkataraman PS, Han BK, Tsang RC, et al. Secondary hyperparathyroidism and bone disease in infants receiving long-term furosemide therapy. Am J Dis Child 1983;137(12):1157–61.

19. Gimpel C, Krause A, Franck P, et al. Exposure to furosemide as the strongest risk factor for nephrocalcinosis in preterm infants. Pediatr Int 2010;52(1):51–6.

20. Robertson CM, Tyebkhan JM, Peliowski A, et al. Ototoxic drugs and sensorineural hearing loss following severe neonatal respiratory failure. Acta Paediatr 2006; 95(2):214–23.

21. Patak RV, Fadem SZ, Rosenblatt SG, et al. Diuretic-induced changes in renal blood flow and prostaglandin E excretion in the dog. Am J Physiol 1979;236(5):F494–500.

22. Miyanoshita A, Terada M, Endou H. Furosemide directly stimulates prostaglandin E2 production in the thick ascending limb of Henle's loop. J Pharmacol Exp Ther 1989;251(3):1155–9.

23. Brion LP, Campbell DE. Furosemide for symptomatic patent ductus arteriosus in indomethacin-treated infants. Cochrane Database Syst Rev 2001;3:CD001148.

24. Lee BS, Byun SY, Chung ML, et al. Effect of furosemide on ductal closure and renal function in indomethacin-treated preterm infants during the early neonatal period. Neonatology 2010;98(2):191–9.

25. Andriessen P, Struis NC, Niemarkt H, et al. Furosemide in preterm infants treated with indomethacin for patent ductus arteriosus. Acta Paediatr 2009;98(5): 797–803.

26. Toyoshima K, Momma K, Nakanishi T. In vivo dilatation of the ductus arteriosus induced by furosemide in the rat. Pediatr Res 2010;67(2):173–6.

27. Green TP, Thompson TR, Johnson DE, et al. Furosemide promotes patent ductus arteriosus in premature infants with the respiratory-distress syndrome. N Engl J Med 1983;308(13):743–8.

28. Yeh TF, Shibli A, Leu ST, et al. Early furosemide therapy in premature infants (less than or equal to 2000 gm) with respiratory distress syndrome: a randomized controlled trial. J Pediatr 1984;105(4):603–9.

29. Belik J, Spitzer AR, Clark BJ, et al. Effect of early furosemide administration in neonates with respiratory distress syndrome. Pediatr Pulmonol 1987;3(4):219–25.

30. Heaf DP, Belik J, Spitzer AR, et al. Changes in pulmonary function during the diuretic phase of respiratory distress syndrome. J Pediatr 1982;101(1):103–7.

31. Bland RD, McMillan DD, Bressack MA. Decreased pulmonary transvascular fluid filtration in awake newborn lambs after intravenous furosemide. J Clin Invest 1978;62(3):601–9.

32. Najak ZD, Harris EM, Lazzara A Jr, et al. Pulmonary effects of furosemide in preterm infants with lung disease. J Pediatr 1983;102(5):758–63.
33. Green TP, Thompson TR, Johnson DE, et al. Diuresis and pulmonary function in premature infants with respiratory distress syndrome. J Pediatr 1983;103(4): 618–23.
34. Green TP, Johnson DE, Bass JL, et al. Prophylactic furosemide in severe respiratory distress syndrome: blinded prospective study. J Pediatr 1988;112(4):605–12.
35. Brion LP, Soll RF. Diuretics for respiratory distress syndrome in preterm infants. Cochrane Database Syst Rev 2008;1:CD001454.
36. Kao LC, Warburton D, Sargent CW, et al. Furosemide acutely decreases airways resistance in chronic bronchopulmonary dysplasia. J Pediatr 1983;103(4):624–9.
37. Patel H, Yeh TF, Jain R, et al. Pulmonary and renal responses to furosemide in infants with stage III-IV bronchopulmonary dysplasia. Am J Dis Child 1985; 139(9):917–9.
38. Engelhardt B, Elliott S, Hazinski TA. Short- and long-term effects of furosemide on lung function in infants with bronchopulmonary dysplasia. J Pediatr 1986;109(6): 1034–9.
39. Stewart A, Brion LP. Intravenous or enteral loop diuretics for preterm infants with (or developing) chronic lung disease. Cochrane Database Syst Rev 2011;9: CD001453.
40. Kugelman A, Durand M, Garg M. Pulmonary effect of inhaled furosemide in ventilated infants with severe bronchopulmonary dysplasia. Pediatrics 1997;99(1): 71–5.
41. Brion LP, Primhak RA, Yong W. Aerosolized diuretics for preterm infants with (or developing) chronic lung disease. Cochrane Database Syst Rev 2006;3: CD001694.
42. Allen LA, Turer AT, Dewald T, et al. Continuous versus bolus dosing of Furosemide for patients hospitalized for heart failure. Am J Cardiol 2010;105(12):1794–7.
43. Luciani GB, Nichani S, Chang AC, et al. Continuous versus intermittent furosemide infusion in critically ill infants after open heart operations. Ann Thorac Surg 1997;64(4):1133–9.
44. Klinge JM, Scharf J, Hofbeck M, et al. Intermittent administration of furosemide versus continuous infusion in the postoperative management of children following open heart surgery. Intensive Care Med 1997;23(6):693–7.
45. van der Vorst MM, Wildschut E, Houmes RJ, et al. Evaluation of furosemide regimens in neonates treated with extracorporeal membrane oxygenation. Crit Care 2006;10(6):R168.
46. Ho KM, Sheridan DJ. Meta-analysis of frusemide to prevent or treat acute renal failure. BMJ 2006;333(7565):420.
47. Moghal NE, Shenoy M. Furosemide and acute kidney injury in neonates. Arch Dis Child Fetal Neonatal Ed 2008;93(4):F313–6.
48. van der Vorst MM, Kist JE, van der Heijden AJ, et al. Diuretics in pediatrics: current knowledge and future prospects. Paediatr Drugs 2006;8(4):245–64.
49. Martinez-Maldonado M, Cordova HR. Cellular and molecular aspects of the renal effects of diuretic agents. Kidney Int 1990;38(4):632–41.
50. Campfield T, Braden G, Flynn-Valone P, et al. Effect of diuretics on urinary oxalate, calcium, and sodium excretion in very low birth weight infants. Pediatrics 1997; 99(6):814–8.
51. Kao LC, Warburton D, Cheng MH, et al. Effect of oral diuretics on pulmonary mechanics in infants with chronic bronchopulmonary dysplasia: results of a double-blind crossover sequential trial. Pediatrics 1984;74(1):37–44.

52. Albersheim SG, Solimano AJ, Sharma AK, et al. Randomized, double-blind, controlled trial of long-term diuretic therapy for bronchopulmonary dysplasia. J Pediatr 1989;115(4):615–20.

53. Kao LC, Durand DJ, McCrea RC, et al. Randomized trial of long-term diuretic therapy for infants with oxygen-dependent bronchopulmonary dysplasia. J Pediatr 1994;124(5 Pt 1):772–81.

54. Stewart A, Brion LP, Ambrosio-Perez I. Diuretics acting on the distal renal tubule for preterm infants with (or developing) chronic lung disease. Cochrane Database Syst Rev 2011;9:CD001817.

55. Hoffman DJ, Gerdes JS, Abbasi S. Pulmonary function and electrolyte balance following spironolactone treatment in preterm infants with chronic lung disease: a double-blind, placebo-controlled, randomized trial. J Perinatol 2000;20(1): 41–5.

56. Dorrington-Ward P, McCartney AC, Holland S, et al. The effect of spironolactone on hirsutism and female androgen metabolism. Clin Endocrinol (Oxf) 1985;23(2): 161–7.

57. Hagadorn JI, Sanders MR, Staves C, et al. Diuretics for very low birth weight infants in the first 28 days: a survey of the US neonatologists. J Perinatol 2011; 31(10):677–81.

Neonatal Blood Pressure Support: The Use of Inotropes, Lusitropes, and Other Vasopressor Agents

Shahab Noori, MD, Istvan Seri, MD, PhD*

KEYWORDS

• Inotropes • Lusitropes • Vasopressors • Hemodynamic
• Hypotension • Shock

The use of inotropes, lusitropes, and vasopressors is common in neonates with cardiovascular compromise.[1,2] Although the understanding of cellular mechanisms of action of these medications is well founded,[3,4] there is little information on their clinically relevant long-term benefits in the neonatal patient population.[5–7] In addition, if not appropriately titrated, these medications may induce abrupt, excessive, and potentially harmful increases in blood pressure and systemic and organ blood flow.[8–11] Thus, in addition to the cardiovascular compromise,[10,11] treatment by suboptimal administration of inotropes, lusitropes, and vasopressors may contribute to short- and long-term morbidities in critically ill preterm and term neonates.[6] Prompt diagnosis of neonatal cardiovascular compromise by state-of-the-art hemodynamic monitoring of blood pressure and systemic and organ blood flow[12] and careful titration of the vasoactive agents to the optimal hemodynamic response[8,13] are thought to be of importance in decreasing mortality and morbidity associated with shock and its treatment in preterm and term neonates.[14,15]

Unfortunately, there is little evidence on what vasoactive medications to use in what patient and when, at what dose to start, how to titrate the drug, and what parameters to monitor.[2,6,16] Because addressing these issues is only possible by opinion- and experience-based reasoning without much evidence at present, this article focuses on describing the documented, developmentally regulated hemodynamic actions of inotropes, lusitropes, and vasopressors, and their short-term hemodynamic benefits and risks. Although there are several reasons to stay away from advocating

Center for Fetal and Neonatal Medicine and the USC Division of Neonatal Medicine, Children's Hospital Los Angeles and the LAC+USC Medical Center, Keck School of Medicine, University of Southern California, 4650 Sunset Boulevard, Mailstop #31, Los Angeles, CA 90027, USA
* Corresponding author. USC Keck School of Medicine, Children's Hospital Los Angeles, 4650 Sunset Boulevard, Mailstop #31, Los Angeles, CA 90027.
E-mail address: iseri@chla.usc.edu

Clin Perinatol 39 (2012) 221–238
doi:10.1016/j.clp.2011.12.010
0095-5108/12/$ – see front matter © 2012 Elsevier Inc. All rights reserved.

experience-based reasoning on the use, benefits, and potential harm of these medications, the notion that experience in medicine might be best defined as "an ability to make a mistake repeatedly with increasing confidence" is one of the reasons with which few would argue.

MECHANISMS OF ACTION OF INOTROPES, LUSITROPES, AND VASOPRESSORS

An inotrope is a manufactured or naturally occurring substance with a primary pharmacologic effect of increasing myocardial contractility. For the classical inotropes (eg, dobutamine) or vasopressor-inotropes (eg, epinephrine and dopamine), the mechanisms of increasing myocardial contractility are primarily based on stimulating α- or β-adrenergic and dopaminergic receptors located on the cell membrane of myocardial cells. Stimulation of these receptors leads to activation of a chain of intracellular events hinging on receptor-specific cyclic adenosine monophosphate (cAMP)–dependent or independent increases in intracellular calcium availability resulting in increased actin–myosin bridge formation and thus contractility (**Fig. 1**).[17]

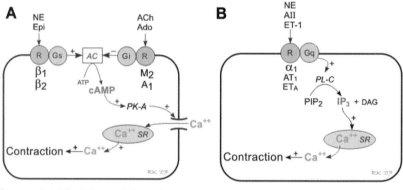

R, receptor; Gs and Gi, stimulatory and inhibitory G-proteins; AC, adenylyl cyclase; PK-A, protein kinase A; SR, sarcoplasmic reticulum; α and β, alpha and beta-adrenoceptors; Epi, epinephrine; NE, norepinephrine; ACh, acetylcholine; M_2, muscarinic receptor; A_1, adenosine (Ado)

R, receptor; Gq, phospholipase C-coupled Gq-protein; PL-C, phopholipase C; PIP_2, phosphatidylinositol biphosphate; IP_3, inositol triphosphate; DAG, diacylglycerol; SR, sarcoplasmic reticulum; NE, norepinephrine; AII, angiotensin II; ET-1, endothelin-1; $α_1$, alpha$_1$-adrenoceptor; AT_1, type 1 angiotensin receptor; ET_A, type A endothelin receptor.

Fig. 1. Mechanisms of cardiomyocyte contraction. (*A*) G_s- and G_i-protein coupled signal transduction. Ligand-induced and receptor-specific activation (β-adrenoreceptor–G_s coupling) or deactivation (muscarinic or adenosine receptor–G_i coupling) of adenylyl cyclase results in increased or decreased cAMP formation, respectively. Increases in cAMP activates protein kinase-A (PK-A) resulting in increased influx of calcium by phosphorylation and activation of L-type calcium channels and enhanced release of calcium by the sarcoplasmic reticulum in the cardiomyocyte leading to increased inotropy, chronotropy, and dromotropy. Activation of G_i-proteins by adenosine and muscarinic receptor stimulation decreases cAMP and decreases calcium entry and release and cell membrane repolarization resulting in decreased inotropy. G_i-protein effects are prevalent mostly in the sinus and atrioventricular (AV) nodes resulting in decreased sinus rate and AV conduction velocity, respectively, with only minimal effects on myocardial contractility. (*B*) IP_3-coupled signal transduction. The IP_3 pathway is linked to activation of $α_1$-adrenoceptors, angiotensin II (AII) receptors, and endothelin-1 (ET-1) receptors and is stimulated by agonist exposure of these receptors coupled to a phospholipase C (PL-C)–linked Gq-protein. Activated PL-C then stimulates formation of inositol triphosphate (IP_3) from phosphatidylinositol biphosphate (PIP_2). Increased IP_3 stimulates calcium release by the sarcoplasmic reticulum resulting in increases in inotropy. (*Modified from* Klabunde RE. Available at: http://www.cvphysiology.com/Blood%20Pressure/BP011a.htm; with permission.)

Another class of inotropes, the phosphodiesterase (PDE) inhibitors (eg, amrinone or milrinone), rather selectively decrease the activity of PDE-III, the enzyme responsible for degradation of cAMP.[18] The resulting increase in intracellular cAMP concentration leads to the chain of events described for the classical inotropes with the end-result of increased myocardial contractility.

A lusitrope is a manufactured or naturally occurring substance that increases the rate of myocardial relaxation. The lusitropic property depends on the compound's ability to reduce intracellular calcium concentration by cAMP-dependent activation of the inward-pumping calcium channels on the sarcoplasmic reticulum, or to promote calcium dissociation from troponin C primarily during diastole.[19,20]

A vasopressor is a manufactured or naturally occurring substance that increases vascular tone. Vascular smooth muscle tone is regulated by complex cellular mechanisms involving a delicate balance between vasodilator and vasoconstrictor factors, and the availability of cytosolic calcium plays a central role in this process (**Fig. 2**). Vasopressors exert their peripheral vasoconstrictive effects primarily through binding to α_1-adrenergic and vasopressin$_{1A}$ (V$_{1a}$) receptors activating the enzyme phospholipase C in the vascular smooth muscle.[21] Phospholipase C in

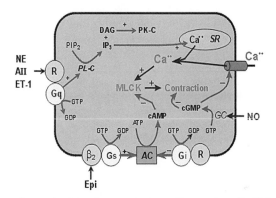

Fig. 2. Regulation of vascular tone in vascular smooth muscle cells. This figure shows the simplified depiction of three pathways of importance in regulation of vascular tone. The phosphatidylinositol (PIP$_2$) pathway is similar to that in the heart with vasopressors (norepinephrine [NE], epinephrine, and dopamine), angiotensin II (AII), and endothelin-I (ET-1) acting by way of the α_1-adrenergic, AII, and ET^A receptors, respectively, to activate phospholipase C (PL-C) to form inositol triphosphate (IP$_3$) and diacylglycerol (DAG). Inositol triphosphate stimulates calcium release from the sarcoplasmic reticulum while DAG activates PK-C contributing to vascular smooth muscle cell contraction. The G$_s$-protein coupled pathway stimulates (receptor coupled with the stimulatory G protein: G$_s$) or inhibits (receptor coupled with the inhibitory G protein: G$_i$) adenylyl cyclase resulting in increased or decreased cAMP formation, respectively. Different vascular beds have a different pattern of α- and β-adrenergic receptor and dopaminergic receptor expression.[3] Increases in cAMP inhibits myosin light chain kinase (MLCK) and decreases phosphorylation of smooth muscle myosin thereby preventing the interactions between actin and myosin and leads to vasodilation. Decreases in cAMP have the opposite effect enhancing the vasoconstrictor tone. The β_2-adrenoceptor–linked mechanism in the vascular smooth muscle cell is different from that in the myocardium. The nitric oxide (NO)–cyclic guanosine monophosphate (cGMP) pathway induces vasodilation by way of the NO-induced activation of guanylyl cyclase (GC) and the resultant increased cGMP formation. cGMP activates the cGMP-dependent protein kinase and potassium channels resulting in inhibition of IP$_3$ formation and calcium entry into the vascular smooth muscle cell. (*Modified from* Klabunde RE. Available at: http://www.cvphysiology.com/Blood%20Pressure/BP011b.htm; with permission.)

turn increases inositol triphosphate leading to release of calcium from the sarco-plasmic reticulum.

Most of the medications used for cardiovascular support in the neonatal intensive care unit have dose-dependent inotropic, lusitropic, and vasopressor effects albeit to a varying degree and, for the compounds exerting their cardiovascular actions by receptor stimulation, with various sensitivity to the cardiovascular adrenergic, dopaminergic, and vascular vasopressin receptors (**Tables 1** and **2**). Discussed next are the developmentally regulated mechanisms of action of these medications, their cardiovascular effects, and the specific cardiovascular pathophysiology and clinical scenarios where each medication might be beneficial.

DOPAMINE

Dopamine is the most commonly used cardiovascular medication in the neonatal intensive care unit. Dopamine exerts its cardiovascular effects by dose-dependent stimulation of the α- and β-adrenergic and dopaminergic receptors and by its serotoninergic actions.[4] In adults and older children, low doses of dopamine (2–4 μg/kg/min) primarily simulate the vascular dopaminergic receptors. Vascular dopaminergic receptors are selectively expressed in the renal, mesenteric, and coronary circulations and to a lesser extent in the pulmonary circulation and the extracranial vessels of the neck and head.[4] At moderate doses (5–10 μg/kg/min), dopamine increases contractility and heart rate by stimulating the cardiac β_1-, β_2-, and α_1-adrenergic and the dopaminergic receptors; at high doses ($\geq$10–20 μg/kg/min) dopamine also increases systemic and probably pulmonary vascular resistance (PVR) by stimulating vascular α_1 receptors.[22,23] Approximately 50% of the positive inotropic effects of dopamine are caused by the dopamine$_2$-receptor stimulation induced release of norepinephrine stored in the peripheral sympathetic nerve endings in the myocardium.[4] Because myocardial norepinephrine stores get depleted within 8 to 12 hours, dopamine, especially in the preterm neonate with decreased myocardial norepinephrine stores, is a less effective positive inotrope in the long run compared with epinephrine.[4]

Because of maturational differences in the expression of the α- and β-adrenergic receptors,[24,25] in neonates without adrenoreceptor downregulation,[26,27] clinical

Table 1
Cardiovascular actions mediated by adrenergic, dopaminergic, and vascular vasopressin receptors

	Adrenergic, Dopaminergic, and Vasopressin Receptors					
	α_1/α_2[a]	β_2	α_1	β_1/β_2	DA$_1$/DA$_2$	V$_{1a}$
	Vascular	Vascular	Cardiac	Cardiac	Vascular/Cardiac	Vascular
Vasoconstriction	++++	0	0	0	0	++++
Vasodilation	0	++++	0	0	++++[b]	0
+Inotropy	0	0	++	++++	+/++	0
+Chronotropy	0	0	0	++++	0	0
Cond. velocity	0	0	0	++++	0	0

Abbreviations: Cond. velocity, conduction velocity; +Chronotropy, positive chronotropy; +Inotropy, positive inotropy.

Estimated relative vascular (vasoconstriction and vasodilation) and cardiac (inotropy, chronotropy, and conduction velocity) effects mediated by the cardiovascular adrenergic (α_1/α_2 and β_1/β_2), dopaminergic (DA$_1$/DA$_1$), and vasopressin (V$_{1a}$) receptor subtypes.

[a] α_2-Receptors cause arterial vasodilation and venous vasoconstriction.

[b] Renal, mesenteric, coronary circulation > pulmonary circulation > extracranial vessels of the neck.

Table 2
Estimated relative cardiovascular receptor stimulatory effects of inotropes, lusitropes, and vasopressors

	Adrenergic, Dopaminergic, and Vasopressin Receptors					
	α_1/α_2	β_2	α_1	β_1/β_2	DA_1/DA_2	V_{1a}
	Vascular	Vascular	Cardiac	Cardiac	Vascular/Cardiac	Vascular
Phenylephrine	++++	0	+	0	0	0
Norepinephrine	++++	0/+	++	++++	0	0
Epinephrine	++++	++++	++	++++	0	0
Dopamine[a]	++++	++	++	+++	++++	0
Dobutamine[b]	+/0	++	++	++++	0	0
Isoprenaline	0	+++	0	++++	0	0
Vasopressin	0	0	0	0	0	++++
PDE-III inhibitors	0	0	0	0	0	0
PDE-V inhibitors	0	0	0	0	0	0

Abbreviations: $\alpha_1/\alpha_2/\beta_1/\beta_2$, subtypes of α- and β-adrenoreceptors; DA, dopamine; DOB, dobutamine; PDE, phosphodiesterase enzyme; PDE-III inhibitors used in neonates, amrinone, milrinone; PDE-V inhibitors used in neonates, sildenafil; V_{1a}, vasopressin receptor expressed in the vasculature.
[a] Dopamine also has serotoninergic actions.
[b] Efficacy of dobutamine is independent of its affinity for adrenoreceptors.

manifestations of vascular α-adrenoreceptor simulation (eg, increased systemic vascular resistance [SVR]) become apparent even at low-to-medium doses.[3,4,28] Therefore, in neonates with escalating dopamine infusion, the pattern of receptor stimulation is first dopaminergic, then α-adrenergic, and finally β-adrenergic (**Fig. 3**).[3,4,28]

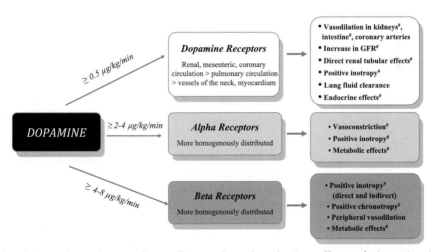

Fig. 3. Dose-dependent cardiovascular, renal, and endocrine effects of dopamine in neonates. Receptor-specific hemodynamic, renal, pulmonary, and endocrine actions of dopamine are shown in the absence of adrenoreceptor downregulation (#denotes the effects demonstrated in preterm neonates). (*Modified from* Seri I. Management of hypotension and low systemic blood flow in the very low birth weight neonate during the first postnatal week. J Perinatol 2006;26:S8–13; with permission.)

Of note is that the hemodynamic effects and the clinical response to dopamine (and other vasopressors and inotropes) is altered by downregulation of adrenergic receptors caused by the critical illness–associated prolonged endogenous and the treatment-associated exogenous receptor stimulation.[27] Furthermore, because cardiovascular adrenergic receptor expression is regulated by corticosteroids,[26] the documented higher incidence of relative adrenal insufficiency[29] also contributes to the observed attenuated hemodynamic response and the development of vasopressor-dependence in preterm and term neonates. These effects are especially seen in patients with prolonged exposure to dopamine and other vasopressors and inotropes.[30] Therefore, pharmacodynamics is more important than established pharmacokinetic data when vasopressors and inotropes are used and their effectiveness considered.[31] In addition, the cardiovascular response to these medications also depends on the developmentally regulated expression and function of the cardiovascular adrenergic and dopaminergic receptors and second messenger systems, and on the dysregulated local production of vasodilators, such as prostaglandins and nitric oxide in patients with a critical illness.

Effect on Systemic Blood Pressure

The efficacy of dopamine in raising blood pressure in hypotensive neonates has been consistently demonstrated. In a randomized controlled trial of dopamine versus hydrocortisone for treatment of hypotension in very-low-birth-weight infants, dopamine was effective in increasing blood pressure 100% of the time.[32] Similarly, randomized controlled trials of dopamine versus dobutamine have demonstrated that dopamine is more effective in increasing blood pressure.[33,34]

Effect on Cardiac Output

Dopamine, when appropriately titrated, has been shown to either increase[35,36] or have no significant effect[33,37] on cardiac output. Padbury and colleagues[35] reported an increase in cardiac output and blood pressure in preterm and term infants after titration of dopamine up to 8 μg/kg/min. The increase in cardiac output is caused by the drug-induced increases in myocardial contractility demonstrated by increased ventricular ejection fraction, even in the 1-day-old very preterm neonate.[38] However, Rozé and colleagues[33] reported an increase in SVR without a significant change in cardiac output in hypotensive preterm infants treated with a dopamine infusion of 12 to 20 μg/kg/min. It is tempting to speculate that, in neonates without significant adrenoreceptor downregulation, the drug-induced increase in SVR at higher doses may attenuate the drug's effect of increased myocardial contractility on cardiac output. Along these lines, in a small subset of preterm infants, higher doses of dopamine resulted in excessive increases in SVR, potentially decreasing cardiac output.[37] These findings point to the importance of establishing an optimum hemodynamic target (pressure and flow); titrating the drug in a step-wise fashion; and the need to monitor systemic blood pressure and blood flow. Overall, the increase in blood pressure observed with dopamine infusion (especially at higher doses) is mainly caused by increases in the SVR, although increases in cardiac output (mainly at moderate doses) also contribute to the rise in blood pressure. It must be remembered, however, that receptor downregulation, relative adrenal insufficiency, and dysregulated vasodilator release modify the "effective dose-range" of dopamine in the given patient and explain the lack of response to conventional doses (2–20 μg/kg/min) in several critically ill neonates. Indeed, findings of a small case series in neonates not responding to conventional doses of dopamine suggest that dopamine at doses of 30 to 50 μg/kg/min increased blood pressure and urine output.[39] However, because the drug might induce significant vasoconstriction at higher doses, administration of high-dose dopamine might result in decreased cardiac output and organ (including brain) blood flow, and therefore blood pressure and systemic and organ blood flow need to be monitored in these critically ill neonates.[12]

Effect on Pulmonary Vascular Bed

Because hypotension commonly occurs during the first few postnatal days when the ductus arteriosus is open, understanding the impact of dopamine on the pulmonary vascular bed is important. For example, if dopamine increased SVR out of proportion to the drug-induced increase in PVR in neonates with a patent ductus arteriosus (PDA), blood pressure would increase but a decrease in systemic blood flow might occur, because the left-to-right shunting through the ductus may also increase. Yet, there are only limited data on the effect of dopamine on the pulmonary vasculature. In hypotensive preterm infants, Liet and colleagues[40] estimated mean pulmonary and systemic blood pressure by assessing the flow velocity through the PDA. Dopamine infusion had variable effects on the ratio of pulmonary-to-systemic blood pressure with half of patients showing an increase and the other half a decrease in the ratio. Relative to SVR, PVR increased in one-half and decreased or did not change in the other half of the studied population. The finding that patients with a low pretreatment pulmonary/systemic blood pressure ratio responded to dopamine primarily with a more pronounced increase in their PVR suggested that hypotensive infants with a significant left-to-right shunt might benefit from dopamine infusion. Indeed, Bouissou and colleagues[41] subsequently found indirect evidence that dopamine decreases left-to-right ductal shunting in hypotensive preterm infants with a hemodynamically significant PDA and thereby improves systemic perfusion. These authors suggested that the increase in superior vena cava (SVC) flow (used as a surrogate of systemic blood flow) and the decrease in cerebral artery resistance index without any change in left ventricular output provided evidence for a decrease in left-to-right ductal shunting. Although this might well be the case, it is also possible that the observed increase in cerebral blood flow (CBF) might have been related to the increase in blood pressure in these critically ill neonates with impaired CBF autoregulation rather than to the decrease in ductal shunting.[9] The limited available data suggest that dopamine has variable effects on the pulmonary vascular bed and in a subset of patients with abnormally increased baseline pulmonary blood flow (ie, neonates with significant left-to-right ductal shunting) dopamine may increase PVR out of proportion to the increase in SVR and thus lead to improved systemic blood flow while raising blood pressure. Along these lines, it is tempting to speculate that the increased pulmonary blood flow in patients with a PDA induces upregulation of pulmonary vasoconstrictive mechanisms, such as α_1 and endothelin receptor expression, as a physiologic response to attenuate pulmonary overcirculation. Dopamine (or other vasopressors) then increases PVR more readily than in patients without preexisting pulmonary overcirculation.

Effect of Dopamine on CBF

Dopamine is thought to be devoid of any direct effect on the cerebral vascular bed.[42] Recent studies in lambs even suggest a possible role for dopamine in the regulation of cerebral flow–metabolism coupling.[43] However, confirmation of these findings is needed before the potential clinical relevance of the drug-associated cerebral flow–metabolism coupling can be further investigated. In hypotensive preterm infants without intact CBF autoregulation, titration of dopamine (or other vasopressors or inotropes) in a stepwise fashion to achieve the "optimal" mean blood pressure resulted in an increase in CBF.[44] Munro and colleagues[45] also demonstrated similar findings and showed that, although blood pressure and CBF increase, CBF autoregulation is not immediately reestablished. Therefore, abrupt and significant elevation in blood pressure induced by the inappropriate use of excessive doses of these vasoactive medications can result in sudden and potentially harmful increases in CBF. In the vulnerable extremely premature neonate, especially after an episode of hypoperfusion, excessive increases in CBF may then lead to reperfusion injury or hemorrhage. Finally, the available very limited information suggests that at least 50 to 90 minutes of relative hemodynamic stability may be required for CBF autoregulation to be reestablished in preterm neonates after a hypotensive episode.[8]

Effect of Dopamine on Mesenteric and Renal Blood Flow

In the human preterm neonate, the selective vasodilatory effects of dopamine on the mesenteric blood flow have not been consistently demonstrated.[42,46] Furthermore, higher doses of dopamine in patients with no significant adrenoreceptor downregulation may result in vasoconstriction of the mesenteric vascular bed.[37] The administration of even low doses of dopamine does not seem to be indicated to selectively increase intestinal blood flow in preterm neonates.

Dopamine has more consistently been shown to increase renal blood flow in preterm neonates.[4,8,42] However, this hemodynamic finding only partially explains the improvement in urine output after starting dopamine infusion in hypotensive neonates. Interestingly, intrarenally produced dopamine, by directly affecting renal microhemodynamics (eg, glomerular filtration rate), tubular epithelial and paracrine, and renal endocrine functions, plays an important regulatory and modulatory role in overall renal function.[4,47] Although discussion of the renal epithelial, paracrine, and endocrine effects of dopamine is beyond the scope of this article, it is important to remember that dopamine causes significant and clinically relevant increases in renal sodium, phosphorous, ammonia, and free-water excretion and decreases in urinary concentrating capacity.[4] The complex renal actions of dopamine may, at least in part, explain the finding that in indomethacin-treated preterm infants with impaired renal perfusion, dopamine increases renal blood flow and urine output.[46] However, because these findings have not been consistently demonstrated, routine use of dopamine to prevent the indomethacin-associated renal dysfunction is not warranted.[48]

Overall, the unique hemodynamic profile of dopamine makes this drug suitable as a first-line medication for the treatment of most forms of neonatal cardiovascular compromise. In addition, the need to carefully titrate the drug and monitor pressure, and directly or indirectly systemic blood flow, and endocrine actions of dopamine need to be kept in mind and further investigated to fully establish the safety and efficacy of this medication in neonates.[4,13] In clinical practice, the drug-induced inhibition of thyroid-stimulating hormone must be kept in mind especially when using dopamine during the first postnatal days.[49,50] Accordingly, the neonatal screen should be repeated once the patient has been off dopamine for at least 12 hours.[4,13,51]

DOBUTAMINE

Because dobutamine has an asymmetric carbon atom, there are two enantiomers of the medication with different affinity for adrenergic receptors.[52] The negative isomer is primarily an α_1-receptor agonist and increases myocardial contractility and SVR. The positive isomer is a β_1- and β_2-receptor agonist causing increases in the myocardial contractility, heart rate, and conduction velocity, and decreases in SVR. In addition, the main metabolite of dobutamine, (+)-3-O-methyl-dobutamine, exerts α_1-receptor inhibitory effects and in itself it decreases myocardial contractility and SVR. Because dobutamine consists of 50% of the positive and negative isomer, the net effects of dobutamine administration are increases in myocardial contractility and, to a lesser extent, heart rate, and either no effect or a decrease in SVR (**Table 3**).[52] As with dopamine, the developmentally regulated differences in vascular α- and β-adrenoreceptor expression affect the cardiac and peripheral vascular response to dobutamine. Because during early development cardiovascular α-adrenergic receptor expression is upregulated while maturation of β-adrenergic receptors lags behind,[24,25] very preterm neonates are likely to respond to dobutamine with attenuated decreases in SVR and thus with more pronounced increase in blood pressure compared with term neonates. However, systematic dose–response studies comparing the cardiovascular effects of dobutamine in preterm neonates with those in term neonates are not available.

The cardiovascular effects of dobutamine are also dose-dependent (**Fig. 4**). At very low doses (2.5 µg/kg/min) no significant hemodynamic effects have been observed in neonates with cardiovascular compromise.[53] However, moderate doses (5–7.5 µg/kg/min) of dobutamine lead to increases in cardiac output, whereas at higher doses (5–20 µg/kg/min) dobutamine increases cardiac output and blood pressure even in hypotensive preterm infants.[33] An additional effect of dobutamine on increasing cardiac output has been demonstrated in hypotensive preterm infants receiving dopamine.[54] In general, dobutamine is more effective than dopamine in increasing cardiac output in neonates with myocardial dysfunction. Although dobutamine at doses of 10 or 20 µg/kg/min was also found to be more effective than dopamine used at the same two doses at increasing low SVC flow in preterm infants during the first postnatal day, even dobutamine had limited efficacy[34] and the clinical relevance of these findings remains unclear. Neonates with myocardial dysfunction respond favorably to dobutamine, as evidenced by increases in cardiac output, minutes after the initiation of the drug infusion followed by increases in organ blood flow hours later.[55] Of note is that higher doses of dobutamine may lead to decreased myocardial compliance potentially affecting ventricular filling especially in patients with myocardial hypertrophy.

Dobutamine is the drug of choice to increase cardiac output in neonates with myocardial dysfunction, and its use likely results in increases in organ blood flow and blood pressure in these patients. However, its effect on organ blood flow may be variable and seems to depend on the underlying pathophysiology. Thus, the hemodynamic response to dobutamine makes the drug's use suitable for clinical situations

Table 3
Mechanisms of action of dobutamine enantiomers and metabolites

| Enantiomers, Metabolites | Pharmacologic Activity | | Heart | | Vasculature |
	Agonist	Antagonist	Force	Rate	Tone
(−) dobutamine	α_1		↑	0	↑
(+) dobutamine	β_1/β_2		↑	↑	↓
(+)-3-O-methyl-dobutamine		α_1	↓	—	↓
(±) dobutamine	$\alpha_1/\beta_1/\beta_2$	α_1	↑↑	↑	0/↓

Adrenergic receptor stimulatory and inhibitory effects of the left (−) and right (+) rotating enantiomers of dobutamine and its major metabolite ((+)-3-O-methyl-dobutamine) are shown. The form of dobutamine used in clinical practice is depicted as (±) dobutamine. $\alpha_1/\alpha_2/\beta_1/\beta_2$ = subtypes of α- and β-adrenoreceptors; ↑, 0, ↓ = increase, no effect, or decrease on myocardial function or vascular tone. The relative effect is indicated by the number of symbols.

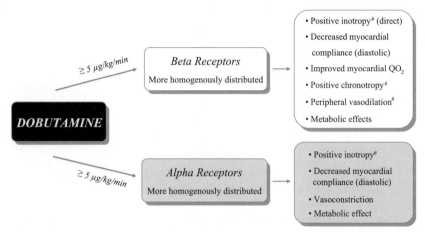

Fig. 4. Dose-dependent cardiovascular effects of dobutamine in neonates. Receptor-specific cardiovascular actions of dobutamine are shown presuming absence of adrenoreceptor downregulation (#denotes the effects demonstrated in neonates). (*Modified from* Seri I. Management of hypotension and low systemic blood flow in the very low birth weight neonate during the first postnatal week. J Perinatol 2006;26:S8–13; with permission.)

where poor myocardial contractility with unchanged or increased SVR is the primary underlying cause of the cardiovascular compromise, such as perinatal asphyxia or the very preterm neonate with poor systemic blood flow and vasoconstriction during the transitional period. In contrast, in conditions with low SVR (eg, vasodilation) as the dominant underlying cause of the hemodynamic disturbance, such as seen in the early stages of septic shock or the very preterm neonate with vasodilatory shock during the transitional period, dobutamine is not the appropriate first drug of choice.[16] However, addition of dobutamine to dopamine in patients with cardiovascular compromise caused by impaired myocardial function and vasodilation is a reasonable approach and may be effective.

EPINEPHRINE

Epinephrine exerts its cardiovascular effects by stimulating the α- and β-adrenergic receptors in a dose-dependent manner (**Fig. 5**). At low doses (0.01–0.1 µg/kg/min) epinephrine primarily stimulates the cardiac and vascular β_1- and β_2-adrenoreceptors receptors leading to increased inotropy, chronotropy, and conduction velocity and peripheral vasodilation (primarily in the muscles), respectively. At doses greater than 0.1 µg/kg/min, epinephrine also stimulates the vascular and cardiac α_1-receptors causing vasoconstriction and increased inotropy, respectively. The hemodynamic effects of vascular α_2-receptor stimulation are less prominent. The net hemodynamic effects of epinephrine administration are significant increases in blood pressure and systemic blood flow caused by the drug-induced increases in SVR and cardiac output. The increase in blood pressure (and possibly cardiac output) increases CBF in hypotensive preterm neonates.[44]

There are limited data on the cardiovascular effects of epinephrine in neonates. The previously cited randomized controlled clinical trial of dopamine versus epinephrine demonstrated that the two medications have similar efficacy in improving blood pressure and increasing CBF in hypotensive preterm infants.[44] However, patients randomized to epinephrine more frequently developed increased serum lactate levels independent of the improvement in their hemodynamic status and hyperglycemia

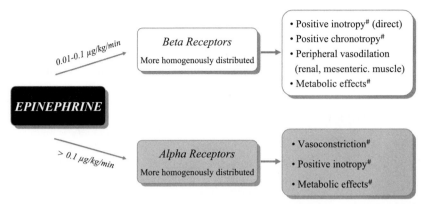

Fig. 5. Dose-dependent cardiovascular effects of epinephrine in neonates. Receptor-specific cardiovascular actions of epinephrine are shown presuming absence of adrenoreceptor downregulation (#denotes the effects demonstrated in neonates). (*Modified from* Seri I. Management of hypotension and low systemic blood flow in the very low birth weight neonate during the first postnatal week. J Perinatol 2006;26:S8–13; with permission.)

requiring insulin treatment.[56] These metabolic effects are most likely explained by the drug-induced stimulation of β_2-adrenoreceptors in the liver and skeletal muscle resulting in decreased insulin release and increases in glycogenolysis leading to increases in lactate production, respectively.

In clinical practice, some neonatologists use epinephrine as the first choice of drug in the treatment of hypotensive neonates with vasodilatory shock with or without myocardial dysfunction. However, most neonatologists use the drug if the patient is unresponsive to higher doses of dopamine (with or without dobutamine). Overall, epinephrine is as effective as dopamine in treating hypotension. However, its metabolic effects need to be kept in mind because the increases in serum lactate limit the use of sequential serum lactate measurements to indirectly follow the changes in the cardiovascular status. The associated hyperglycemia might require initiation of insulin administration. Also, because epinephrine is a potent vasoconstrictor, extreme caution is warranted when titrating and weaning the drug and on syringe changes dictated by pharmacy or nursing protocols. However, the significant effects of epinephrine on the vascular tone and myocardial contractility make it an effective choice for the treatment of conditions where low vascular resistance with or without impaired myocardial contractility is the primary underlying cause of the cardiovascular compromise, such as in septic shock or certain cases with asphyxia-associated hemodynamic compromise.

VASOPRESSIN

Vasopressin has widespread physiologic effects, although its primary physiologic role is regulation of extracellular osmolality.[57] The vascular effects of vasopressin occur by stimulation of the G protein–coupled V_{1a} and V_2 receptors expressed in the cardiovascular system.[57] The V_{1a} and V_2 receptors induce vasoconstriction and vasodilation by activation of the IP_3 and cAMP pathways, respectively. The potent vasoconstrictive effects of vasopressin dominate the cardiovascular response when it is used as an infusion.[57]

Vasopressin administration has been suggested to be beneficial in vasodilatory shock and deficiency of endogenous vasopressin production in adults[58] and children with septic shock[59] and infants and children after cardiac surgery for congenital heart disease (CHD).[60] In these studies on patients unresponsive to conventional vasopressors, a relative hypersensitivity to vasopressin administration has been found. Several case reports in a small number of hypotensive preterm and term neonates unresponsive to conventional vasopressors have reported mostly beneficial effects of vasopressin or terlipressin, a long-acting vasopressin agonist. For a thorough review of the literature on this subject, the reader is referred to the relatively recent review by Meyer and colleagues.[61] Because terlipressin has also been reported to decrease pulmonary artery pressure in animal models of hypoxic pulmonary constriction,[62] a recent case report describes its use and systemic and pulmonary effects in a neonate with congenital diaphragmatic hernia and pulmonary hypertension.[63] It is clear that more information from prospective observational and randomized controlled trials is needed before vasopressin use in neonates with vasopressor-resistant shock can be recommended. At present, low-dose hydrocortisone is the drug of choice in clinical practice in neonates with vasopressor-resistant shock, although hydrocortisone administration is not without potential side effects especially in the very preterm neonate in the immediate postnatal period.[30,64]

MILRINONE

Milrinone is a selective PDE-III inhibitor and thus it exerts its cardiovascular effects through the inhibition of cAMP degradation. By increasing the concentration of cAMP, milrinone enhances myocardial contractility, promotes myocardial relaxation, and decreases vascular tone in the systemic and pulmonary vascular beds. Given this intriguing profile of cardiovascular actions, milrinone has been most commonly used in the postoperative care of patients with CHD to treat low cardiac output state[65] and in near-term and term neonates with persistent pulmonary hypertension of the neonate (PPHN) as an adjunct to inhaled nitric oxide (iNO).[66,67]

There are very limited data on the cardiovascular effects of milrinone in preterm and term neonates. The only randomized controlled clinical trial of milrinone performed in neonates evaluated the effects of the medication on preventing low SVC flow in extremely preterm infants.[68] This well-designed study did not provide evidence for beneficial effects of milrinone administration, because the incidence of low SVC flow was similar in the treatment and placebo groups. Furthermore, milrinone-treated subjects had an increased incidence of tachycardia, low blood pressure, and hemodynamically significant PDA. Comparing with a historical control group, findings of a recent study suggest that milrinone administration immediately after ligation of the ductus arteriosus in preterm infants with relatively low cardiac output might reduce hemodynamic instability during the first 24 hours after the procedure.[69] Given that myocardial dysfunction is common after PDA ligation,[70] the inotropic and lusitropic properties of milrinone are likely responsible for the observed beneficial effects.

It remains unclear whether milrinone exerts significant myocardial effects immediately after delivery in the human neonate. According to studies in developing animals, PDE-IV rather than PDE-III is the most active enzyme responsible for cAMP metabolism in the fetal heart.[71] The findings that milrinone has a poor inhibitory effect on PDE-IV and upregulation of PDE-III and downregulation of PDE-IV expression only start at birth[71] explain why it takes 3 to 7 days after delivery until the inotropic effects of milrinone can convincingly be demonstrated in the immature animal model.[71,72]

Other than the potential benefits of milrinone in improving cardiac output, the medication may also have beneficial effects in the treatment of PPHN especially in cases unresponsive to iNO. In a small case series of nine term infants with PPHN unresponsive to iNO, oxygenation index significantly improved within a few hours after starting milrinone.[73] Recent findings explain, at least in part, the cellular basis of the enhanced responsiveness to milrinone in neonates with PPHN unresponsive to iNO.[74] Contrary to endogenous nitric oxide, exogenous (inhaled) nitric oxide upregulates PDE-III in the smooth muscle cells of the pulmonary vasculature resulting in a decrease or loss of the cAMP-dependent vasodilatory mechanisms.[74] Addition of milrinone to iNO has been proposed to restore pulmonary vasodilatory mechanisms dependent on cAMP; both the cyclic guanosine monophosphate (nitric oxide–dependent) and cAMP vasodilatory systems become operational, potentially resulting in increased pulmonary vasodilation and improvement in oxygenation in these patients.

Because none of the cardiovascular effects of milrinone (inotropy, lusitropy, and pulmonary vasodilation) has been convincingly demonstrated in neonates without CHD, further well-designed studies on milrinone in neonates with primary myocardial dysfunction and PPHN are urgently needed.

LEVOSIMENDAN

Levosimendan exerts its positive inotropic effects by enhancing binding of calcium to troponin C. Calcium binding to troponin C induces a conformation change in the troponin complex, which results in the uncovering of the myosin binding-site on actin and thereby making it accessible to myosin.[75] The calcium-sensitizer effect of this medication is unique because the other more commonly used inotropes exert their effects either through increases in intracellular cAMP concentration or by the inositol triphosphate-induced increases in intracellular calcium availability (see **Fig. 1**). In addition, by activating the ATP-sensitive potassium channels, levosimendan also has vasodilatory properties. Similar to that of milrinone, the drug's hemodynamic profile of positive inotropy and peripheral vasodilation is especially beneficial in patients with myocardial dysfunction, because the reduction in the afterload contributes to improvements in cardiac output.

Levosimendan is a relatively new cardiovascular medication used primarily in adults with congestive heart failure.[76] Recently, its use in postoperative care of infants with CHD has been reported.[77,78] However, the experience with this medication in preterm or term neonates is limited and appropriately designed clinical trials are needed to establish the benefits and describe the risks of levosimendan use in neonates without CHD.

SUMMARY

A solid understanding of the mechanisms of action of cardiovascular medications used in clinical practice along with efforts to develop comprehensive hemodynamic monitoring systems to improve the ability to accurately identify the underlying pathophysiology of cardiovascular compromise are essential in the management of neonates with shock. This article reviews the mechanisms of action of the most frequently used cardiovascular medications in neonates. Because of paucity of data from controlled clinical trials, evidence-based recommendations cannot be made for the clinical use of these medications. That said, it is suggested that careful titration of the given medication with close monitoring of the cardiovascular response using echocardiography and a combination of the recently developed technologies[12] if available might improve the effectiveness and decrease the risks associated with administration of these medications. Although there is evidence for short-term hemodynamic benefits of cardiovascular supportive care in neonates when inotropes, lusitropes, and vasopressors or a combination of these medications is used tailored to the underlying pathophysiology of the cardiovascular compromise, the impact of these medications on the clinically most relevant long-term outcome measures is not well understood.[6,10,79,80]

REFERENCES

1. Al-Aweel I, Pursley DM, Rubin LP, et al. Variations in prevalence of hypotension, hypertension, and vasopressor use in NICUs. J Perinatol 2001;21(5):272–8.
2. Kluckow M, Seri I. Clinical presentations of neonatal shock: the VLBW infant during the first postnatal day. In: Kleinman CS, Seri I, editors. Hemodynamics and cardiology. Neonatal questions and controversies. Philadelphia: Saunders Elsevier; 2008. p. 147–77.
3. Seri I. Management of hypotension and low systemic blood flow in the very low birth weight neonate during the first postnatal week. J Perinatol 2006;26:S8–13.
4. Seri I. Cardiovascular, renal and endocrine actions of dopamine in neonates and children. J Pediatr 1995;126:333–44.
5. Fanaroff JM, Wilson-Costello DE, Newman NS, et al. Treated hypotension is associated with neonatal morbidity and hearing loss in extremely low birth weight infants. Pediatrics 2006;117:1131–5.
6. Barrington KJ. Hypotension and shock in the preterm infant. Semin Fetal Neonatal Med 2008;13:16–23.
7. Noori S, Seri I. Etiology, pathophysiology, and phases of neonatal shock. In: Kleinman CS, Seri I, editors. Hemodynamics and cardiology. Neonatal questions and controversies. Philadelphia: Saunders Elsevier; 2008. p. 3–18.
8. Seri I, Rudas G, Bors ZS, et al. The effect of dopamine on renal function, cerebral blood flow and plasma catecholamine levels in sick preterm neonates. Pediatr Res 1993;34:742–9.
9. Greisen G. Autoregulation of vital and nonvital organ blood flow in the preterm and term neonate. In: Kleinman CS, Seri I, editors. Hemodynamics and cardiology. Neonatal questions and controversies. Philadelphia: Saunders Elsevier; 2008. p. 19–38.
10. du Plessis AJ. The role of systemic hemodynamic disturbances in prematurity-related brain injury. J Child Neurol 2009;24:1127–40.
11. O'Leary H, Gregas MC, Limperopoulos C, et al. Elevated cerebral pressure passivity is associated with prematurity-related intracranial hemorrhage. Pediatrics 2009;124:302–9.
12. Soleymani S, Borzage M, Seri I. Hemodynamic monitoring in neonates: advances and challenges. J Perinatol 2010;30(Suppl 1):S38–45.
13. Seri I. Circulatory support of the sick newborn infant. Semin Neonatol 2001;6: 85–95.
14. Goldstein RF, Thompson RJ, Oehler JM, et al. Influence of acidosis, hypoxaemia, and hypotension on neurodevelopmental outcome in very low birth weight infants. Pediatrics 1995;95:238–43.
15. Martens SE, Rijken M, Stoelhorst GM, et al. Is hypotension a major risk factor for neurological morbidity at term age in very preterm infants? Early Hum Dev 2003; 75:79–89.
16. Evans N. Which inotrope for which baby? Arch Dis Child Fetal Neonatal Ed 2006; 9:F213–20.
17. Zheng M, Zhu W, Han Q, et al. Emerging concepts and therapeutic implications of beta-adrenergic receptor subtype signaling. Pharmacol Ther 2005;108: 257–68.

18. Endoh M. The therapeutic potential of novel cardiotonic agents. Expert Opin Investig Drugs 2003;12:735–50.
19. Johnson RG Jr. Pharmacology of the cardiac sarcoplasmic reticulum calcium ATPase-phospholamban interaction. Ann N Y Acad Sci 1998;853:380–92.
20. Morgan JP, Perreault CL, Morgan KG. The cellular basis of contraction and relaxation in cardiac and vascular smooth muscle. Am Heart J 1991;121:961–8.
21. Kellum JA, Pinsky MR. Use of vasopressor agents in critically ill patients. Curr Opin Crit Care 2002;8:236–41.
22. Goldberg LI. Cardiovascular and renal actions of dopamine: potential clinical applications. Pharmacol Rev 1972;24:1–29.
23. D'Orio V, el Allaf D, Juchmès J, et al. The use of low doses of dopamine in intensive care medicine. Arch Int Physiol Biochim 1984;92:S11–20.
24. Felder RA, Eisner GM, Montgomery SB. Renal alpha-adrenergic receptors in canine puppies. Pediatr Res 1980;14:619–25.
25. Vapaavouri EK, Shinebourne EA, Williams RL, et al. Development of cardiovascular responses to autonomic blockade in intact fetal and neonatal iambs. Biol Neonate 1973;22:177–88.
26. Davies AO, Lefkowitz RJ. Regulation of beta-adrenergic receptors by steroid hormones. Annu Rev Physiol 1984;46:119–30.
27. Ruffolo RR Jr, Kopia GA. Importance of receptor regulation in the pathophysiology and therapy of congestive heart failure. Am J Med 1986;80:67–72.
28. Seri I, Tulassay T, Kiszel J, et al. Cardiovascular response to dopamine in hypotensive preterm neonates with severe hyaline membrane disease. Eur J Pediatr 1984;142:3–9.
29. Fernandez EF, Watterberg KL. Relative adrenal insufficiency in the preterm and term infant. J Perinatol 2009;29(Suppl 2):S44–9.
30. Seri I, Tan R, Evans J. The effect of hydrocortisone on blood pressure in preterm neonates with pressor-resistant hypotension. Pediatrics 2001;107:1070–4.
31. Padbury JF. Neonatal dopamine pharmacodynamics: lessons from the bedside. J Pediatr 1998;133:719–20.
32. Bourchier D, Weston PJ. Randomised trial of dopamine compared with hydrocortisone for the treatment of hypotensive very low birthweight infants. Arch Dis Child Fetal Neonatal Ed 1997;76:F174–8.
33. Rozé JC, Tohier C, Maingueneau C, et al. Response to dobutamine and dopamine in the hypotensive very preterm infant. Arch Dis Child 1993;69:59–63.
34. Osborn D, Evans N, Kluckow M. Randomized trial of dobutamine versus dopamine in preterm infants with low systemic blood flow. J Pediatr 2002;140:183–91.
35. Padbury JF, Agata Y, Baylen BG, et al. Dopamine pharmacokinetics in critically ill newborn infants. J Pediatr 1987;110:293–8.
36. Lundstrøm K, Pryds O, Greisen G. The haemodynamic effects of dopamine and volume expansion in sick preterm infants. Early Hum Dev 2000;57:157–63.
37. Zhang J, Penny DJ, Kim NS, et al. Mechanisms of blood pressure increase induced by dopamine in hypotensive preterm neonates. Arch Dis Child Fetal Neonatal Ed 1999;81:F99–104.
38. Clark SJ, Yoxall CW, Subhedar NV. Right ventricular performance in hypotensive preterm neonates treated with dopamine. Pediatr Cardiol 2002;23:167–70.
39. Perez CA, Reimer JM, Schreiber MD, et al. Effect of high-dose dopamine on urine output in newborn infants. Crit Care Med 1986;14:1045–9.
40. Liet JM, Boscher C, Gras-Leguen C, et al. Dopamine effects on pulmonary artery pressure in hypotensive preterm infants with patent ductus arteriosus. J Pediatr 2002;140:373–5.

41. Bouissou A, Rakza T, Klosowski S, et al. Hypotension in preterm infants with significant patent ductus arteriosus: effects of dopamine. J Pediatr 2008;153: 790–4.
42. Seri I, Abbasi S, Wood DC, et al. Regional hemodynamic effects of dopamine in the sick preterm neonate. J Pediatr 1998;133:728–34.
43. Wong FY, Barfield CP, Horne RS, et al. Dopamine therapy promotes cerebral flow-metabolism coupling in preterm infants. Intensive Care Med 2009;35:1777–82.
44. Pellicer A, Valverde E, Elorza MD, et al. Cardiovascular support for low birth weight infants and cerebral hemodynamics: a randomized, blinded, clinical trial. Pediatrics 2005;115:1501–12.
45. Munro MJ, Walker AM, Barfield CP. Hypotensive extremely low birth weight infants have reduced cerebral blood flow. Pediatrics 2004;114:1591–6.
46. Seri I, Abbasi S, Wood DC, et al. Regional hemodynamic effects of dopamine in the indomethacin-treated preterm infant. J Perinatol 2002;22:300–5.
47. Aperia AC. Intrarenal dopamine: a key signal in the interactive regulation of sodium metabolism. Annu Rev Physiol 2000;62:621–47.
48. Barrington K, Brion LP. Dopamine versus no treatment to prevent renal dysfunction in indomethacin-treated preterm newborn infants. Cochrane Database Syst Rev 2002;3:CD003213.
49. Seri I, Tulassay T, Kiszel J, et al. Effect of low dose dopamine infusion on prolactin and thyrotropin secretion in preterm infants with hyaline membrane disease. Biol Neonate 1985;47:317–22.
50. De Zegher F, Van Den Berghe G, Devlieger H, et al. Dopamine inhibits growth hormone and prolactin secretion in the human newborn. Pediatr Res 1993;34:642–5.
51. Seri I, Somogyvary Z, Hovanyovszky E, et al. Developmental regulation of the dopamine-induced inhibition of pituitary prolactin release in the human preterm neonate. Biol Neonate 1998;73:137–44.
52. Noori S, Friedlich P, Seri I. Pharmacology review: the use of dobutamine in the treatment of neonatal cardiovascular. Neo Rev 2004;5:e22–6.
53. Martinez AM, Padbury JF, Thio S. Dobutamine pharmacokinetics and cardiovascular responses in critically ill neonates. Pediatrics 1992;89:47–51.
54. Lopez SL, Leighton JO, Walther FJ. Supranormal cardiac output in the dopamine- and dobutamine-dependent preterm infant. Pediatr Cardiol 1997;18:292–6.
55. Robel-Tillig E, Knüpfer M, Pulzer F, et al. Cardiovascular impact of dobutamine in neonates with myocardial dysfunction. Early Hum Dev 2007;83:307–12.
56. Valverde E, Pellicer A, Madero R, et al. Dopamine versus epinephrine for cardiovascular support in low birth weight infants: analysis of systemic effects and neonatal clinical outcomes. Pediatrics 2006;117:e1213–22.
57. Dyke PC II, Tobias JD. Vasopressin: applications in clinical practice. J Intensive Care Med 2004;19:220–8.
58. Landry DW, Levin HR, Gallant EM, et al. Vasopressin deficiency contributes to the vasodilation of septic shock. Circulation 1997;95:1122–5.
59. Rodríguez-Núñez A, López-Herce J, Gil-Antón J, et al, RETSPED Working Group of the Spanish Society of Pediatric Intensive Care. Rescue treatment with terlipressin in children with refractory septic shock: a clinical study. Crit Care 2006; 10:R20.
60. Rosenzweig EB, Starc TJ, Chen JM, et al. Intravenous arginine-vasopressin in children with vasodilatory shock after cardiac surgery. Circulation 1999;100(Suppl 19): II182–6.
61. Meyer S, Gortner L, McGuire W, et al. Vasopressin in catecholamine-refractory shock in children. Anaesthesia 2008;63:228–34.

62. Walker BR, Haynes J Jr, Wang HL, et al. Vasopressin-induced pulmonary vasodilation in rats. Am J Physiol 1989;257:H415–22.

63. Stathopoulos L, Nicaise C, Michel F, et al. Terlipressin as rescue therapy for refractory pulmonary hypertension in a neonate with a congenital diaphragmatic hernia. J Pediatr Surg 2011;46:e19–21.

64. Cole C. The preterm neonate with relative adrenal insufficiency and vasopressor-resistant hypotension. In: Kleinman CS, Seri I, editors. Hemodynamics and cardiology. Neonatal questions and controversies. Philadelphia: Saunders Elsevier; 2008. p. 195–207.

65. Chang AC, Atz AM, Wernovsky G, et al. Milrinone: systemic and pulmonary hemodynamic effects in neonates after cardiac surgery. Crit Care Med 1995; 23:1907–14.

66. Bassler D, Kreutzer K, McNamara P, et al. Milrinone for persistent pulmonary hypertension of the newborn. Cochrane Database Syst Rev 2010;11:CD007802.

67. Farrow KN, Steinhorn RH. Phosphodiesterases: emerging therapeutic targets for neonatal pulmonary hypertension. Handb Exp Pharmacol 2011;204:251–77.

68. Paradisis M, Evans N, Kluckow M, et al. Randomized trial of milrinone versus placebo for prevention of low systemic blood flow in very preterm infants. J Pediatr 2009;154:189–95.

69. Jain A, Sahni M, El-Khuffash A, et al. Use of targeted neonatal echocardiography to prevent postoperative cardiorespiratory instability after patent ductus arteriosus ligation. J Pediatr 2011. [Epub ahead of print].

70. Noori S, Friedlich P, Seri I, et al. Changes in myocardial function and hemodynamics following ligation of the ductus arteriosus in preterm infants. J Pediatr 2007;150:597–602.

71. Akita T, Joyner RW, Lu C, et al. Developmental changes in modulation of calcium currents of rabbit ventricular cells by phosphodiesterase inhibitors. Circulation 1994;90:469–78.

72. Artman M, Kithas PA, Wike JS, et al. Inotropic responses change during postnatal maturation in rabbit. Am J Physiol 1988;255:H335–42.

73. McNamara PJ, Laique F, Muang-In S, et al. Milrinone improves oxygenation in neonates with severe persistent pulmonary hypertension of the newborn. J Crit Care 2006;21:217–22.

74. Chen B, Lakshminrusimha S, Czech L, et al. Regulation of phosphodiesterase 3 in the pulmonary arteries during the perinatal period in sheep. Pediatr Res 2009; 66:682–7.

75. Toller WG, Stranz C. Levosimendan, a new inotropic and vasodilator agent. Anesthesiology 2006;104:556.

76. Dickstein K, Cohen-Solal A, Filippatos G, et al. ESC Committee for Practice Guidelines (CPG). ESC guidelines for the diagnosis and treatment of acute and chronic heart failure 2008: the Task Force for the diagnosis and treatment of acute and chronic heart failure 2008 of the European Society of Cardiology. Developed in collaboration with the Heart Failure Association of the ESC (HFA) and endorsed by the European Society of Intensive Care Medicine (ESICM). Eur J Heart Fail 2008;10:933–89.

77. Lechner E, Moosbauer W, Pinter M, et al. Use of levosimendan, a new inodilator, for postoperative myocardial stunning in a premature neonate. Pediatr Crit Care Med 2007;8:61–3.

78. Bravo MC, López P, Cabañas F, et al. Acute effects of levosimendan on cerebral and systemic perfusion and oxygenation in newborns: an observational study. Neonatology 2011;99:217–23.

79. Noori S, Stavroudis T, Seri I. Systemic and cerebral hemodynamics during the transitional period after premature birth. Clin Perinatol 2009;36:723–36.

80. Pellicer A, del Carmen Bravo M, Madero R, et al. Early systemic hypotension and vasopressor support in low birth weight infants: impact on neurodevelopment. Pediatrics 2009;123:1369–76.

Anesthesia and Analgesia in the NICU

R. Whit Hall, MD

KEYWORDS

• Anesthesia • Analgesia • NICU • Pain management
• Infant newborn • Infant premature

Pain management is increasingly recognized as an integral part of effective management of vulnerable babies in the neonatal intensive care unit (NICU). Traditionally, neonates have not been accorded the same respect for pain as have their older counterparts because pain, as defined by the International Association for the Study of Pain, is "always subjective." Babies requiring intensive care are unable to express discomfort. Furthermore, preterm neonates in particular do not have the strength to protest like older children or even term neonates. The parents, who would advocate for their babies, are often asked to wait outside the NICU while painful procedures are being performed (despite evidence that pain can be mitigated by parental involvement[1]). Furthermore, neonates do not fill out satisfaction surveys or express displeasure as a result of being exposed to painful stimuli, making them at risk for inadequate pain treatment.

Before 1980, pain in the newborn period was infrequently recognized or treated.[2] Because the gold standard of pain assessment is self-reporting, which is clearly not possible in the newborn period, clinicians can only measure pain indirectly. Animal and human studies have documented that neonatal pain is associated with short- and long-term adverse consequences.[3,4] Furthermore, the enhanced survival of extremely low-birth-weight babies makes them more susceptible to the effects of pain and stress because of increased exposure. Indeed, one study documented that neonates less than 32 weeks' gestation were exposed to 10 to 15 painful procedures per day, up to 22 procedures per day in the first 2 weeks of life,[5] and most of these procedures were untreated.[6] Clinicians advocating pain relief continue to struggle. A recent study by Carbajol and colleagues[7] has documented the increased occurrence and lack of treatment of neonatal pain in almost 80% of newborns in intensive care.

Analgesia and sedation in the NICU has been fraught with controversy because of concern about the safety of these drugs in the neonatal population, lack of adequate

Supported in part by NCRR Grant 20146.
Division of Neonatology, University of Arkansas for Medical Sciences, Slot 512B, 4301 West Markham, Little Rock, AR 72205, USA
E-mail address: hallrichmanw@uams.edu

Clin Perinatol 39 (2012) 239–254
doi:10.1016/j.clp.2011.12.013
0095-5108/12/$ – see front matter © 2012 Elsevier Inc. All rights reserved.

pharmacokinetic and pharmacodynamic data in this population, difficulty in pain assessment, and lack of long-term neurodevelopmental assessment of survivors for the pain experienced in the neonatal period.[8–11] Legitimate concern about safety has led to more governance for moderate sedation privileges for clinicians caring for neonates and more emphasis on obtaining consent for sedation,[12] leading to road-blocks to giving sedation to neonates undergoing painful procedures. Furthermore, individual differences and decreased morphine metabolism in younger gestational age neonates may lead to the rapid development of tolerance and accumulation of the drug in extremely preterm neonates.[13] Thus, the use of sedation and analgesia in the neonatal population although extremely important, must be done safely and effectively (**Table 1**).

In a practical sense, every NICU should have a program to reduce pain for the NICU patient. This program should include a comprehensive approach, as shown in **Fig. 1**. A stepwise approach should begin with avoidance of painful procedures as much as possible, followed by nonpharmacologic and then pharmacologic methods for pain relief. Because the projected pain is expected to become more severe, increasingly potent drugs (with increasing complications) should be used. An effective pain relief program also provides education for all healthcare providers.[27,28]

NEONATAL PAIN ASSESSMENT

Pain assessment has been termed the "fifth vital sign" by the Joint Commission for the Accreditation of Hospitals. However, the gold standard is self-reporting, obviously not possible in neonates. Therefore, several pain assessment tools (>40 and still counting) have been developed for this purpose.[10] Pain assessment is based on physiologic (heart rate, blood pressure, respiratory rate, and oxygen saturation) and behavioral (facial action, body movements, and cry) measures. Behavioral measures are more pain specific,[29] whereas physiologic measures are more indicative of stress and not as specific for pain.[30] Unfortunately, there is poor correlation between these two measurements,[31] and neonatal pain assessment remains controversial. Furthermore, preterm neonates exhibit differential responses to pain as evidenced by the different pain scores in the Premature Infant Pain Profile, one of the pain assessment tools commonly used in NICUs.[32] Clearly, the metabolic cost of mounting a robust response to pain for an extremely preterm neonate is not worth the energy expenditure given the limited energy reserves.[33]

Table 1
Balance between treatment for pain and concerns regarding treatment

Reasons to Treat for Pain	Concerns Regarding Treatment
Beneficial short-term effects (less ventilator asynchrony, splinting, faster intubation,[14] decreased morbidity especially after surgery[15])	Adverse short-term effects (hypotension, respiratory depression, prolonged ventilator dependence,[16,17] intraventricular hemorrhage[18])
Beneficial long-term effects (improved response to pain,[19] downregulation of the hypopituitary-adrenal axis[20])	Prolonged metabolism of opioids and benzodiazepines[21]
Less stress associated with pain[22]	Hyperalgesia[23]
Decreased neuronal cell death in the presence of pain[24]	Enhanced neuronal cell death[25]
Compassion[26]	Unknown effects of commonly used drugs

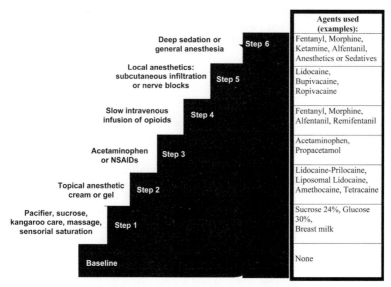

The following table summarizes the agents used:

Step	Method	Agents used (examples):
Step 6	Deep sedation or general anesthesia	Fentanyl, Morphine, Ketamine, Alfentanil, Anesthetics or Sedatives
Step 5	Local anesthetics: subcutaneous infiltration or nerve blocks	Lidocaine, Bupivacaine, Ropivacaine
Step 4	Slow intravenous infusion of opioids	Fentanyl, Morphine, Alfentanil, Remifentanil
Step 3	Acetaminophen or NSAIDs	Acetaminophen, Propacetamol
Step 2	Topical anesthetic cream or gel	Lidocaine-Prilocaine, Liposomal Lidocaine, Amethocaine, Tetracaine
Step 1	Pacifier, sucrose, kangaroo care, massage, sensorial saturation	Sucrose 24%, Glucose 30%, Breast milk
Baseline		None

Fig. 1. Stepwise approach for the management of acute pain in neonates.

Almost all pain assessment scores have been developed for acute pain in neonates, but chronic pain is common and important for neonatal assessment. Assisted ventilation, necrotizing enterocolitis, and postsurgical trauma are all chronic painful conditions in need of treatment. To date, only two pain assessment tools have been validated for chronic neonatal pain: the Neonatal Pain and Discomfort Scale[34] and the Echelle Douleur Inconfort Nouveau-Ne Scale.[35] Although there are advocates for each of these pain scales, it is more important for providers to become familiar with at least one scale that can be used to assess acute and chronic pain and assess neonates of different gestational ages.

NONPHARMACOLOGIC METHODS

Nonpharmacologic pain treatment in neonates has been clearly demonstrated to relieve mild to moderate pain. The best studied techniques include nonnutritive sucking (with and without sucrose); breastfeeding; swaddling; kangaroo care (skin-to-skin contact); and massage therapy. Nonnutritive sucking and sucrose work by increasing endogenous endorphins. Although sucrose has been shown to enhance effectiveness, they have both been shown to decrease crying time and improve pain scores after acute mild pain, such as heel-stick pain.[36–38] Sucrose is efficacious in reducing the pain from single events, such as retinopathy of prematurity screening,[39,40] oral gastric tube insertion,[41] and heel lance.[42] However, sucrose is controversial when given repeatedly, possibly leading to adverse long-term outcomes.[43] Kangaroo care, which was first used in developing countries to decrease neonatal mortality, has also been shown to relieve neonatal pain. Kangaroo care decreases the pain associated with single procedures, such as heel lance,[44,45] but the magnitude of the effect is unknown.[46] Swaddling decreases acute mild-to-moderate pain, such as the pain associated with heel-lance procedures.[47] Massage therapy has been inadequately studied; however, it has shown promise in ameliorating heel-stick pain[48] and it is effective in multisensorial stimulation.[49] Nonpharmacologic techniques are safe and have demonstrated effectiveness in relieving mild-to-moderate neonatal pain associated with single procedures. These methods generally require parental involvement; thus, family centered care in the NICU should be encouraged to ameliorate neonatal pain.

PHARMACOLOGIC METHODS
Opioids

Opioids are commonly used in modern NICUs.[50] They provide procedural pain relief, such as for intubation premedication[51–53]; relief from chronic pain, such as necrotizing enterocolitis[54]; and ventilation.[16,55,56] Several studies and reviews have pointed to the conclusion that they should be used selectively. A recent Cochrane review found insufficient evidence to recommend routine use of opioids in mechanically ventilated newborns.[56] The Cochrane review looked at pain scales, and overall found that a significant effect on pain was found in the treatment group. No significant effect was found in favor of the treatment group with respect to neonatal mortality; duration of ventilation; neurodevelopmental outcome, short-term and long-term; incidence of severe intraventricular hemorrhage (IVH); any IVH; and periventricular leukomalacia (PVL). Given the likely long-term adverse consequences associated with the chronic pain and stress of mechanical ventilation, it is reassuring that short-term adverse effects are not more common in the opioid-treated groups.

Morphine

Morphine is the most frequently used opioid analgesic in all ages, and is the most commonly used drug for analgesia in ventilated neonates.[50] Morphine has a slow onset of analgesia. Its mean onset of action is 5 minutes and the peak effect is at 15 minutes. It is metabolized in the liver into two active compounds: morphine-3-glucuronide and morphine-6-glucuronide. The former is an opioid antagonist, and the latter is a potent analgesic. Preterm infants mostly produce morphine-3-glucuronide, which explains why after 3 to 4 days of morphine therapy, the infant develops tolerance.[57] Side-effects of morphine include hypotension in neonates with pre-existing hypotension and gestational age less than 26 weeks,[17] prolonged need for assisted ventilation, and increased time to reach full feeds.[16,55] Others have suggested that morphine may have a specific effect on pulmonary mechanics, possibly caused by undefined direct toxicity, such as histamine release or bronchospasm.[58] Although commonly used, there is controversy as to whether morphine is effective in the treatment of acute pain.[59]

Two large randomized studies have compared morphine with placebo in neonates. A randomized controlled trial conducted in the Netherlands compared the analgesic effect of morphine with placebo infusions for the duration of 7 days in 150 newborns who received mechanical ventilation. The findings of this study suggested that routine morphine infusion in preterm newborns who received ventilatory support neither improved pain relief nor protected against poor neurologic outcome, defined as severe IVH, PVL, or death within 28 days.[55] The Neurologic Outcomes and Preemptive Analgesia in Neonates trial included ventilated preterm neonates from 16 centers in the United States and Europe. It compared the effect of morphine with placebo infusions, after a loading dose, on the neurologic outcomes of the ventilated neonates. The results suggested that continuous morphine infusion did not reduce early neurologic injury in ventilated preterm neonates, defined as severe IVH, PVL, or death.[16,60] Hypotension did occur more frequently in the morphine versus the placebo group.

One study assessed the long-term outcome at 5 to 6 years of prematurely born children (<34 weeks of gestation) who by randomization received morphine in the neonatal period to facilitate mechanical ventilation. This study looked at children from two trials. The first one included 95 infants who were randomly assigned to receive morphine alone, pancuronium alone, or morphine and pancuronium. The second trial included 21 infants who received morphine and 20 infants who received placebo. Each child was assessed using three scales: the full scale Weschler Preschool and Primary Scale of Intelligence, the Movement Assessment Battery for Children, and the Child Behavior Checklist. There were no adverse effects found on intelligence, motor function, or behavior.[61]

Fentanyl

Fentanyl is an opioid analgesic that is 50 to 100 times more potent than morphine.[62] It is used frequently because of its ability to provide rapid analgesia.[63] It may be used as a slow intravenous push every 2 to 4 hours or as a continuous infusion. Tolerance may develop and withdrawal symptoms may occur after 5 days or more of continuous infusions.[62] In a masked randomized controlled trial, a single dose of fentanyl given to ventilated preterm newborns significantly reduced pain behaviors and changes in heart rate. It also increased growth hormone levels.[64] In another study, fentanyl provided the same pain relief as morphine but with fewer side effects.[65] In other studies, fentanyl use resulted in lower heart rates, behavioral stress scores, and pain scores compared with placebo; however, the infants receiving fentanyl required higher ventilator rates and peak inspiratory pressures at 24 hours.[66] Fentanyl may also be used transdermally in patients with limited intravenous access. Side effects of fentanyl include bradycardia, chest wall rigidity, and opioid tolerance after prolonged therapy.

Methadone

Methadone is a potent analgesic with a rapid onset of action and prolonged effect.[63] It has minimal side effects, high enteral bioavailability, and a low cost.

Other opiates

Other opiates include the short-acting drugs sulfentanil, alfentanil, and remifentanil. All are useful for short procedures, such as intubation. Sulfentanil and alfentanil are metabolized by the liver, which is immature in preterm neonates resulting in increased levels with repeated infusions, especially in preterm neonates.[67] Remifentanil, however, is rapidly cleared by plasma esterases and is unaffected by the maturity of the liver enzyme system, making it attractive for short neonatal surgery or other procedures when rapid recovery is anticipated (**Table 2**).[67]

Benzodiazepines

The benzodiazepines are anxietolytic drugs that have limited analgesic effect but are commonly used in NICUs to produce sedation, muscle relaxation, and provide amnesia (in older patients), but they provide little analgesia. This class of drugs inhibits γ-aminobutyric acid A receptors.[68] The main complications include myoclonic jerking, excessive sedation, respiratory depression, and occasional hypotension.

Midazolam

The most commonly used benzodiazepine in the NICU is midazolam. When administered with morphine, it has been shown to provide better sedation than morphine alone in ventilated patients, without adverse effects.[69] The minimal effective dose for most neonates is 200 µg/kg with a maintenance dose of 100 µg/kg/h.[70] Although it can be given orally, the bioavailability is only half that of intravenous midazolam in neonates.[71] Intranasal midazolam has been shown to be effective for fundoscopic

Table 2
Summary of opiate drugs

Drug	Advantages	Disadvantages
Morphine	Potent pain relief Better ventilator synchrony Sedation Hypnosis Muscle relaxation Inexpensive	Respiratory depression Arterial hypotension Constipation, nausea Urinary retention Central nervous system depression Tolerance and dependence Long-term outcomes not studied Prolonged ventilator use
Fentanyl	Fast acting Less hypotension	Respiratory depression Short half-life Quick tolerance and dependence Chest wall rigidity Inadequately studied
Remifentanyl	Fast acting Degraded in the plasma Unaffected by liver metabolism	

examinations in older children, but this mode of delivery has not been tested in neonates.[72] One recent review found no apparent clinical benefit of midazolam compared with opiates in mechanically ventilated neonates.[73] Furthermore, midazolam was associated with worse short-term adverse effects (death, severe IVH, or PVL) in the NOPAIN trial compared with morphine alone.[18] Midazolam seems to provide sedative effects in mechanically ventilated neonates, but it should be used with caution because of reported adverse effects, particularly when used alone. The decreased number of γ-aminobutyric acid A receptors in neonates compared with adults may contribute to the neonate's risk of neuroexcitability and clonic activity that resembles and, in some cases may be, seizure activity.[74] Finally, metabolism for these drugs occurs through glucuronidation (hydroxymidazolam) in the liver, and there is potential for decreased bilirubin metabolism, especially in asphyxiated or preterm newborns. Its half-life is only 30 to 60 minutes, but it may be prolonged in preterm and sick neonates. Thus, pharmacokinetic and pharmacodynamic data are unreliable in sick neonates and drug levels correlate poorly with sedative effects, so it should be titrated using a validated pain scale.[75,76] Although there are relatively few studies to support the use of midazolam in neonates, it is common practice to use this drug as a sedative for ventilated neonates and for procedural pain.[77] A Cochrane report described only three trials using this drug, which could not be combined for analysis because of different tools used to assess sedation.[78] There are some concerns regarding the use of midazolam in neonates. One study reported an increased incidence of adverse short-term effects (IVH, PVL, or death) and a longer hospital stay associated with midazolam.[18] Finally, midazolam has been associated with benzyl alcohol exposure.[79] There have been no long-term studies describing benefit or harm with midazolam. It has been shown (along with morphine) to adhere to the tubing in patients on extracorporeal membrane oxygenation, increasing dosing requirements by 50% in those patients.[80]

Lorazepam

Lorazepam has also been used in the intensive care nursery. Because it is a longer-acting drug than midazolam with a duration of action of 8 to 12 hours, it does not have to be given as a drip or as frequently. It has been used successfully for seizure control in neonates who are refractory to phenobarbital and phenytoin despite its potential neuronal toxicity.[81] It has been associated with propylene glycol exposure (**Table 3**).[79]

Barbiturates

Phenobarbital

Phenobarbital is usually considered the drug of choice for seizure control. Despite animal evidence for antinociception, it is often used for analgesia.[82] It is also used in conjunction with opioids for sedation,[16] although there is little recent evidence that it is effective. Classically, it has been used for neonatal abstinence syndrome, but recent work by Ebner and coworkers[83] demonstrates that opiates shorten the time required for treatment. However, because of its anticonvulsant effects, phenobarbital is an attractive adjunct for patients with seizures.

Chloral Hydrate

Chloral hydrate is commonly used in neonatal intensive care when sedation, particularly sleep, is required without analgesia. It is commonly used for radiologic procedures, electroencephalography, echocardiography, and dental procedures in older patients. It is converted to trichloroethanol, which is also metabolically active.[84] A recent retrospective review found an increased incidence of apnea and desaturation in term neonates less than 1 month and in preterm neonates less than 60 weeks postconceptual age who underwent magnetic resonance imaging.[85] Thus, this drug should be used with caution in preterm and young term neonates.

Propofol

Propofol has become popular as an anesthetic agent for young children, but it has not been studied extensively in neonates.[86–88] One study compared propofol with morphine, atropine, and suxamethonium for intubation and found that propofol led

Table 3 Benzodiazepines		
Drug	**Advantages**	**Disadvantages**
Benzodiazepines	Better ventilator synchrony Antianxiety Sedation Hypnosis Muscle relaxation Amnesia Anticonvulsant	No pain relief Arterial hypotension Respiratory depression Constipation and nausea Urinary retention Myoclonus Seizures Central nervous system depression Tolerance and dependence May interfere with bilirubin Metabolism Propylene glycol and benzyl alcohol exposure
Midazolam	Most studied benzodiazepine Quickly metabolized	Short acting
Lorazepam	Longer acting Better anticonvulsant	More myoclonus reported
Diazepam		Not recommended in the neonate

to shorter intubation times, higher oxygen saturations, and less trauma than the combination regimen in neonates.[89] However, propofol should be used with caution in young infants because clearance is inversely related to neonatal and postmenstrual age. There is significant interindividual variability in the pharmacokinetics of propofol in that population[90] and its use has led to transient decreases in heart rate and oxygen saturation and more prolonged (60 minutes) hypotension.[91]

Ketamine

Ketamine is a dissociative anesthetic that provides analgesia, amnesia, and sedation. Ketamine has been studied and used extensively in older children,[92] but there have been few studies in newborns. Ketamine causes mild increases in blood pressure and heart rate, decreases in respiratory drive, and mild bronchodilation[93] with minimal effects on cerebral blood flow,[94] making it an attractive choice for some unstable hypotensive neonates requiring procedures, such as cannulation for extracorporeal membrane oxygenation.[94] Doses for effective pain management of the pain caused by endotracheal suctioning in ventilated neonates were 2 mg/kg in one Finnish study.[95] It has also been shown to decrease inflammatory cell death in the presence of pain in immature rodents in the author's laboratory, which would also make it attractive for preterm neonates, although this has not been shown in human studies.[96] Despite these theoretical advantages, ketamine is a potent anesthetic with minimal study in neonates. As such, it should only be used for highly invasive procedures.

Acetaminophen

Acetaminophen acts by inhibiting the cyclooxygenase (COX) enzymes in the brain, and it has been well studied in newborns.[54] It is useful for mild pain, in conjunction with other pain relief, or after circumcision.[97]

Local Anesthetics

Lidocaine

Lidocaine inhibits axonal transmission by blocking Na^+ channels. Lidocaine is commonly used for penile blocks for circumcisions. In this circumstance, its use has demonstrated effectiveness in decreasing pain response to immunizations as long as 4 months after circumcision compared with neonates who received placebo.[19] Compared with a dorsal penile root block or eutectic mixture of local anesthetics cream, the ring block has been shown to be the most effective means of pain relief for circumcision.[98]

Topical anesthetics

Topical anesthetics have demonstrated effectiveness for certain types of procedural pain, such as venipuncture,[99] lumbar puncture,[100] or immunizations.[101] Complications include methemoglobinemia and transient skin rashes.[102] In preterm neonates with thin skin the concern for methemoglobinemia is accentuated.

Unfortunately, topical anesthetics have not been effective in providing pain relief for the heel prick, one of the most common skin-breaking procedures, because of increased skin thickness.[103] Newer topical anesthetics include 4% tetracaine and 4% liposomal lidocaine. Although the newer agents have a shorter onset of action, they are no more effective.

COMMON PROCEDURES

Common neonatal procedures and advantages and disadvantages of pain relief are summarized in **Table 4**.

Table 4
Summary of procedures and recommendations for pain relief

Procedure	Drugs	Advantages of Treatment	Disadvantages of Treatment	Other Comments
Mechanical ventilation[16,55,56,65]	Fentanyl (1–3 µg/kg), morphine (0.1 mg/kg), midazolam (0.1–0.2 mg/kg)	Improved ventilator synchrony, lower pain scores	Prolonged time on assisted ventilation, prolonged time to full feeds, increased bladder catheterization, hypotension	Use sedation as needed, not pre-emptively; Midazolam associated with adverse short-term effects in NOPAIN Trial
Circumcision[98,102]	Lidocaine (1 mL), Eutectic mixture of local anesthetics	Less pain response up to 4 months postprocedure	Allergic reaction, bruising at injection site	Ring block is more effective than dorsal penile nerve root block
Heel lance[103]	Sucrose	Shorter crying, less changes in heart rate	None	Eutectic mixture of local anesthetics cream is not effective
Venipuncture, arterial puncture, and lumbar puncture[100,101]	Topical anesthetic (eutectic mixture of local anesthetics), sucrose	Lower premature infant pain profile scores, less crying	Local reaction, rare methemoglobinemia	Other nonpharmacologic treatments effective
Intubation[52,53,89,104,105]	Morphine 0.1 mg/kg, fentanyl 1–3 µg/kg, remifentanyl 1 mg/kg, midazolam 0.2 mg/kg, propofol 2–6 mg/kg, ketamine 1 mg/kg, suxamethonium 2 mg/kg	Shorter time to intubation, less trauma, less desaturation, better maintenance of vital signs	None	No accepted premedication Opiates most common class used
More invasive procedures, such as cannulation for extracorporeal membrane oxygenation[106,107]	Propofol 2–6 mg/kg, ketamine 1 mg/kg, fentanyl 1–3 µg/kg	Maintenance of cardiovascular stability	Questionable neurotoxicity with ketamine	Ketamine may be neuroprotective
Postsurgical pain[108]	Fentanyl 1–3 µg/kg, morphine 0.1 mg/kg, acetaminophen 15 mg/kg	Lowered neuroendocrine response, faster recovery	Respiratory depression, hypotension with opiates	Acetaminophen for mild pain only
Endotracheal suctioning[70,109]	Midazolam 0.2 mg/kg, morphine 0.1 mg/kg, fentanyl 1–3 µg/kg	Anxietolytic	Respiratory depression, hypotension, dependence	Usually not treated
Imaging (magnetic resonance imaging)[110]	Chloral hydrate 50–100 mg/kg	Sedation	Respiratory depression, hypotension	Chloral hydrate provides sedation only

FUTURE DIRECTIONS
Nonsteroidal Anti-inflammatory Drugs

Nonsteroidal anti-inflammatory drugs are used extensively for pain relief in children and adults but they are mainly used for patent ductus arteriosus closure in neonates. They act by inhibiting the COX enzymes (COX-1 and COX-2) responsible for converting arachidonic acid into prostaglandins, thus producing their analgesic, antipyretic, and anti-inflammatory effects.[63] The analgesic effects of nonsteroidal anti-inflammatory drugs have not been studied in neonates, although ibuprofen and indomethacin have been studied for use in patent ductus arteriosus closure. Concern about side effects of renal dysfunction, platelet adhesiveness, and pulmonary hypertension has limited their study for this indication.[73,111,112] However, ibuprofen has demonstrated beneficial effects on cerebral circulation in human studies[113] and beneficial effects on the development of chronic lung disease in baboon experiments,[114] making it an attractive analgesic in preterm neonates.

Nonpharmacologic Methods

Nonpharmacologic approaches, such as acupuncture and music, may be effective, but their use in acute pain relief needs further research.[115] Music has beneficial effects on mothers, but it has not yet been shown to consistently relieve pain.[116] Acupuncture has been studied extensively in older children and adults but it has not yet been studied in neonates.[117] Acupuncture, especially electroacupuncture, has great potential to relieve neonatal pain, but it has also been inadequately studied.[118]

Quality Improvement Approach

A suggested approach to evidence-based recommendations for the treatment of neonatal pain includes the following:

1. Recognition of neonatal pain as a valid concern
2. Recognition of acute procedural and chronic neonatal pain in need of treatment
3. Validated assessment tool for neonatal pain
4. Educational resources for caregivers and parents in the NICU
5. Protocolized stepwise treatment plan for the procedures and conditions encountered in the NICU using nonpharmacologic and pharmacologic approaches to treatment
6. Continued auditing to ascertain appropriate treatment for neonatal pain
7. A well-planned program of coordination, facilitation, and using local champions and project teams to elicit a beneficial change in practice.[119]

REFERENCES

1. Meaney MJ. Maternal care, gene expression, and the transmission of individual differences in stress reactivity across generations. Annu Rev Neurosci 2001;24:1161–92.
2. Anand KJ, Hall RW. Controversies in neonatal pain: an introduction. Semin Perinatol 2007;31(5):273–4.
3. Anand KJ, Hickey PR. Pain and its effects in the human neonate and fetus. N Engl J Med 1987;317(21):1321–9.
4. Fumagalli F, Moteni R, Racagni G, et al. Stress during development: impact on neuroplasticity and relevance to psychopathology. Prog Neurobiol 2007;81(4):197–217.

5. Cignacco E, Hamers J, van Lingen RA, et al. Neonatal procedural pain exposure and pain management in ventilated preterm infants during the first 14 days of life. Swiss Med Weekly 2009;139(15-16):226–32.

6. Barker DP, Rutter N. Exposure to invasive procedures in neonatal intensive care unit admissions. Arch Dis Child Fetal Neonatal Ed 1995;72(1):F47–8.

7. Carbajal R, Rousset A, Danan C, et al. Epidemiology and treatment of painful procedures in neonates in intensive care units. JAMA 2008;300(1):60–70.

8. Jacqz-Aigrain E, Burtin P. Clinical pharmacokinetics of sedatives in neonates. Clin Pharmacokinet 1996;31(6):423–43.

9. Anand KJ, Aranda JV, Berde CB, et al. Summary proceedings from the neonatal pain-control group. Pediatrics 2006;117(3 Pt 2):S9–22.

10. Ranger M, Johnston CC, Anand KJ. Current controversies regarding pain assessment in neonates. Semin Perinatol 2007;31(5):283–8.

11. Whitfield MF, Grunau RE. Behavior, pain perception, and the extremely low-birth weight survivor. Clin Perinatol 2000;27(2):363–79.

12. American Academy of Pediatrics, American Academy of Pediatric Dentistry, Coté CJ, et al; Work Group on Sedation. Guidelines for monitoring and management of pediatric patients during and after sedation for diagnostic and therapeutic procedures: an update. Pediatrics 2006;118(6):2587–602.

13. Saarenmaa E, Neuvonen PJ, Rosenberg P, et al. Morphine clearance and effects in newborn infants in relation to gestational age. Clin Pharmacol Ther 2000;68(2):160–6.

14. VanLooy JW, Schumacher RE, Bhatt-Mehta V. Efficacy of a premedication algorithm for nonemergent intubation in a neonatal intensive care unit. Ann Pharmacother 2008;42(7):947–55.

15. Anand KJ. The stress response to surgical trauma: from physiological basis to therapeutic implications. Prog Food Nutr Sci 1986;10(1-2):67–132.

16. Anand KJ, Hall RW, Desai N, et al. Effects of morphine analgesia in ventilated preterm neonates: primary outcomes from the NEOPAIN randomised trial [see comment]. Lancet 2004;363(9422):1673–82.

17. Hall RW, Kronsberg SS, Barton BA, et al. Morphine, hypotension, and adverse outcomes in preterm neonates: who's to blame? Pediatrics 2005;115(5):1351–9.

18. Anand KJ, Barton BA, McIntosh N, et al. Analgesia and sedation in preterm neonates who require ventilatory support: results from the NOPAIN trial. Neonatal Outcome and Prolonged Analgesia in Neonates [erratum appears in Arch Pediatr Adolesc Med 1999;153(8):895]. Arch Pediatr Adolesc Med 1999; 153(4):331–8.

19. Taddio A, Katz J, Ilersich AL, et al. Effect of neonatal circumcision on pain response during subsequent routine vaccination. Lancet 1997;349(9052):599–603.

20. Grunau RE, Weinberg J, Whitfield MF. Neonatal procedural pain and preterm infant cortisol response to novelty at 8 months. Pediatrics 2004;114(1):e77–84.

21. Anand KJ, Anderson BJ, Holford NHG, et al. Morphine pharmacokinetics and pharmacodynamics in preterm and term neonates: secondary results from the NEOPAIN trial. Br J Anaesth 2008;101(5):680–9.

22. Grunau RE, Haley DW, Whitfied MF, et al. Altered basal cortisol levels at 3, 6, 8 and 18 months in infants born at extremely low gestational age. J Pediatr 2007; 150(2):151–6.

23. Bekhit MH. Opioid-induced hyperalgesia and tolerance. Am J Ther 2010;17(5): 498–510.

24. Bhutta AT, Venkatesan AK, Rovnaghi CR, et al. Anaesthetic neurotoxicity in rodents: is the ketamine controversy real? Acta Paediatr 2007;96(11):1554–6.

25. Zou X, Patterson TA, Divine RL, et al. Potential neurotoxicity of ketamine in the developing rat brain. Toxicol Sci 2009;108(1):149–58.

26. Anand KJ, Hall RW. Love, pain, and intensive care. Pediatrics 2008;121(4): 825–7.

27. Schultz M, Loughran-Fowlds A, Spence K. Neonatal pain: a comparison of the beliefs and practices of junior doctors and current best evidence. J Paediatr Child Health 2010;46(1-2):23–8.

28. Polkki T, Korhonen A, Laukkala S, et al. Nurses' attitudes and perceptions of pain assessment in neonatal intensive care. Scand J Caring Sci 2010;24(1): 49–55.

29. Craig KD, Whitfield MF, Grunau RV, et al. Pain in the preterm neonate: behavioural and physiological indices [erratum appears in Pain 1993;54(1):111]. Pain 1993;52(3):287–99.

30. Stevens BJ, Johnston CC. Physiological responses of premature infants to a painful stimulus. Nurs Res 1994;43(4):226–31.

31. Johnston CC, Stevens BJ, Yang F, et al. Differential response to pain by very premature neonates. Pain 1995;61(3):471–9.

32. Stevens B, Johnston C, Petryshen P, et al. Premature infant pain profile: development and initial validation. Clin J Pain 1996;12(1):13–22.

33. Barr RG. Reflections on measuring pain in infants: dissociation in responsive systems and honest signalling. Arch Dis Child Fetal Neonatal Ed 1998;79(2): F152–6.

34. Hummel P, Puchalski M, Creech SD, et al. Clinical reliability and validity of the N-PASS: neonatal pain, agitation and sedation scale with prolonged pain. J Perinatol 2008;28(1):55–60.

35. Debillon T, Bureau V, Savagner C, et al. Pain management in French neonatal intensive care units. Acta Paediatr 2002;91(7):822–6.

36. Corbo MG, Mansi G, Stagni A, et al. Nonnutritive sucking during heelstick procedures decreases behavioral distress in the newborn infant. Biol Neonate 2000;77(3):162–7.

37. Gibbins S, Stevens B, Hodnett E, et al. Efficacy and safety of sucrose for procedural pain relief in preterm and term neonates. Nurs Res 2002;51(6):375–82.

38. Mitchell A, Waltman PA. Oral sucrose and pain relief for preterm infants. Pain Manag Nurs 2003;4(2):62–9.

39. O'Sullivan A, O'Connor M, Brosnahan D, et al. Sweeten, soother and swaddle for retinopathy of prematurity screening: a randomised placebo controlled trial. Arch Dis Child Fetal Neonatal Ed 2010;95(6):F419–22.

40. Sun X, Lemyre B, Barrowman N, et al. Pain management during eye examinations for retinopathy of prematurity in preterm infants: a systematic review. Acta Paediatr 2010;99(3):329–34.

41. Kristoffersen L, Skogvoll E, Hafstrom M. Pain reduction on insertion of a feeding tube in preterm infants: a randomized controlled trial. Pediatrics 2011;127(6): e1449–54.

42. Johnston CC, Filion F, Campbell-Yeo M, et al. Enhanced kangaroo mother care for heel lance in preterm neonates: a crossover trial. J Perinatol 2009;29(1): 51–6.

43. Holsti L, Grunau RE. Considerations for using sucrose to reduce procedural pain in preterm infants. Pediatrics 2010;125(5):1042–7.

44. Cong X, Ludington-Hoe SM, McCain G, et al. Kangaroo care modifies preterm infant heart rate variability in response to heel stick pain: pilot study. Early Hum Dev 2009;85(9):561–7.

45. Freire NB, Garcia JB, Lamy ZC. Evaluation of analgesic effect of skin-to-skin contact compared to oral glucose in preterm neonates. Pain 2008;139(1):28–33.

46. Warnock FF, Castral TC, Brant R, et al. Brief report: maternal kangaroo care for neonatal pain relief: a systematic narrative review. J Pediatr Psychol 2010;35(9): 975–84.

47. Morrow C, Hidinger A, Wilkinson-Faulk D. Reducing neonatal pain during routine heel lance procedures. MCN Am J Matern Child Nurs 2010;35(6):346–54 [quiz: 354–6].

48. Jain S, Kumar P, McMillan DD. Prior leg massage decreases pain responses to heel stick in preterm babies. J Paediatr Child Health 2006;42(9):505–8.

49. Bellieni CV, Bagnoli F, Perrone S, et al. Effect of multisensory stimulation on analgesia in term neonates: a randomized controlled trial. Pediatr Res 2002;51(4): 460–3.

50. Hall RW, Boyle E, Young T. Do ventilated neonates require pain management? Semin Perinatol 2007;31(5):289–97.

51. Whyte S, Birrell G, Wyllie J. Premedication before intubation in UK neonatal units [see comment]. Arch Dis Child Fetal Neonatal Ed 2000;82(1):F38–41.

52. Roberts KD, Leone TA, Edwards WH, et al. Premedication for nonemergent neonatal intubations: a randomized, controlled trial comparing atropine and fentanyl to atropine, fentanyl, and mivacurium. Pediatrics 2006;118(4):1583–91.

53. Sarkar S, Schumacher RE, Baumgart S, et al. Are newborns receiving premedication before elective intubation? J Perinatol 2006;26(5):286–9.

54. Menon G, Anand KJ, McIntosh N. Practical approach to analgesia and sedation in the neonatal intensive care unit. Semin Perinatol 1998;22(5):417–24.

55. Simons SH, van Dijk M, van Lingen RA, et al. Routine morphine infusion in preterm newborns who received ventilatory support: a randomized controlled trial. JAMA 2003;290(18):2419–27.

56. Bellu R, de Waal KA, Zanini R. Opioids for neonates receiving mechanical ventilation. Cochrane Database Syst Rev 2008;1:CD004212.

57. Anand KJ. Pharmacological approaches to the management of pain in the neonatal intensive care unit. J Perinatol 2007;27(Suppl 1):S4–11.

58. Levene M. Morphine sedation in ventilated newborns: who are we treating? [comment]. Pediatrics 2005;116(2):492–3.

59. Carbajal R, Lenclen R, Jugie M, et al. Morphine does not provide adequate analgesia for acute procedural pain among preterm neonates. Pediatrics 2005; 115(6):1494–500.

60. Bhandari V, Bergqvist LL, Kronsberg SS, et al. Morphine administration and short-term pulmonary outcomes among ventilated preterm infants [see comment]. Pediatrics 2005;116(2):352–9.

61. MacGregor R, Evans D, Sugden D, et al. Outcome at 5-6 years of prematurely born children who received morphine as neonates. Arch Dis Child Fetal Neonatal Ed 1998;79(1):F40–3.

62. Mitchell A, Brooks S, Roane D. The premature infant and painful procedures. Pain Manag Nurs 2000;1(2):58–65.

63. Anand KJ, Hall RW. Pharmacological therapy for analgesia and sedation in the newborn [erratum appears in Arch Dis Child Fetal Neonatal Ed 2007;92(2):F156; note dosage error in text]. Arch Dis Child Fetal Neonatal Ed 2006;91(6): F448–53.

64. Guinsburg R, Kopelman BI, Anand KJ, et al. Physiological, hormonal, and behavioral responses to a single fentanyl dose in intubated and ventilated preterm neonates. J Pediatr 1998;132(6):954–9.

65. Saarenmaa E, Huttunen P, Leppaluoto J, et al. Advantages of fentanyl over morphine in analgesia for ventilated newborn infants after birth: a randomized trial [see comment]. J Pediatr 1999;134(2):144–50.

66. Orsini AJ, Leef KH, Costarino A, et al. Routine use of fentanyl infusions for pain and stress reduction in infants with respiratory distress syndrome [see comment]. J Pediatr 1996;129(1):140–5.

67. Berde CB, Jaksic T, Lynn AM, et al. Anesthesia and analgesia during and after surgery in neonates. Clin Ther 2005;27(6):900–21.

68. Blumer JL. Clinical pharmacology of midazolam in infants and children. Clin Pharmacokinet 1998;35(1):37–47.

69. Arya V, Ramji S. Midazolam sedation in mechanically ventilated newbons: a double blind randomized placebo controlled trial [see comment]. Indian Pediatr 2001;38(9):967–72.

70. Treluyer JM, Zohar S, Rey E, et al. Minimum effective dose of midazolam for sedation of mechanically ventilated neonates. J Clin Pharm Ther 2005;30(5): 479–85.

71. de Wildt SN, Kearns GL, Hop WC, et al. Pharmacokinetics and metabolism of oral midazolam in preterm infants. Br J Clin Pharmacol 2002;53(4):390–2.

72. Altintas O, Karabas VL, Demirci G, et al. Evaluation of intranasal midazolam in refraction and fundus examination of young children with strabismus. J Pediatr Ophthalmol Strabismus 2005;42(6):355–9.

73. Aranda JV, Carlo W, Hummel P, et al. Analgesia and sedation during mechanical ventilation in neonates. Clin Ther 2005;27(6):877–99.

74. Chess PR, D'Angio CT. Clonic movements following lorazepam administration in full-term infants. Arch Pediatr Adolesc Med 1998;152(1):98–9.

75. Ahsman MJ, Hanekamp M, Wildschut ED, et al. Population pharmacokinetics of midazolam and its metabolites during venoarterial extracorporeal membrane oxygenation in neonates. Clin Pharmacokinet 2010;49(6):407–19.

76. de Wildt SN, de Hoog M, Vinks AA, et al. Pharmacodynamics of midazolam in pediatric intensive care patients. Ther Drug Monit 2005;27(1):98–102.

77. Benini F, Farina M, Capretta A, et al. Sedoanalgesia in paediatric intensive care: a survey of 19 Italian units. Acta Paediatr 2010;99(5):758–62.

78. Ng E, Taddio A, Ohlsson A. Intravenous midazolam infusion for sedation of infants in the neonatal intensive care unit. Cochrane Database Syst Rev 2003; 1:CD002052.

79. Shehab N, Lewis CL, Streetman DD, et al. Exposure to the pharmaceutical excipients benzyl alcohol and propylene glycol among critically ill neonates. Pediatr Crit Care Med 2009;10(2):256–9.

80. Bhatt-Meht V, Annich G. Sedative clearance during extracorporeal membrane oxygenation. Perfusion 2005;20(6):309–15.

81. McDermott CA, Kowalczyk AL, Schnitzler ER, et al. Pharmacokinetics of lorazepam in critically ill neonates with seizures. J Pediatr 1992;120(3):479–83.

82. Gonzalez-Darder JM, Ortega-Alvaro A, Ruz-Franzi I, et al. Antinociceptive effects of phenobarbital in "tail-flick" test and deafferentation pain. Anesth Analg 1992;75(1):81–6.

83. Ebner N, Rohrmeister K, Winklbaur B, et al. Management of neonatal abstinence syndrome in neonates born to opioid maintained women. Drug Alcohol Depend 2007;87(2-3):131–8.

84. Mayers DJ, Hindmarsh KW, Gorecki DK, et al. Sedative/hypnotic effects of chloral hydrate in the neonate: trichloroethanol or parent drug? Dev Pharmacol Ther 1992;19(2-3):141–6.

85. Litman RS, Soin K, Salam A. Chloral hydrate sedation in term and preterm infants: an analysis of efficacy and complications. Anesth Analg 2010;110(3): 739–46.

86. Disma N, Astuto M, Rizzo G, et al. Propofol sedation with fentanyl or midazolam during oesophagogastroduodenoscopy in children. Eur J Anaesthesiol 2005;22(11):848–52.

87. Rigby-Jones AE, Nolan JA, Priston MJ, et al. Pharmacokinetics of propofol infusions in critically ill neonates, infants, and children in an intensive care unit. Anesthesiology 2002;97(6):1393–400.

88. Jenkins IA, Playfor SD, Bevan C, et al. Current United Kingdom sedation practice in pediatric intensive care. Paediatr Anaesth 2007;17(7):675–83.

89. Ghanta S, Abdel-Latif ME, Lui K, et al. Propofol compared with the morphine, atropine, and suxamethonium regimen as induction agents for neonatal endotracheal intubation: a randomized, controlled trial [see comment]. Pediatrics 2007;119(6):e1248–55.

90. Allegaert K, Peeters MY, Verbesselt R, et al. Inter-individual variability in propofol pharmacokinetics in preterm and term neonates. Br J Anaesth 2007;99(6): 864–70.

91. Vanderhaegen J, Naulaers G, Van Huffel S, et al. Cerebral and systemic hemodynamic effects of intravenous bolus administration of propofol in neonates. Neonatology 2010;98(1):57–63.

92. Green SM, Denmark TK, Cline J, et al. Ketamine sedation for pediatric critical care procedures. Pediatr Emerg Care 2001;17(4):244–8.

93. Chambliss CR, Anand KJ. Pain management in the pediatric intensive care unit. Curr Opin Pediatr 1997;9(3):246–53.

94. Betremieux P, Carre P, Pladys P, et al. Doppler ultrasound assessment of the effects of ketamine on neonatal cerebral circulation. Dev Pharmacol Ther 1993;20(1-2):9–13.

95. Saarenmaa E, Neuvonen PJ, Huttunen P, et al. Ketamine for procedural pain relief in newborn infants. Arch Dis Child Fetal Neonatal Ed 2001;85(1):F53–6.

96. Anand KJ, Soriano SG. Anesthetic agents and the immature brain: are these toxic or therapeutic? [see comment]. Anesthesiology 2004;101(2):527–30.

97. Howard CR, Howard FM, Weitzman ML. Acetaminophen analgesia in neonatal circumcision: the effect on pain. Pediatrics 1994;93(4):641–6.

98. Lander J, Brady-Fryer B, Metcalfe JB, et al. Comparison of ring block, dorsal penile nerve block, and topical anesthesia for neonatal circumcision: a randomized controlled trial [see comment]. JAMA 1997;278(24):2157–62.

99. Garcia OC, Reichberg S, Brion LP, et al. Topical anesthesia for line insertion in very low birth weight infants. J Perinatol 1997;17(6):477–80.

100. Kaur G, Gupta P, Kumar A. A randomized trial of eutectic mixture of local anesthetics during lumbar puncture in newborns. Arch Pediatr Adolesc Med 2003; 157(11):1065–70.

101. Gradin M, Eriksson M, Holmqvist G, et al. Pain reduction at venipuncture in newborns: oral glucose compared with local anesthetic cream [see comment]. Pediatrics 2002;110(6):1053–7.

102. Taddio A, Stevens B, Craig K, et al. Efficacy and safety of lidocaine-prilocaine cream for pain during circumcision [see comment]. N Engl J Med 1997; 336(17):1197–201.

103. Larsson BA, Norman M, Bjerring P, et al. Regional variations in skin perfusion and skin thickness may contribute to varying efficacy of topical, local anesthetics in neonates. Paediatr Anaesth 1996;6(2):107–10.

104. Pereira e Silva Y, Gomez RS, Barbosa RF, et al. Remifentanil for sedation and analgesia in a preterm neonate with respiratory distress syndrome [see comment]. Paediatr Anaesth 2005;15(11):993–6.
105. Knolle E, Oehmke MJ, Gustorff B, et al. Target-controlled infusion of propofol for fibreoptic intubation. Eur J Anaesthesiol 2003;20(7):565–9.
106. Singh A, Girotra S, Mehta Y, et al. Total intravenous anesthesia with ketamine for pediatric interventional cardiac procedures. J Cardiothorac Vasc Anesth 2000; 14(1):36–9.
107. Oklu E, Bulutcu FS, Yalcin Y, et al. Which anesthetic agent alters the hemodynamic status during pediatric catheterization? comparison of propofol versus ketamine [see comment]. J Cardiothorac Vasc Anesth 2003;17(6):686–90.
108. Bouwmeester NJ, Hop WC, van Dijk M, et al. Postoperative pain in the neonate: age-related differences in morphine requirements and metabolism. Intensive Care Med 2003;29(11):2009–15.
109. Simons SH, van Dijk M, Anand KS, et al. Do we still hurt newborn babies? A prospective study of procedural pain and analgesia in neonates. Arch Pediatr Adolesc Med 2003;157(11):1058–64.
110. McCarver-May DG, Kang J, Aouthmany M, et al. Comparison of chloral hydrate and midazolam for sedation of neonates for neuroimaging studies [see comment]. J Pediatr 1996;128(4):573–6.
111. Allegaert K, Cossy V, Debeer A, et al. The impact of ibuprofen on renal clearance in preterm infants is independent of the gestational age. Pediatr Nephrol 2005;20(6):740–3.
112. Ohlsson A, Walia R, Shah S. Ibuprofen for the treatment of patent ductus arteriosus in preterm and/or low birth weight infants. Cochrane Database Syst Rev 2008;1:CD003481.
113. Naulaers G, Delanghe G, Allegaert K, et al. Ibuprofen and cerebral oxygenation and circulation. Arch Dis Child Fetal Neonatal Ed 2005;90(1):F75–6.
114. McCurnin D, Seidner S, Chang LY, et al. Ibuprofen-induced patent ductus arteriosus closure: physiologic, histologic, and biochemical effects on the premature lung. Pediatrics 2008;121(5):945–56.
115. Golianu B, Krane E, Seybold J, et al. Non-pharmacological techniques for pain management in neonates. Semin Perinatol 2007;31(5):318–22.
116. Lai HL, Chen CJ, Peng TC, et al. Randomized controlled trial of music during kangaroo care on maternal state anxiety and preterm infants' responses. Int J Nurs Stud 2006;43(2):139–46.
117. Wu MT, Sheen JM, Chuang KH, et al. Neuronal specificity of acupuncture response: a fMRI study with electroacupuncture. Neuroimage 2002;16(4):1028–37.
118. Woo YM, Lee MS, Nam Y, et al. Effects of contralateral electroacupuncture on brain function: a double-blind, randomized, pilot clinical trial. J Altern Complement Med 2006;12(8):813–5.
119. Spence K, Henderson-Smart D. Closing the evidence-practice gap for newborn pain using clinical networks. J Paediatr Child Health 2011;47(3):92–8.

Index

Note: Page numbers of article titles are in **boldface** type.

Clin Perinatol 39 (2012) 255–267
doi:10.1016/S0095-5108(12)00010-3
0095-5108/12/$ – see front matter © 2012 Elsevier Inc. All rights reserved.

perinatology.theclinics.com

Moving?

Make sure your subscription moves with you!

To notify us of your new address, find your **Clinics Account Number** (located on your mailing label above your name), and contact customer service at:

Email: journalscustomerservice-usa@elsevier.com

800-654-2452 (subscribers in the U.S. & Canada)
314-447-8871 (subscribers outside of the U.S. & Canada)

Fax number: 314-447-8029

Elsevier Health Sciences Division
Subscription Customer Service
3251 Riverport Lane
Maryland Heights, MO 63043

*To ensure uninterrupted delivery of your subscription, please notify us at least 4 weeks in advance of move.